THE PEOPLE'S Cancer GUIDE BOOK

by Ronald E. Aigotti, M.D.

Practical Information to
Help You Understand Cancer;
Its Causes, Early Detection, Prevention,
Symptoms, Stages, Treatments,
and Cure.

FIRST EDITION 1995

Printings 1 2 3 4 5

ISBN 0-9648656-0-2

LCCN 95-076465

Dedicated to the memory of Sue Morgan-Messaglia, August 16, 1987. She faced the most feared disease in history. . . without fear.

ACKNOWLEDGMENTS

The author wishes to express his gratitude to all those who contributed to the completion of this work both in spirit and actual assistance in its writing. Undoubtedly my initial thanks must go to my wife, Barbara, for tolerating all of my hours of separation and isolation spent in formulating and drafting this manuscript. Secondly, to her as well my children, Diane, Julianne, Matthew and Mia goes my appreciation for their suggestions and encouragement to continue and persevere.

Without the technical advice and suggestions of my writing colleagues, critics and friends--Sue Antonovitz, Myrna Stainer, John Houghton and Dr. Brian Rolfe--surely this composition would have lacked whatever it has in the way of substance and style. For this I shall be eternally in their debt and always available to their needs.

Special thanks, also, to Sister Marjorie Packer, C.S.C. for her expert proofreading skill and medical scientific knowledge as a graduate nurse.

Lastly, I owe a great deal to Mr. James Bowers for the structure, format and design of this finished transcript.

Contents

The People's Cancer Guide Book

Introduction

The following information and advice has resulted from a combination of my almost thirty years in the field of clinical medicine. The last twenty of those years were spent specifically in dealing with the group of diseases called cancer and my interaction with cancer patient's and their families. This experience also includes many years of study of the broad subject of cancer from a scientific, clinical, psycho-social and practical view point. It is not my intention that this work be encyclopedic in its scope or infallible in its judgments. Rather it is hoped that it will instruct and inform the reader about the clearly known as opposed to the speculated concepts about cancers and how the ordinary person on the street can deal with them.

If the reader is searching for an erudite volume brimming over with scientific fact and technical data about cancer this is the wrong book. There will be very little, if any, technical jargon, biological theory and the like. Instead, what the reader will find is a down to earth description of cancer, and its definition, cause, prevention, diagnosis (detection) and treatment. Wherever possible, all information is expressed in common language. Wherever technical terms must be used, those terms will also be defined in plain language. If the author has failed to do this at any point, he apologizes because there are rare instances where this may not be possible. For example the adrenal glands have no simpler name that I have ever heard.

This treatise was written with essentially one purpose in mind: i.e., to reduce the mortality, and the suffering caused by this group of diseases. And such a reduction is possible even in light of our present day limitations regarding our knowledge of the causes and cures for these diseases.

This author believes that the reduction of mortality and suffering is attainable because—as has been true throughout the ages—the greatest impediment to the conquering of all diseases has been the lack of understanding and knowledge about that disease which can produce uncontrollable, paralyzing fear. The product of such fear has not resulted in the avoidance of the disease by the public. On the contrary, it has produced a terror which causes a reluctance to seek professional help early enough to produce a cure.

It is my hope that this volume will remove this paralyzing fear and instill in its place a respect and a reasonable concern for the presence of or possible presence of cancer which will then lead to the more rational response; namely, the seeking professional help as early as possible.

It has been estimated, and I believe realistically, that 80%-85% of all cancers could be cured if detected and treated early enough in the natural course of the disease. In my twenty years practicing medical oncology (cancer medicine) the most common reason stated for waiting before seeking treatment—as long as six years in my personal practice experience—has been, "I didn't come sooner because everybody knows you can't cure any cancer." Nothing could be farther from the truth. Over the years it has become patently obvious that the major reason for such statements has been the uncontrolled fear of the worst. A fear which is engendered by a lack of understanding and general misinformation about this group of diseases. There are two main sources of this misinformation: the use of hearsay information from friends, relatives, the mass media and the lay press; and a failure of the medical profession and its agencies to disseminate the appropriate information to the general public.

It is my most sincere hope and intention that this work will help, at least partially, to correct this sad state of affairs.

Part One

Understanding Cancer

Chapter 1

Definitions and Non-Definitions

Widespread confusion now exists when discussing the group of diseases known as cancer. To avoid this confusion, much of the following text is devoted to defining this group of diseases. An equally large number of words are used to define what cancers 'are not.' This is an extremely important point because it is not possible to rationally discuss any subject when one party is discussing apples specifically, and the other is discussing in terms of fruits in general. This has been the most common pitfall in discussions between physician and patient.

Both the reader and the health professionals must recognize that there is no single disease or abnormality called 'cancer.' Rather, there is a large heterogeneous group of conditions called 'the cancers.' In the western hemisphere this amounts to over 270 different types of cancers—including one hundred or so in North America—which have been identified, described, and studied. Therefore, it is inappropriate to discuss *a cure for cancer* when we should be discussing a cure or treatment for a particular 'type of cancer.' In many instances the same kind of cancer in different persons might be treated in different, yet successful ways. Therefore, to look for a universality or a **'treatment of choice,'** world wide or even nation wide, is not realistic.

We must now begin to think of cancers as a heterogeneous mixture of maladies, each with its own characteristics. Only then will we begin to understand that there will probably never be a single *magic bul-*

let which will cure or treat all kinds of cancer. We should not be discouraged by this statement, however. Throughout the history of medical science, this has usually been the case. The sole exception is in the prevention of some diseases by immunizations—such as Poliomyelitis, Diphtheria, Tetanus, etc. But prevention is not the same as treatment or cure.

The definition of cancer: There are as many definitions for cancer as there are scientists, oncologists and other professionals who deal with cancer. The precise cause or causes of many diseases are often not known. The most precise definitions of any disease in medical science is possible when based on the known causative agent(s).

Technical and highly scientific descriptions, however, are beyond the scope of this work and not the intention of this author. Wherever possible, descriptions and definitions will be given in simple and useful terms. The usefulness of a definition should be derived from the fact that it provides the reader with a practical guide in helping them decide whether they might have the disease and when to seek professional help for appropriate treatment. It should not drive the reader away from that professional help.

I offer what I believe is a simple and useful definition of cancer. Cancers are a group of diseases characterized by uncontrolled and disorderly growth of human cells which could lead to illness and eventual death if not appropriately treated.

Please note the absence of the following words—either stated or implied—in this definition: malignant, terminal, hopeless, incurable, untreatable. These terms were excluded intentionally because they have no place in a general definition for a mixed group of maladies. These modifying terms should be applied only after the individual type of cancer and the extent of its activity have been determined. Only then are they appropriate.

Unfortunately, many readers presume that these characteristics are already inherent in the diagnosis of cancer. As a result, many do not present themselves to a physician early enough to effect a cure. You must not make such inaccurate assumptions and allow fear to divert you from the proper course of action.

These qualifying terms will first be defined from the standpoint of medical and oncology practice. Then they will be contrasted with the common misconceptions of the reader and the general public.

Malignant: In reference to medical diseases in general, the term malignant means a condition which universally leads to a fatal outcome. On the other hand, in cancer medicine the word malignant is always added as a qualifier to a pathology report of a biopsy of tissue taken from the patient. When applied in this manner the word malignant is used to alert your physician to the fact that further, more extensive action and treatment is needed to cure this condition. If more aggressive action is not undertaken it is highly likely the clinical situation could lead to the death of the patient. This otherwise frightful term has no other meaning.

The word malignant is not, in and of itself, a prediction for the outcome of any cancer. The true prognosis, mortality rate and treatability of any cancer requires much more information before your physician can formulate such predictions for anyone. And even then, at best, these predictions can only come in the form of averages and percentages.

As for the other qualifiers—hopeless, untreatable, terminal, etc.- these are essentially useless words to the physician and individual affected by cancer. Only with further clinical information obtained through other testing can your physician outline the basic facts every individual patient has the right to know in order to ask some very pertinent questions. And those questions are: what kind of cancer do I have; can it be treated and how, and at what cost in terms of pain, discomfort and life-style changes; what are the chances of curing or arresting it; and how long can one expect to live and what quality of life will I have; and last, but equally vital, what are the answers to these same questions if I choose not to have any treatment at all?

After the reader finishes reading this book they should be able to ask intelligent, meaningful, practical questions to obtain these important pieces of information from their physician.

The following section is devoted to naming and identifying many of the words and phrases used by physicians, and other paramedical professionals, to evade the word *cancer.* These are used not with the intention of deceiving but because of the professional individual's discomfort in handling the difficult task of using the word, *cancer.* Often it is a reflection of the difficulty the professionals have in facing the reality of their own vulnerability and inevitable mortality. They are, after all, human beings, too.

The use of the following terms is acceptable, and even preferable, when a diagnosis of cancer has not yet been established through a biopsy or by some other means. But these terms are not acceptable when discussing a patient's cancer once it is has been clearly diagnosed.

Tumor: Strictly speaking a *tumor* is simply defined as a swelling or a localized enlargement without any real additional meaning. For example, abscesses, warts, corns, bunions or cysts are, by definition, tumors. Malignancy or benignity (its opposite) is not inherent in the term, tumor. This is, unfortunately, the most commonly used synonym even within the medical profession. But the lay person should not settle for this term when talking to their physician about their specific clinical situation.

Mass: A mass is a large collection of tissue where one would not be expected to be found. It is commonly used as an early designation when first discovered by the physician's examining hands or, when seen on an x-ray.

Lesion: The word lesion is a vague term used to designate a indefinite abnormality. Therefore, an ulcer in the mouth or on the skin is a lesion and an abnormal shadow seen on x-ray examination is a lesion also.

Growth: This designation most frequently used in the phrase, *abnormal growth.* It is a totally useless term once biopsy material is obtained and interpreted by the pathologist.

The following terms are a number of impressive, high technology words and phrases often heard used when professionals discuss a cancer case. They should never be accepted by the patient when they are discussing their specific cancer with their doctor. These include: *mitotic changes; anaplastic growth; aggressive growth; anaplastic le-*

sion; carcinomatous process; malignant process; malignant growth; neoplasm; neoplastic growth; and so on.

The next group of words are not so high tech-sounding but are equally meaningless: 'a bit of cancer'; 'just a small cancer or small amount of cancer'; 'a touch of cancer'; 'a little cancer.'

And finally, the most common known designation and probably the most feared word in the English language:

Cancer: The word cancer is itself derived from the original Latin word for crab. It was initially used by pathologists early in medical history when performing autopsies. When cancers were discovered and viewed by the naked eye they often had the appearance of a crab with its larger central portion with tentacles radiating out from the edges. Thus the designation was coined as a descriptive one. Cancer is no longer an accurate term in the light of contemporary knowledge since there are many types of cancer that never take on the appearance of the crab—leukemia and myeloma, for example. Nevertheless, the word is too ingrained in our culture to be displaced. Let it suffice for me to endeavor to clarify its meaning and, it is hoped, to remove the fear-filled stigma the word carries with it for those so afflicted.

But the final diagnosis when revealed to the patient or the family must not end there because the diagnosis alone does nothing to answer the four basic questions stated above: i. e., what must be done next? what chance is there of it being cured or controlled? how is it best treated and at what costs? what is life expectancy with and without treatment? The details of these points will be delved into more deeply in the following pages.

In conclusion, it must be made clear that at this point none of the information given you thus far says anything—explicit or implied—about your individual prognosis.

Chapter 2

Naming of the Cancers

At the outset you should be made aware of the fact that names and titles are not needed to answer 'the four basic questions'; but patients do have the right to know them, if they so desire. It is, however, strongly urged to make no assumptions or conclusions from them. It is the physician's job to help interpret their meaning and significance as they apply to the patient.

Organ of Origin: This is the most commonly used and easily recognized method of naming cancers. It indicates the organ in which the cancer was first discovered or the organ from which it most likely arose. Therefore, Breast Cancer, Lung Cancer, Stomach Cancer, Colon Cancer are terms that imply the cancer started or was first discovered in that organ. It is called the 'Primary Cancer Site' or simply, the 'Primary Cancer.' Some confusion can arise when the cancer has spread to other organs, but this will be discussed and clarified later in this text.

Tissue of Origin: The most complex and confusing designations, for the cancers arise from this method of terminology. Of course, they are useful for physicians and scientists to communicate with each other around the world. But these serve no useful purpose to the ordinary person. They will be touched upon here so that they can be recognized and discarded without any fear of missing something important.

Human cancers arise from one of two types of tissue: they are epithelium (skin-like); or connective tissue such as bone, muscle and the like.

If epithelial in origin, they are called carcinomas; if connective tissue in origin they are called sarcomas. As one can see, the suffix -oma is added to both terms as a standard procedure. The reason it is added is not important, at least not outside of scientific circles. But they will at least be recognized by the reader. Both are malignant cancers, but as already discussed, we have learned the term, malignant, has little predictive use by itself.

There is a misconception that the suffix—*oma*— always indicates malignancy or cancer. It does not. Many medical conditions have this same suffix and they are not malignant or even cancers. This misconception should be discarded immediately. It only leads to more confusion.

This final list of designations are most often used as modifiers for the basic names of cancers. They add only clutter. The following are only a few examples.

Adenocarcinoma - simply indicates that the cancer contains elements of glandular structures (thus the prefix, adeno-). Thus, any organ that contains glands can develop an adenocarcinoma, i.e., Adenocarcinoma of the Stomach; Adenocarcinoma of the Lung, and so on.

Other modifiers in this category are Epidermoid, Squamous Cell, Bronchogenic, Undifferentiated, Poorly differentiated, Small Cell, Large Cell, Osteogenic, Hepatocellular, and on, and on they go into infinity.

These also should be set aside for the same reason as the others. They do not help the affected person get answers to the four basic questions in a specific case.

The reader can ask for, of course, and has the right to know the full title of the cancer that is present, as long as they do not make any assumptions about its meaning from the name itself. With the availability of so called, "Medical Encyclopedias," it is easy to look up the title and definition of any disease. These can be imprecise and very general. Many of these books discuss several hundred common disease entities and several thousand symptoms. Cancer is only one of these many entities. It is hoped that this book is more precise and specific by giving adequate definitions and explanations of terms, dealing with only one entity, cancer. Even if this is accomplished, it is still advised that this book be used only as a guide. Any major decisions or interpretations should still be made with the advice and counsel of a physician.

Chapter 3

Causes of Cancer

Again we begin with a definition of terms to make for easy discussion.

In medical science a direct, simple, precise causative agent is not currently known for many diseases. When it is known, it is the purest and most ideal way of naming a disease. Examples are Tuberculosis, in which the exact group of bacteria (called Tubercle Bacillus) that causes this condition is known. Another is Pneumococcal (Pneumococcus Bacillus) Pneumonia, and so on. It is called the 'Causative Agent.'

In most diseases, however, what is known is only some of the predisposing factors, risk factors, inciting agents, and other imprecise, indirect, vague factors. This is especially true for cancer. From reading the mass-media and lay-press, one easily gets the impression there are cancer causing substances all around us. This just isn't so.

The so called 'cancer causing chemicals' have only been found guilty in either occupational exposure or in only certain susceptible individuals. Even smoking tobacco is only considered a risk factor but it is a very powerful risk factor. It is probably the most potent, high-risk cancer causing agent known.

The following is a list of factors that increase the risk of cancer. They are divided into 'known risk factors,' 'suspected risk factors,' and 'unproven or mythical factors.' But note, they are only *risk factors* and not known causes.

Known Risk Factors:

Age - age over 50 years is associated with a higher incidence of almost all cancers. It doesn't mean that all, or even most, people who live past age 50 will develop cancer. Nor does it imply that people under 50 cannot get cancer. Cancer does, however, have a lower incidence in the under-age-50-group.

Asbestos - with *occupational* exposure and *cigarette smoking* there is a 5 fold increase in the risk of a special kind of lung cancer called mesothelioma. Emphasis is placed on occupation and smoking. It should also be noted that not all types of lung cancer have an increased occurrence in these circumstances, only a specific kind called mesothelioma. There is no convincing evidence that occasional limited exposure to asbestos, such as in buildings and homes, is unequivocally a risk factor.

Cigarette Smoking - produces a clear cut, tenfold increase in the risk of lung cancer; and it is a strongly suspected risk factor also in bladder cancer, throat cancer, esophagus cancer and others.

Cigar and Pipe Smoking, Chewing Tobacco - is associated with a markedly increased risk of cancers of the mouth, tongue, lip, voice box and esophagus.

Medications:

D.E.S.- (known also as diethylstilbestrol) if used by a mother during pregnancy increases the risk of cancer of the vagina in their daughters.

Estrogen Used in Menopause - increases the risk of cancer of the endometrium (the lining of the inside of the Uterus).

Inheritance or Family History - this has been demonstrated to increase the risk of breast cancer in women who have a history of breast cancers in their mother, sisters, and daughters.

Colon cancers have also been shown to have an inheritance risk factor. There is no demonstrated cross inheritance, which means there is no known increased risk of lung cancer because a parent has had breast cancer, or skin cancer, for example. A general family or inheritable predisposition to cancer is postulated but has not been proven.

Industrial Chemicals - only occupational exposure to agents such as benzene, nickel, chromates, asbestos and others has been implicated. Again the emphasis is on occupational, which means a steady high rate of exposure over an extended period of time. In other words, it is a question of total cumulative doses of these substances. Casual or occasional exposure has not been demonstrated to increase cancer risks.

Radiation or X-Ray Exposure –Therapeutic exposure to high doses of radiation, especially at a young age, has been related to an increased risk of cancer of the thyroid, of leukemia and of sarcomas. The points to be emphasized here are *therapeutic* and *high doses*. Therapeutic, means when radiation, x-ray, radium, cobalt and other nuclear agents are used to treat specific diseases. Therefore, the amount of exposure used in diagnostic x-rays, as used to detect or diagnose diseases, has a very low to insignificant risk especially with contemporary, highly technologically developed x-ray equipment.

Sun Light - with prolonged exposure or frequent overexposure, there is an increased risk of some kinds of skin cancer, especially without sunscreen protection.

Unproven or Mythical Causes:

The following list can never be anything but incomplete, since many of the items listed are propagated by word of mouth and not by scientific investigation.

Bumps, bruises, pinches and other forms of minor injury. This idea may have started from the fact that some patients discover a lump or mass—most commonly a breast lump in woman—after such a minor injury and, therefore, conclude that it actually caused the cancer. More than likely the cancer existed for some time before the injury. Many of these swellings are more sensitive to pain than normal tissue. This would naturally draw more attention to them when minor trauma occurs. And the automatic reflex reaction we all have to sudden, minor injury is to reach for and examine the area. Thus, the lump is discovered and the injury blamed.

It stands to reason that if this myth were true, then people in occupations associated with many daily minor injuries—professional athletes, carpenters, laborers, etc.,—would have a much higher incidence of cancer. But this has not been shown to be the case in comparative studies of cancer incidence.

Contagion - This myth states that cancer is a communicable disease, much like measles, tuberculosis, chicken pox, etc. This has also not stood up under the tests of scientific scrutiny.

Although true 'clusters' of certain kinds of cancer—Leukemia and Hodgkin's Disease, for example—have been reported for decades, it has never been demonstrated that a communicable agent is the common factor. If this were the case, logic would indicate that cancer would have a higher occurrence rate among physicians, nurses and other health care personnel; spouses and other family members sharing a household with a cancer patient, etc. No doubt there are many anecdotal reports of such cases, but they are few and far between. I have encountered this situation on only two occasions in my experience with several hundred cases of cancer of all types.

Other occasional sensationalized mythical causes are included: fluoridated water; vitamin deficiencies; deficiencies of other unproven substances such as krebiozin, laetrile or amygdalin, etc.

It is appropriate at this point to make some statements about animal cancers as they are utilized in research and in screening industrial and other chemical substances for cancer risk.

Unfortunately, the public has been misled by sensationalized reports that the relationship between human cancers and animal cancers is an absolute one, meaning that if a certain cancer occurs in an animal of any type, that exactly the same type of cancer can be produced in humans. Even less correct is the idea that if a cancer is successfully treated or cured in an animal, by any agent, that the same agent will work in humans.

By and large, when scientists inject human cancer cells into animals, instead of growing they are rejected by the animals. The reverse is also true. As a matter of fact, when human cancers are injected into human volunteers, the volunteer recipients do not develop cancer. These are exactly the reasons that cancer research has been so tedious and slow. The lack of a reliable, predictable laboratory model is still missing in cancer research.

To illustrate this, for example, when new cancer drugs are screened for usefulness in human breast cancer, they are tested in mice—not with mouse breast cancer—but with a special kind of leukemia.

These are two cancers that have little in common. It was simply and accidentally noted that drugs which were effective in treating the mouse leukemia happened to be effective in human breast cancer. No one can deny that this is a useful and effective research model but it is purely an accidental one.

This is one of the reasons premature conclusions based on animal cancer are unwarranted and unproductive. Sadly, the general public has been so misinformed about this relationship that the fear of cancer and the misconception that cancer causing substances are all around us, in our food, in our water and in our air, that many people are driven away from physicians and medical facilities.

Chapter 4

Symptoms and Signs of Cancer

Definitions: As usual, before discussing what signals to look for to alert one to the possibility of cancer, we must define our language.

Simply stated, a symptom is a change, an experienced abnormality, or other clue the person receives from their body, telling them that something is wrong. That he is sick. Obvious things such as pain, bleeding, abnormal lumps, fever, and so on, immediately come to mind. These are the clues the individual himself perceives through his own senses and powers of observation.

On the other hand, a sign is an abnormality detected or perceived by the senses of a trained observer such as a doctor or nurse; or a laboratory test, or an x-ray abnormality detected by routine or indicated testing.

Time is taken to describe these two terms and their meanings, to urge that you not be concerned with using them by their proper scientific names when reporting a problem. The doctor will not be interested in whether or not you can use the proper jargon or precise descriptive terms. If you hurt, say so. If you have only a soreness or tenderness or discomfort, say it that way. Don't look to see if the doctor will approve of your terminology because it is not significant. What is significant is that you know something is not right and you know that you are not your usual self. It is always best to put things in your own words—everyday, common words are enough.

Even if you cannot put it into real terms, say so. Did you ever wonder why in medical jargon there are so many terms with vague meanings? There are words such as malaise, euphoria, rigors, debility and so on. These words were coined out of necessity, in a futile attempt to describe the nondescript. Many of the modifiers used were invented for the same purpose, such as; common, very common, not uncommon, uncommon but not rare, local, focal, regional, sectional, mild, moderate, severe, moderately severe, almost never, nearly always, and so on. Even its language must be vague and imprecise. This is not by choice or design. Mother Nature has not blessed our profession or human biology with enough consistencies to enable it to state that two plus two always equals four.'

Therefore, don't be concerned with being able to tell your problem in precise terms. Physicians don't expect them because they are trained to interpret the principle of the complaints, not the clear cut letter of them. Medical clinical science is made up of more grays than blacks-and-whites, even in the light of today's more or less exact technology. There it is, another one of those vague qualifiers. Yes, it even applies to our wonderful technology.

Now for the clues one can use to suspect they are sick—or at least decide to seek professional advice. The term, *clues*, was deliberately used because that is what a physician really does. He interprets and investigates clues. The more commonly used term 'signals' was avoided because it sounds and reads too much like the word 'sign' discussed above.

Also note these are designated as clues to illness and not as clues to cancer. That's because there is no single clue or group of clues that is unique to cancer. And the reverse is also true. There has never been a clue (symptom or sign) that has not been the first and only clue to the presence of a cancer. Throughout medical history several disease entities have been designated as 'the great imitator.' Among them were syphilis and tuberculosis. They earned the distinction because they were the ravages of their era and until a precise means of diagnosing them became available every sign and symptom was suspect and possible. Today cancer is at the top of that list.

But what about the highly publicized 'seven warning signs of cancer?' These are probably helpful, but they are hardly specific. In talking to lay people over the years of practice, many are surprised that physicians do not have these committed to memory. The reason is they are mixed in their minds, inconspicuously, with dozens of other signals which are equally significant. Many are not even sure the number 'seven' is correct.

Why is time taken to make this point, you might ask. There are two reasons. First, to avoid the false sense of security patients derive from not having any of these seven signals; second, to remove the fear that goes with the assumption that these are indeed surefire evidence of cancer. The result, too often, has been that in both situations the individual does not visit a physician early enough to achieve a cure.

The only clue that comes closest to being moderately specific is the appearance of a lump, swelling or mass. But, out of a hundred patients who present to their doctors with body lumps, perhaps 5% have a chance of having a cancer. It is true that the location of the mass will produce higher suspicion in the physician's mind that a cancer is much more likely. For example, lumps in the breast are highly suspicious, but lumps on the arms or legs are very unlikely to be cancers. Why? Because doctor know that cancers of the extremities are relatively rare compared to cancers of the internal organs, the breast, the throat, and so on.

These points are not emphasized to decrease the usefulness of these signals but to indicate that they are helpful because they are the most common clues to the most common types of cancers, by actual number and percentages, occurring in the western hemisphere, but not because they are specific for cancer, nor are they exclusively limited to cancer.

If there are not truly reliable guide posts for a layperson to suspect that they might have cancer, then what shall you use to help you decide to seek a physician's help? It is best not to think in terms of what your diagnosis might be, but instead, to think in terms of having an abnormality that needs investigation. Do not think in terms of specialists immediately, but start with a good general physician such as a family practitioner, general internist, or gynecologist in the case of adults; and pediatricians and family practitioners in the case of children. All physicians, whether specialists or not, are trained to have a high index of suspicion for the possibility of cancer and to know how to pursue its diagnosis. If one is not satisfied with the physician's investigation of the problem or his conclusion they are, of course, free to seek the advice of a specialist. And they owe it to themselves to do so if they are not confident or comfortable with the results.

Since the seven warning signals have received such wide attention and are so familiar to the public they are discussed and their precise meaning elaborated upon. They are discussed to put them into proper perspective while taking the liberty of adding some clues that the author feels are useful.

A change in bowel or bladder habits: The first usually listed is a change in bowel or bladder habits. These two should be separated and discussed individually. This is done in the following paragraphs.

A change in bowel habits should be more clearly characterized as a sudden, major and sustained change in bowel habits in either direction. This signifies that both diarrhea and constipation may be important. Most people are aware of the significance of constipation but not of diarrhea, especially bloody diarrhea. The problem with the simple term *constipation* arises with people who have been intermittently constipated most of their adult lives. It you try to think of this in quantitative terms, it becomes more clear. For example, if you have had to use a laxative, suppository or enema once or twice every few months and now it is suddenly required once or twice every week or two, this is a significant quantitative change. Its significance increases when it is accompanied by blood in the stool or a black tar-like stool, and weight loss.

In discussing diarrhea quantification and duration are also important. Who among us has not had episodes of this problem, off and on throughout our lives, especially after ingesting some excessively spicy foods or during the intestinal flu season? These are normal or expected situations. But the individual who suddenly has recurring diarrhea every month, or even two or three weeks must be on the alert.

Again this is especially important when gross amounts of red blood are present or when the stool is jet black in color. They should be alerted to the need to see a physician. The first concern of the person should not be cancer but that he requires medical attention.

Although the odds are high that these clues are *not* due to cancer, a check on the symptoms is mandatory. If the physician shrugs them off, seek another opinion.

Even the phrase 'change in bowel habits' is fraught with too many pitfalls. What if the frequency, quantity and the form of the bowel movements are normal but they contain blood most of the time? The appearance of bloody stools is highly significant, no matter what the circumstances, and should be investigated by a doctor.

In discussing change in bladder habits clear-cut guidelines are even more difficult to state, especially in adult males, and in females over the age of fifty. The problem of frequent night time urination, uncontrolled loss of urine, passing only small amounts of urine several times a day, burning or discomfort on urination, are all very non-specific and most often not suggestive of cancer.

The one exception to clues in the urinary tract in the passage of grossly bloody urine, or pink tinged urine. Although, in the majority of cases cancer will not be the cause, it should be regarded as highly suspicious. Thorough examination of the urinary tract in males, plus the reproductive system in females, must be undertaken.

Coughing & hoarse voice: Unrelenting cough and hoarseness of the voices are also listed together. They should be discussed separately so it does not give the impression they indicate the same kinds of cancers. They do not. Also, it might create the idea that both symptoms must occur together to be significant. This is also not the case. Anatomically speaking, they are remotely related since they are both part of the respiratory tract but they should not be thought of in the same functional way. Coughing suggest some kind of lung problem, and hoarseness suggests throat or voice box difficulties. This is the more correct and more useful way to think of these signs.

Coughing should also be qualified and quantified since it is such a common symptom, especially among smokers. And it is the smokers group that we are trying to focus on since they have the greatest likelihood of getting lung cancers, besides many other cancers and other non-cancerous disease.

Coughing that is chronic (long lasting), even if intermittent, and is most difficult to subdue even with treatment is highly suspicious. Everyone has tried to suppress a cough with home remedies such as using cough drops, hard candy, steam inhalation, over-the-counter proprietary cough medicines, and so on, which often help temporarily. But the unrelenting cough, especially if accompanied by shortness of breath, chest pain, and a sensation of choking, is so obviously abnormal we can all recognize it. The significance increases markedly when there is blood—bright red or dark red—in the sputum (phlegm) produced.

Rationalizing away the cough as just a 'smokers cough'—as if that made it all right— or as a summer cold, or winter cold, or allergy-spring cold, or a fall cold that has lasted several weeks—are the most common evasions people use. A good rule of thumb is that an ordinary, innocuous virus or allergy cold will never last more than 10 to 14 days.

It is usually the fear of the worst and the unknown, at this point, that drives people away from their physician. It is exactly this kind of rationalization and fear that this book will try to dispel. Please read on, especially under the section which discusses lung cancer and its prevention.

Hoarseness: Here is a clue that is entirely a *horse* of a different color, if you'll pardon the pun. It is most often suggestive of disease of the vocal cords or the throat. An important point is that it does not necessarily mean cancer of the vocal cords or throat.

Since we have all experienced a temporary deepening of the pitch or tone of our voice, we know that it usually clears in a short time even without medical treatment. This benign type of hoarseness nearly always disappears within 7 to 10 days. If it does not clear spontaneously, and in a short time, or if it is accompanied by difficulty in swallowing, difficulty in breathing or weight loss, then medical attention and examination is mandatory.

However, there are many more causes of hoarseness that are minor or at least not cancerous. And the overwhelming chances are that cancer is not the cause of this clue. Using the above guidelines should help the reader decide when to seek their physician's advice. But, when in doubt, get it checked out.

Thickening or lump in the breast: Now we come to one of the most feared and publicized early clues to cancer. The publicity given this point is good and useful. The fear it engenders is not good and must be dealt with and dispelled, because it keeps people from seeing their physician. Too many patients will ignore a lump in the breast for as long as ten years before seeing a physician. The reasons given usually are words to the effect—"I knew it was cancer and that I didn't have a chance" or "I knew nothing could be done and I wouldn't live long." The fact that they didn't develop any distressing symptoms, such as pain, for the first 9 or10 years, or didn't succumb, illustrates how wrong that rationalization was. The person obviously had a slow growing, non-aggressive cancer which could have been treated effectively and perhaps even cured. The point is that even if the patient were right in the diagnosis, the conclusions about treatment were wrong. Even large, long-standing breast cancers can and are being cured by surgery alone, or with combinations of surgery, radiation therapy and chemotherapy.

The second point to be made is that even though breast cancer is the first suspicion the physician will have, the odds are greater that the lump is *not* a breast cancer. Benign, innocuous conditions are still more common than breast cancer, no matter what the lump is like or how long it has been present. So always—and you will notice throughout this book that absolutes are rarely used—'always' seek the advice of a physician.

Additional facts that should alert someone to the possibility of breast cancer are the following: a previous history of breast cancer in the patient; a history of breast cancer in first degree,(mother,sisters and/or daughters) female members of the patient's family; and a patient who has had her first pregnancy after the age of thirty five or has had no pregnancies at all. All these factors increase one's risk of developing breast cancer. They *do not* guarantee that one will inevitably develop the disease.

But avoiding the physician is not the appropriate, rational way to react and thus ignore the predisposition to breast cancer. Regular self-examination of the breast, yearly checkups by a physician, and frequent mammography are 'must do's' for people so predisposed.

The phrase "or elsewhere" is usually added to the above statement about lumps or thickening discovered in the breast by the subject. This may be useful as a signal but it is too general and too vague. Visible or 'feel-able' cancers will be discussed under the dissertations of the individual cancers given in the following pages.

Testicular masses: A more specific and easily examined area which should also raise one's level of concern is a lump or swelling in the testicle(s). Again, the likelihood is that a cancer is not the cause of this change, but it is still an abnormality and must be investigated. This is especially true if it is an entirely new lump, or is a previously noted mass which has increased in size. Also, as in assessing all lumps or masses, they need not be painful, sore or tender to be abnormal, since most testicular cancer masses are painless (as is true for many cancer masses in the early stages).

Skin changes: Here, two of the seven warning signals should be combined into one. They are listed separately as 'an obvious change in a wart or mole' and 'a sore that does not heal.' The reason for combining them is that most 'sores' that a person can see will rarely be found anywhere other than on the skin. Most other sores that are cancers are not easily visualized by the person. Occasionally a sore in the mouth, on the lips, on the tongue or on the very edge of the opening into the nostrils are found by the subject. But these are rare situations and are not as likely to be cancerous growths as some other changes. Also, they are more appropriately discussed under cancers of the mouth and lips.

Before beginning a discussion about the signals arousing suspicion of skin cancer, one important point will be clarified. Here is an area where the public should never fail to seek medical advice because of the high degree of curability (90-95%) of skin cancers and the ease of the treatment (outpatient, minor surgery); the low risk of death from this cancer; and the ease of self-surveillance of the skin.

With the single exception of malignant melanoma—the rarest kind of skin cancer— all other forms of skin cancer are virtually 99% cured with simple removal, usually by minor surgery. They can often be removed in the doctor's office or in an outpatient surgery unit. Even malignant melanoma is often curable if completely removed, early.

According to most surveys, skin cancer accounts for less than two percent of cancer deaths in the United States, and these are mostly due to the highly malignant melanoma form. These facts are emphasized to reduce the fear which is rampant regarding skin cancer and encourage people to seek early medical help for skin abnormalities.

Addressing the statement, "an obvious change in a wart or mole and a sore that does not heal," the qualifiers, 'gross changes' and 'relatively recent and/or rapid changes' should be added.

These qualifiers are added because practically all skin growths change over the years, but they do so very slowly and subtly. The viewpoint that, over-emphasis and excess awareness will bring the patient in earlier or that more people will seek medical examination, even if the warning is exaggerated, is not valid. It simply magnifies the excessive fear mentioned earlier. My personal practical experience has not borne out this viewpoint of over-emphasis. On the contrary, it appears that the fear of "deadly skin cancer" has caused more people to delay treatment. Fear is a weapon that does not work in cancer prevention.

Indigestion and difficulty swallowing: These two signals are usually grouped together as one, although they are quite different in their origins and meaning. Presumably they are joined because they are usually symptoms of trouble in the digestive system.

Difficulty in swallowing, which is discussed first, may be a too general and non-descript term. More specific and inclusive might be phrases such as; pain on swallowing food, liquids or even saliva; inability of food or liquids to pass a point in the passage to the stomach; inability to swallow any foods that are not soft or liquid in consistency; fear of eating, with its resultant weight loss, because of experienced difficulty in the passage of food. To put it very simply, swallowing should be an effortless, almost unconscious act, with no real awareness or distress. If it becomes so, the reader should seek medical examination and advice.

Such a constellation of symptoms indicate abnormalities in the throat itself; in the structures in the neck that impinge on the throat (such as the thyroid gland); in the swallowing tube leading to the stomach (esophagus); along the course of the esophagus as it passes through the chest cavity (containing the lungs, heart and other structures); the stomach itself, or the junction between the esophagus and the stomach.

Obviously, the assessment of such a wide variety of structures will be a major challenge to the physician's abilities, and will require much testing.

Again, as in all symptoms and signs, none of the above are specific for cancer. The overwhelming statistical chances are that cancer is not the cause but, nevertheless, the symptoms must be investigated. Therefore, the reader must not jump to any conclusions but instead they should seek professional help.

Indigestion: Here is another term which is particularly troublesome to define and discuss because of its vagueness and non-specificity. Certainly, the intention in initiating the term was to call attention to cancers involving the digestive system. However, the most common cancer of this system is, by far, in the colon, which was covered by the discussion of 'change in bowel habits,' which is its most common clue. The other organs of the digestive system— namely stomach, liver, pancreas, gall bladder and small intestines—will usually have pain as their most frequent sign of trouble. Therefore, the preferred terms are, pain, discomfort, soreness, tenderness or cramping in the abdominal area at any time. These may occur spontaneously and not only follow eating or drinking.

Unusual bleeding or discharge: These two terms satisfy a need for brevity but are too general and vague. Presumably they were intended to alert the public to the sudden onset of spontaneous bleeding from natural body orifices such as, rectum, vagina, mouth, urinary tract, gums, nose, ears,and the like. Specifying these locations would eliminate the common kinds of bleeding after minor injury from a wound of the skin, nails, etc.

Therefore, assuming that bleeding and discharge from these sites is what is meant, these terms are qualified in the following ways. The word 'discharge' is changed to mean bright red, bloody discharge, or blood tinged discharge, or a brown-black discharge which indicates old, dried blood. These more meaningful and descriptive characteristics eliminate the confusion regarding some normal discharges that occur naturally.

The material discharged from these natural body openings—normally or abnormally—are limited to colors that are close to either white, yellow, blood red or burgundy, brown (old blood) and occasionally green. By and large, the colors of blood-red, pink or brown are the colors which raise the suspicion of cancer as the possible underlying cause. The other colors are more indicative of infection or inflammation of some kind and are infrequently a sign of cancer.

Least likely among these locations to indicate a serious problem is nasal bleeding. This is rarely a signal of cancer primarily because cancer of the nasal passages is relatively uncommon. The one exception is in certain forms of leukemia (erroneously referred to as 'cancer of the blood') and then there are other more specific signals for this affliction. Therefore, it is better to de-emphasize nose bleeds as a useful clue for cancer. Nevertheless, nose bleeds should be investigated by a physician since there is always a cause for this abnormality, although they are seldom serious or life threatening causes.

Bleeding or bloody discharge from the ears and penis (urethra) also fit in the category of rare signs indicative of cancer but, they should be investigated.

Bleeding from the mouth can be interpreted in a variety of ways. The most significant is the actual coughing of blood which can arise from many organs and structures that lead to the mouth. These include: the mouth structures themselves (such as gums, tongue, palate, etc.); the posterior nasal passages; from the intestinal tract as vomiting blood; the throat or the lungs. Each of these areas will be covered under the appropriate discussions of the various cancers based on their location in the body. Suffice it here to say, that, coughing of blood from the lungs portends the most ominous of possibilities namely, cancer of the lung.

Cancer of the colon, rectum or anus, of course, may be signaled by the presence of bloody bowel movements, spontaneous rectal bleeding or black tar-colored stools. These areas have already been discussed in previous passages under, 'changes in bowel habits.'

Moving on to the very important subject of vaginal bleeding it is necessary to try to clarify this commonly confusing situation. It is not required for the patient to be certain whether the bleeding seen is arising from the vagina or the anus before seeing their physician. This is, of course, extremely important to the physician in determining the ultimate cause of the problem. However, the patient should tell the physician that they are not certain where the bleeding arose so that he is not misled away from one area or the other. The physician is now alerted to the need to investigate both of the possible anatomic areas. The close proximity of the vaginal opening to the anal opening can easily cause this dilemma. But the patient should not be embarrassed to admit this uncertainty to the doctor. He realizes the difficulty and he has certainly dealt with it before.

Vaginal bleeding is an extremely important topic for discussion for two basic reasons. First, cancer of the cervix—which frequently causes this symptom—is highly curable if caught early. Second, because the anatomical area is so accessible to examination and routine surveillance. The phrase, *'relative ease,'* is used with tongue-in-cheek. Since, as a male I cannot state this is an easy or not an unpleasant examination to undergo. By relative ease I mean that the examination is of low risk to the patient, is inexpensive, is very helpful and very accurate and does not require hospitalization or sophisticated equipment. These are the desirable characteristics of the Pap smear. Also, it affords the physician the rare opportunity to directly visualize the area of concern without need for x-rays, blood test, exploratory surgery, etc.

A great deal of difficulty arises from trying to define what is considered 'abnormal or unusual' vaginal bleeding in the menstruating female. However, this difficulty never arises in the minds of females who no longer have any vaginal bleeding because they have passed menopause, or have had surgical removal of the uterus (i.e., Hysterectomy). Whether the cervix or ovaries were also removed is not germane to the problem since vaginal bleeding, whether normal or abnormal, can only occur when the uterus is present regardless of the status of the ovaries. Therefore, all vaginal bleeding in all post-menopausal or post-hysterectomy persons requires medical attention. Cancer may not be, and most likely is not, the cause of the bleeding but it is still an abnormal occurrence in post-menopausal women and hysterectomized women.

Defining 'unusual vaginal bleeding' is perplexing in the female during the active menstrual era of her life, but it is even more difficult at the beginning of her menstrual life (menarche) and near the end of it (menopause). At both these ends of the menstrual spectrum vaginal bleeding is usually erratic and irregular.

The usual guidelines given for seeking medical advice include: spotting between menstrual periods; starting to have bleeding again after having stopped for several days; bleeding for more than one's usual length of days; marked increase in the amount of bleeding—best judged by a increase in number of pads used each day, or the passage of large clots; bleeding or spotting that continues, non-stop, throughout the month; marked increase in the amount of pain or cramps experienced during the menstrual period; or the appearance of any unusual or previously inexperienced symptom during an otherwise normal menstrual period.

For many women patients the common misconceptions are: the bleeding must be massive (hemorrhage) to be significant; there must be severe pain accompanying the other change(s) in the pattern; or, since they generally feel well and are not 'sick,' they cannot have a serious problem. None of these changes need accompany abnormal bleeding for it to be significant. The absence of these symptoms may produce a false sense of security. Thus, they may have caused a significant and, sometimes, a fatal delay in diagnosis and treatment.

Miscellaneous signals: Included in this list are some useful signals not usually listed in lay publications.

Weight loss, which is otherwise unexplained and unintentional, is an extremely common and generally, non-specific symptom of many diseases. But it can also be indicative of an active cancer. Some explanation of the term *'weight loss'* is needed. This is not to say that controlling one's weight by dieting or that loosing too much weight can cause cancer. Nor does it mean that if you are 'slightly' overweight you are less likely to develop cancer. On the contrary, there is now beginning to appear some research evidence that cancers are more common and more difficult to diagnose in the obese person. What is referred to is the unexplained, unintentional loss of significant amounts (10% of ideal) of body weight. In other words a loss of body weight despite a normal or even increased caloric intake.

However, this is not an argument in support of the claim that a vitamin deficiency is necessarily a cause of cancer. It also does not imply that taking extra large, or 'mega-doses' of vitamins will protect one from developing cancer. In spite of what we were all told by our beloved mothers and grandmothers, if you're a little chubby it does not mean you are healthier or safer from disease—any disease. Well nourished does not mean over-nourished or over-vitaminized. It means a well balanced diet containing all four basic food groups.

What is considered a 'significant amount' of weight loss? In general, physicians believe that any weight loss greater than 10% of one's usual body weight—over an intermediate period of time (1 to 12 months)—must have a cause. One of those possible causes is cancer.

As with most of the other signals, a non-cancerous cause is statistically more likely but cancer must be considered high on the list.

Summary statement about specific signals: In summary it must be emphasized that there are no universally specific signals which *always* mean cancer is present. Nor are there any *universally mandatory* signals that one must experience to have cancer.

There has never been, nor is there now, any sign or symptom, or group of these (called a syndrome), which has not been experienced by at least some cancer patients. In addition, medical science has not found a signal which reliably excludes or confirms the presence of cancer. A capable physician is aware of this fact and has it tucked away in the back of his brain-files. He rules out or rules in the possibility of cancer with appropriate examinations and testing.

The way cancer produces illness and causes death: Although this seems a gruesome and distasteful topic it is important to discuss and clarify because it also keeps people from seeking early medical attention.

When one hears the statement that someone has "died a terrible death from cancer," or simply that someone has died from cancer, it is automatically assumed that this is undoubtedly the most painful or uncomfortable way to die. Well, to put it frankly, dead is dead. The cause in itself is not important after the fact. However, the mode of death and duration of illness are important.

Studies have shown, and it has been borne out by practical experience, the majority of cancer patients do not experience any significant pain during the course of their illness. And just as importantly, most do not have a painful death. On the contrary, most cancer patients—that is 80% or greater—lapse into a coma. Coma is a painless, anxiety-free state of unconsciousness similar to anesthesia. One might ask, "isn't coma painful?". No coma is not painful. Coma is defined in Webster's dictionary as-a state of deep and prolonged unconsciousness. And in a popular medical dictionary as—an unconsciousness from which the patient cannot be aroused by any stimulus. These stimuli include the sensation of pain, hunger, anxiety, fear,etc. Many have even come to consider it a God-sent, spontaneous type of general anesthesia with freedom from all discomforts. Relatively speaking, this is not necessarily the most uncomfortable way to die. Thus, the mistaken fear of facing the most "horrible form of death" can cause people to neglect their symptoms and miss the chance for a cure.

While it is true that some forms of cancer are accompanied by excruciating kinds of pain—which is also true of many other non-cancerous diseases—the majority of cancer patients do not experience it.

Mechanisms of cancer symptoms: Since the specific mechanisms which cause symptoms are discussed under each cancer type in later chapters, only some general points are made here.

There are several general mechanisms which produce cancer symptoms and signs. These are: local compression of surrounding organs and structures; destruction of distant structures or alteration of an organs normal functions; alteration of the patients natural immunity and resistance to infections; visible and/or detectable alterations in normal anatomy or appearance; and lastly, production by the cancer of hormones, chemicals or other toxic substances which cause the abnormal changes.

All of the above mechanisms can be produced locally at the original site of the cancer, or at a location away from the original growth when the cancer spreads (metastasizes). These are also the ways in which cancer finally takes the life of the patient.

Common examples of the above mechanisms are given below.

Local Compression: Difficulty in swallowing caused by a cancer obstructing or pressing on the esophagus. Examples; Cancer of throat, thyroid, esophagus, stomach, lung, etc.

Damage to Local Structures: Abnormal bleeding such as coughing blood from a lung cancer caused by the cancer growing into and destroying the integrity of a blood vessel. Other similar examples of cancers that cause bleeding by a similar mechanism; cancer of the lung, colon, stomach, uterine cervix, sinus, etc.

Destruction of an Organ: Spontaneous or traumatic bone fractures caused by a cancerous growth destroying the integrity of a otherwise normal bone. Examples: cancer of the breast that has spread to bone; cancers that have spread from elsewhere to other organs—such as spread to the kidney, liver, heart, brain, etc.

Alteration of the Function of an Organ: Shortness of breath caused by destruction of a lung by a lung cancer is typical of a cancer that has destroyed its organ of origin. Other similar examples; Cancer of the lung, brain, liver, kidney, ovary, etc.

Impairment of Immunity and Increased Susceptibility to Infection: A variety of cancers cause a decrease in the amount of immunity inducing proteins manufactured by the body and/or a decrease in the number, and the function of white blood cells which fight infection. Examples; Leukemia, Myeloma, Hodgkin's Disease involving bone marrow, Stomach Cancer that has spread to the liver, etc.

Visible Changes in Anatomy or Physical Appearance: Lumps or masses in the breast, testicles and other visible parts of the body; skin moles, sores or other lesions; enlarged lymph nodes in the neck or groin. Examples; breast cancer, skin cancer, Hodgkin's disease, etc. In addition, through profound weight loss and malnutrition many cancers produce the general appearance of ill-health called emaciation.

Production of Toxins and Hormones: Such mechanisms explain some of the many non-specific symptoms of cancer such as loss of appetite, fever, general feeling of malaise (illness), weakness of muscles, anemia, depression, easy fatigability, weight loss, etc. The production of such toxins or hormones explains the peculiar way in which cancer outside of the digestive system—as bone cancer in an extremity—can cause profound loss of appetite and weight.

Chapter 5

Incidence and Mortality of Cancer

The actual statistics for the occurrence rate and mortality of cancer are readily available to anyone upon request from the National Institutes of Health and the National Cancer Institute. Therefore, no attempt is made here to quote these figures or to reproduce the many charts and graphs of these facts. It is the writer's intention to put these figures in their proper perspective and indicate their true meaning relative to the other causes of death in America.

Also, it is not intended, in anyway, to minimize or de-emphasize cancer as a significant cause of mortality and suffering in the United States. The only desire is to alleviate the excessive fear caused by a distortion of facts which gives the impression everyone is dying from cancer and it must be feared above all other diseases.

In actual fact, cancer is the second leading cause of death in the U.S. and is exceeded by the much more prevalent general group called the *Heart and Vascular Diseases*. Even then, these cancer deaths statistics do not include the very common and nonfatal forms of skin cancer or non-invasive cancer (in situ) of the uterine cervix. The National Cancer Institute does not even feel the need to include them in the statistics of causes of death in the United States because they have so little effect of mortality. Therefore, the figures are skewed and the actual incidence of cancers will far exceed the number of lives it threatens.

Probably more importantly, the disproportionate fear of death from cancer often overshadows *the true leading* cause of death in Americans—Arteriosclerosis ("Hardening of the Arteries"). This single entity, when lumped together instead of being listed under its separate manifestations--heart disease, hypertension, stroke and kidney failure—easily accounts for close to 50% of all deaths in the United States.

When listed separately as Heart Disease, Cerebrovascular Disease, Arteriosclerosis and Aortic Aneurysm—all of which are caused by Arteriosclerosis—these account for approximately 1 million deaths yearly. Whereas, cancer is expected to cause about 520,000 deaths in 1995. The figures acquire even more significance when it is realized that Arteriosclerosis is even more preventable than cancers. A change in dietary habits and personal life styles can save many more lives than appreciated.

The primary purpose here, again, is to discuss cancers and not American health, disease prevention and causes of death in general. But since uncontrolled fear of cancer is a major impediment to its early diagnosis and treatment, if the people need fear any disease, statistically, arteriosclerosis is more appropriate.

Experience has shown this writer that fear is not an effective method in defeating or preventing any disease. Accurate knowledge and understanding are the most effective ideal weapons in our arsenal. These weapons must be widely disseminated to be used to their ultimate effectiveness.

Part Two

The Diagnosis of Cancer

Chapter 6

Diagnosis of Cancer

Defining and clarifying terms for better understanding is the best way to begin. Too often the term 'diagnosis' is considered some mystical, magical method the physician uses to conjure up a cause for a medical problem. According to one medical dictionary it is defined as: "the art and action of determining the nature of the disease" causing the patient's problem. Put simply, it means the use of conventional scientific methodology and rational deduction to reach a conclusion as to the disease producing the problem.

However, in the case of cancer, much more is required to reach such a conclusion. The extra step is the obtaining of a biopsy or an actual piece of the diseased tissue—a small portion of flesh, if you will—to be examined under the microscope. In this way, and in only this way can the diagnosis of cancer be clearly established. At least, it is the only means of establishing the diagnosis beyond any reasonable doubt.

Of course, accomplishing a diagnosis cannot ordinarily be accomplished in a matter of minutes, and seldom even within hours or, on occasion, even days. Certainly, after the first visit to the physician the reader cannot reasonably expect to have the diagnosis confirmed. Three stages are followed in the process of establishing a diagnosis. These stages are, **(1) the Initial Impression, (2) the Clinical (Working) Diagnosis, (3) the Final (Pathological) Diagnosis.** Each of these steps is discussed in the order in which they will occur, for clarity. As a result of this orderly discussion the reader will now understand the process and what can be expected from it.

Why even bother with these time consuming steps? Why not proceed directly to obtaining the biopsy? Sometimes this is possible with abnormalities or lesions which are easily accessible, such as the Pap smear by pelvic examination in the female, or by office biopsy of a skin lesion. However, often the material for biopsy is not easily accessible and can be obtained only with significant risk and requires hospitalization for safety. Under these circumstances there are now several ways to obtain the needed tissue for diagnosis. The careful, competent physician now proceeds in a logic, step wise manner to choose the proper method of biopsy.

Beginning with the safest, least painful, and least traumatic procedure, the physician then progresses to the more difficult means of obtaining the biopsy. Sometimes the safer procedure also yields the lowest rate of positive results but it seems reasonable to avoid any hazard to the patient, whenever possible. If the simple collection of a sample of sputum, or scraping from a mouth lesion help to avoids surgical biopsy, it is worth the short delay.

The question of so called *delay* deserves comment. Frequently the patient feels that time is of such major essence and that diagnosis must be established within days or even hours. While time is important, a rapid diagnosis within days or hours is seldom, if ever, of critical import. Even the so called 'very aggressive cancers' take weeks to months to progress and threaten life. The performance of a biopsy can be a fatal procedure for the patient who has serious complications from other illnesses such as heart disease or lung disease. The physician first treats these problems to reduce the risk of fatality to the lowest level. Therefore, time must be taken to improve the general health status of the subject.

The basic medical axiom, "first, doctor, be sure to cause no harm," is a reflection of this philosophy. Decades of clinical experience in managing cancer cases has demonstrated that a cautious, step wise approach has not caused undue risk of the cancer progressing rapidly. The old cliche—haste makes waste—is very appropriate to medical diagnosis.

Now getting back to the three stages in the diagnostic process; initial impression, clinical (working) diagnosis, final (pathological) diagnosis.

The **initial impression** is the educated guess(es) the physician makes after he has completed his initial basic and simple examination. Simple and basic means those things the physician does using his five senses and the simple instruments found in every doctor's office. The blood pressure cuff, stethoscope, thermometer and ophthalmoscope are examples of these instruments.

However, before placing a hand or instrument on the patient a meticulous, complete examination begins with a series of pointed and specific questions—known as the medical history. In fact, as much time, if not more, should be spent asking these questions as is spent in actual physical examination. It is an inherent part of a complete examination. It is more appropriately called the **'Medical History and Physical Examination.'** Together they form an indispensable part of the careful, comprehensive evaluation of any case.

Therefore, do not become impatient with your physician during this questioning period. At times the questions seem irrelevant and unimportant but having confidence in your doctor includes trusting that he knows what is useful, even if it seems trivial. If this confidence in his judgement is not there, it is best the reader choose another physician.

After the series of, seemingly boring and unnecessary, questions with their appropriate answers obtained the actual laying on of hands can begin. After any and all significant abnormalities are noted and recorded the physician may ask more questions in reference to any abnormal findings uncovered.

All these findings and answers to questions are then formulated to reach an **initial impression,** i.e.; what is most likely causing the symptoms. More often than not, however, this preliminary information leads to a list of two or three possibilities(called the 'differential diagnosis') which are considered most likely to be present. Just as often it is decided which particular organ system is diseased, i.e., the digestive system (stomach, colon, gallbladder, etc.), the respiratory system (lungs, throat, sinuses, etc.). The next step is to proceed with testing of each of the suspected areas. In perhaps 20% of instances the physician might confess that he cannot even make a rough estimate of the cause of the problem with the information presently available. The doctor should be willing to discuss such a dilemma with the patient at this point. She should reveal her impressions and where her analysis is leading her. If she doesn't, ask him. The patient has the right to know.

The **History and Physical** examination are now complete and the process moves to the next stage in the evaluation. Take note that no laboratory testing or x-rays have been carried out up to this point. Special emphasis is placed on this because many readers believe a thorough 'physical' is synonymous with a large amount of testing. This is simply not the case. A simple office biopsy at this point may be all that is required to establish the diagnosis. The physician is the best judge of what constitutes a **Complete Physical** because there is no one infallible formula. The judgement and experience of the physician becomes most important here, not a universal formula or computer printout.

All of these bits of information are now fed into the doctor's *fleshy computer*—called the brain, which contains an ingredient no computer has, namely, experience. Now through logic she chooses some specific and some general kinds of laboratory tests and x-rays. Keep in mind, at this point cancer may or may not even be on the list of possibilities, or it may be very low on the list. It depends on the historical facts obtained from the questions and on the signs (anatomical abnormalities) found on the physical examination.

The **Clinical (Working) Diagnosis** results from the assessment of the combined information obtained from the first two steps; the history and physical examination, and the initial laboratory tests and x-rays. At this time the doctor has some specific ideas and precise disease entities he is strongly considering. This may still comprise a list of possibilities but the list should now be shorter and more specific.

As an example, the following combination of facts is a common clinical situation. A history of coughing blood, shortness of breath and weight loss is reported by a cigarette smoker. Abnormal sounds are heard in the lungs on physical examination of the chest and an abnormal shadow is seen on a chest x-ray. These findings, however, do not exclusively lead to a diagnosis of lung cancer but they are strong evidence for it. Among others diseases, these symptoms can be caused by lung abscess, chronic pneumonia, tuberculosis, bronchitis, emphysema, etc.

When the information is digested and analyzed by the physician, the next step can be taken to reach the **Final (Pathological) Diagnosis,** namely, the biopsy. A pathologist then examines the biopsy under the microscope after some special processing and staining. He then determines if the specimen is or is not cancerous.

Chapter 7

The Definitive Diagnosis of Cancer

The Biopsy

I'm sure the physician will have discussed with the reader the reasons it was decided a biopsy was necessary. Also, the risk versus the benefits should have been pointed out. If these points were not discussed, be sure to ask. You have the right to know and need to know these answers before proceeding.

Several characteristics of the biopsy are worth discussing before undertaking the procedure.

When the physician suggests a biopsy be taken he is still not necessarily implying that cancer is present. The biopsy is also useful for diagnosing many other noncancerous diseases. In many cases it is the only way to accurately diagnose many maladies not even remotely related to cancer but which can mimic it.

Therefore, hasty conclusions should not be made by the reader when a biopsy is suggested. Although cancer may be the physician's number one consideration at this point it cannot be established as the 'final diagnosis' until that biopsy is obtained and interpreted.

Exactly what is a biopsy and how is it obtained? Most important, besides clarifying what a biopsy *is,* it is equally important to know what it *is not*, what it can do and cannot do, and other pertinent facts.

A biopsy is a collection of cells obtained from the living body by a variety of methods which allow a pathologist to examine those cells under a microscope (and by other means) to determine what disease the abnormal tissue represents.

What a biopsy *is not*, : It is not perfect; it cannot tell the future or give a prognosis; it is not a death warrant; it cannot tell the extent of the disease throughout the body; it does not mean a hopeless outcome; it does not mean that cure or effective treatment is not available.

The biopsy is just like any other test used in medical diagnosis in that it is not infallible. It is not 100% accurate no matter who reads it. There are false positives and false negatives. There are also many situations where no conclusion at all can be reached from examining the biopsy. Ordinarily, a repeat of the biopsy will be recommended. When this occurs the reader should not surmise that the professionals involved were incompetent. The most prestigious of medical centers have inconclusive results. It is simply the nature of the test. This is precisely the reason medical science is considered as inexact. Natural human biology, and its abnormal variant called pathology, follows very few rules. And even those few are not followed consistently.

Pathology is a science practiced by human beings who examine thousands of biopsy specimens and, therefore, as humans they are not infallible. With enough training and experience they can examine a biopsy specimen and reach a reasonable conclusion—most of the time. But it is very much like beauty, or ugliness in the case of disease. It is all in the eye of the beholder and, thus, open to a variety of interpretations. And, naturally, there are some disagreements on the interpretation. Therefore, a biopsy which is inconclusive should not cause the reader an undue amount of distress. It is not a reflection of incompetency or carelessness. It is simply the nature of the science. Most often a repeat biopsy, in the near future or after a short period of observation, will settle the issue.

The biopsy is *not* a means of making a prediction (prognosis), at least not by itself—there are a few exceptions to this statement which are outlined in future chapters. There are occasional instances when the biopsy is the most reliable means of indicating prognosis but it is seldom the *only* means.

If the physician gives the patient a copy of the final pathology report—and you have a right to it, if you so desire, but you really don't need it to ask some basic questions—it may contain words such as Malignant, Invasive, Class V, Aggressive, Infiltrating, etc. As discussed elsewhere these terms are not of any value to you, the patient. They do not indicate your future outcome. These are words and phrases which help the physician decide on a course of action. He then conducts other tests to determine your Clinical Stage of the cancer and, thus, arrives at a choice of treatment and the case's prognosis—and the patient's chances of survival or cure. These are discussed in detail in due course.

In summary, the pathologist decides if the biopsy is a cancer but that is all he determines. The pathologist is not a clinical practitioner, meaning he does not, ordinarily, treat any patients and is not trained to do so. Your physician, or the specialist he designates, determines the extent of the cancer and then makes a judgement regarding prognosis and treatment.

We are now at the point at which the histological type of the cancer is assigned to the biopsy. Words such as carcinoma, sarcoma, adenocarcinoma, etc. are assigned to the tissue examined. These terms were defined and discussed in prior sections.

It was pointed out that these terms indicated malignant change, which only means that the physician must act aggressively to effect a cure but this term is not a death warrant.

Other qualifying terms may also be applied to the biopsy report, such as; invasive, class I, II or III, aggressive, penetrating, etc. These also are only terms of utility. They alert the physician to the need for aggressive therapy.

Evasive Terms: The physician not accustomed to handling the word frequently might be reluctant to use the term CANCER. Instead, evasive words might be used such as neoplasm, malignant growth, anaplastic cells, serious growth, tumor, and the like. As has been stated, these are chosen because the physician knows the immediate conclusions reached in the patient's mind and the fear engendered by the word cancer. But now, after thoroughly defining and discussing it, it is clear what the word cancer does and does not mean. Therefore, ask your physician in a straightforward manner if he is referring to cancer or not. Once that hurdle is cleared everyone can relax and proceed to the more pertinent facts about staging, treatment plan, risk versus benefit, cure rates, survival rates, etc. Remember these cannot be determined by the biopsy alone.

Chapter 8

Methods of Obtaining a Biopsy

The means of obtaining the biopsy are extremely varied and are based on the clinical situation, the location of the possible cancer, the age of the patients and their general medical condition, etc. As a thorough and competent professional your physician has already completed the history and physical examination; performed and interpreted preliminary blood, urine, sputum and other basic tests; has already done preliminary x-ray examinations and is now ready to approach the area to be biopsied.

There are three distinct ways the biopsy specimen may be obtained. These are classified as **(1) Non-invasive, (2) Semi-invasive, and (3) Invasive.** These three divisions indicate whether or not the natural integrity of the body has to be penetrated to obtain the specimen.

Non-invasive is a method of obtaining cells from a naturally occurring body opening without breaking through the tissue. This method would include, for example; a Pap smear from the female uterine cervix, collecting sputum through induced or spontaneous coughing, gently scraping some cells from the lining of certain structures such as stomach, mouth, throat or nasal passages. But the major point is that natural body cavities are *not* penetrated by needles or surgery. These means of testing pose no major risk to the subject and, therefore, are somewhat ideal methods. Unfortunately, the positive yield or chances of obtaining a conclusive answer to the diagnostic dilemma by this method is not perfect and not many cancers are accessible via this means.

Semi-invasive studies means actual penetration of some body cavity and thereby breaking down some natural defenses to obtain a piece of tissue or to aspirate (suction out) some cells. Examples of such approaches include a needle biopsy of an organ, i.e., liver, lung, kidney, breast, etc. These procedures have a moderately higher risk for complications, and even rarely death, but are still lower in risk and mortality than actual surgery.

The invasive methods include all surgical means of obtaining a biopsy. The natural skin, and other barriers of the body, are actually opened and penetrated to reach the suspicious area for biopsy. The procedure includes biopsy by excision of a tumor mass, an entire organ, or diseased area to be examined by the pathologist. Examples are: excisional breast biopsy; abdominal surgery; chest cavity surgery; brain surgery; excisional removal of lymph nodes in the neck, groin and other areas; bladder and prostate surgery.

Regardless of the technique the physician chooses it must be discussed in detail with the patient and family before proceeding. If discussion of this information is not volunteered, ask your physician to outline the plan. You do have the right to know, you must know these facts, to make a rational judgement along with the physician's expert advise regarding such an important choice. The reader should avoid any preconceived judgements before discussing these options, although the author realizes that this is sometimes difficult. The physician can give a reasonable, logical explanation why it was decided to proceed in a specific manner. If your doctor refuses to discuss the reasons for the choice it is best to seek a second opinion.

Now that it has been established that a biopsy or cell sample is the only reliable way to establish the diagnosis of cancer, how does the doctor decide what and where to biopsy? On the surface, the choice appears simple and obvious, and on occasion, it is. But more often than not it is a very difficult choice for the physician to make. His expertise, training, wisdom, and experience are put to a major test in making the decision. Indeed, any automaton can push a computer button and order every test and x-ray known to medical science without any rhyme or reason. Not only does this make the cost of medical diagnosis excessive, but it also endangers many people by subjecting them to hazardous and unnecessary testing.

The only situations where the site of biopsy is obvious are in the cases of suspicious lesions directly visible to the physician with the unaided eye. Examples of such situations are; skin growths, abnormalities in the mouth, nasal passages, vagina, and the cervix of the uterus. However, most cancers are of the internal variety and can only be biopsied with some degree of risk. Therefore, to justify the risk the physician gathers some clues to strongly support his suspicion of cancer and its location. The basic, logical steps your physician first learned in medical school are used to gather the clues. The doctor then progresses up a rational path paved with caution, scientific reasoning, safety and cost effectiveness to a logical choice.

The *medical history* followed by the basic *physical examination* is the first indispensable step to be taken. Basic, common and readily available blood tests, urine tests, and x-rays usually follow. After the baseline information is obtained, the possibility of a biopsy and how best to obtain it follows.

There are great many words written and spoken regarding the perfect universal *Cancer Test(s)*. The truth is that there is (are) no such test(s). We all dream and pray for a safe, simple, inexpensive and easy to apply test to screen large numbers of people for any and all kinds of cancer, but none exists at the present time. This statement also includes all of the unproven blood, urine, electronic and other tests claiming to have such universal capabilities. The subject of unfounded claims for treatment and diagnosis will be discussed in more detail later.

In going through the process of eliminating possible diagnoses many different scientific tools are used to examine the structure and function of the internal organs. Blood and urine tests are utilized for this specific purpose but not necessarily to diagnose cancer. They are used to test a wide variety of organs for evidence of abnormal function or structure. As an example, the commonly used general blood profile—also known as the Chemistry Profile, SMA 12, 21, etc.,—is such a test. It helps to detect abnormalities of the liver, kidneys, pancreas, heart, lungs, and almost every other internal organ, directly or indirectly. But, it is *not* a cancer test. It simply directs the physician down the most likely diagnostic path.

The same can be stated for: the routine blood cell count—an actual numerical count of blood cells; the routine urine analysis (mistakenly thought to test only for diabetes); the chest x-ray, which not only visualizes the structure of the lungs but also of the heart, large blood vessels, lymph nodes, bones, ribs, and the air passages.

Many other x-rays are used to study the structure of other internal organs. Another example is the barium studies, a liquid that is swallowed or inserted through an enema tube, to examine most of the length of the intestinal tract. Harmless dyes can be administered either by mouth or by injection to visualize countless structures including kidney, gallbladder, liver, circulatory system, etc. Ingenious ways have been devised to improve the imaging of these techniques such as scans, tomograms, CAT (Computerized Axial Tomography) scan, and so on.

An extremely highly technological method called Magnetic Resonance Imaging (MRI) has been developed to enhance the ability of examining otherwise inaccessible internal structures while eliminating even the small hazards of dyes and radiation exposure from radioactive contrast substances. The patient is not subjected to even one particle of radiation by this technique.

Ultrasonic imaging (echogram or sonogram) is another technique developed for the same purpose and with the same advantages; that is, examination of internal structures without dyes or radiation exposure. The technique is even safe enough to examine the developing fetus inside the uterus of the mother.

Make no mistake about it, however, none of these tests actually make a diagnosis of cancer... because they do not provide the mandatory sample of tissue or cells required to make such a diagnosis. They simply help to direct the physicians attention to the area most likely to provide the necessary specimen.

Methods of Obtaining the Biopsy Specimen:

There are any number of ways of obtaining the necessary tissue for a diagnosis but your physician proceeds in a logical way to do so. What he should consider first is the ease of performing the test with as little discomfort to the patient as possible; second, the safety of the method to minimize the risk of mortality or permanent disability is ascertain; third, the accuracy of the method; and last, the relative cost are major concerns.

One of the easiest and safest methods of obtaining cells is to simply collect and examine any of the bodies natural secretions for cancerous changes. A prime example is the simple procedure of collecting and examining coughed sputum for cancer cells. But, unfortunately the method has very limited utility.

There are three basic methods which are utilized to obtain a specimen: simple scraping or brushing of cells from the surface of the lesion; snipping or pinching off a small piece of the tissue; or actual surgical excision under local or general anesthesia. These approaches range in magnitude from a simple office procedure with no risks to major surgery with very high risks. Obviously, every attempt is made to avoid the last method, if at all possible, especially if the patient has other serious complicating medical conditions.

Brushings or Scrapings: the common and well known "Pap' test best exemplifies this method. Cells are scraped from the surface of the uterine cervix, the vaginal walls, and aspirated as secretions from the opening in the cervix which are expelled by the lining of the uterus when performing the test. Lesions which may be visible to the physician on pelvic examination can also be snipped off with minor discomfort, great safety and high yield accuracy

Other approaches used to obtain scrapings include a variety of endoscopic procedures. Endoscopy means the insertion of a tube (scope) into a natural body passage through which the physician directly visualizes the suspicious area and, either brushes some cells off or snips off a portion of tissue. Such samples are commonly obtained from the colon via a colonoscope; from the stomach via a gastroscope;

from the colon via a colonoscope; from the stomach via a gastroscope; from the larynx via a laryngoscope; from the bronchial tubes of the lungs via a bronchoscope; etc. The principal advantages of these methods are the physician's ability to actually see the area being biopsied, and the lower risk to the subject in avoiding major surgery.

Another means of approaching a suspicious lesion is the needle biopsy and some of its variations. The disadvantages of the needle method include, the moderately increased danger and discomfort to the patient; and the slightly greater cost; and the inability to directly visualize the lesion. The last drawback is partially overcome by the operator guiding the needle to the precise area under fluoroscopy or, more recently, via the CAT scan. In this needle biopsy method an actual piece of tissue is removed, as opposed to an aspiration of cells, which makes the accuracy of the method greater.

Some needle biopsy methods are totally *blind* and without visualization but these are very safe procedures which have a high degree of accuracy and do not require general anesthesia. The list of these methods consists of such procedures as, bone marrow aspiration, bone marrow biopsy, lumbar punctures, and other internal organ needle biopsies.

The final method, actual surgical excision, is frequently fraught with the greatest risk of mortality. But this statement is true only when a major body cavity is entered or when general anesthesia is required. The major body cavities include the head or cranial cavity (neurosurgery), the chest cavity (thoracic surgery), the abdominal cavity (abdominal surgery), the pelvis in the female (gynecological surgery), or the pelvis in the male (genito-urological surgery).

The surgeon who is to perform the operation or the primary care physician should discuss the hazards of procedure and the reasons why this approach is necessary before proceeding.

There are, of course, simple and safe means of surgical excision of a cancer such as removal of skin lesions; snaring of polyps via the colonoscope; and the like.

In certain disease situations abnormal fluid is produced in large quantities by the body as a manifestation of that disease. Often the fluid is safely, painlessly removed and examined for cancer cells.

Chest (pleural) fluid, and abdominal fluid (also known as ascites) are examples which readily come to mind.

Surgery for diagnostic biopsy is different than surgery for therapeutic or curative purposes. In the first instance the surgery is performed solely for clarifying an unclear diagnosis. It is a means of obtaining the necessary sample of tissue but is not necessarily part of the treatment and does not eliminate the need for further therapy. There are occasions when the surgical removal of an entire organ for biopsy is also part of the treatment of the cancer. But not always. The reader should not consider this surgery as treatment unless so stated by the physician. If the patient has any doubts about this point they should ask their physician before the surgery is performed.

After the biopsy specimen is obtained and interpreted as being a cancer the next steps can be taken but only after certain details of this process are discussed with the patient.

These steps are collectively known as the *staging process*. Without this most important process a rational prediction of curability (prognosis) and a sensible treatment plan *cannot* be made. Staging simply means examining other organs of the body most commonly affected by a specific type of cancer to determine if they are indeed involved with the disease. This process exists because medical science has come to recognize that cancer is most often a systemic, generalized disease and not a locally limited process. The recognition of this fact is one of the single most, and most unheralded, advancements in the field of cancer medicine. And now, all physicians and the public must think of cancer as a generalized, systemic illness. Realization of this systemic principle explains why surgery alone has failed to cure many cancers which were heretofore considered to be localized.

Readers take note of the emphasis on the statement made above that *the prognosis and the treatment plan cannot* logically follow *without* the completed staging process. The following chapter will describe and define the staging process in detail.

Therefore, after the completion of the biopsy or removal of the cancer the physician is *not* finished and he *cannot* answer many, if any of the reader's questions in the areas of prognosis, treatment choice, and so on.

Chapter 9

The Staging of Cancer

Staging is generally divided into two types: pathological staging and clinical staging.

Clinical staging means nonsurgical testing to detect the presence of any spread of the cancer to any other organ or tissue. Testing may included further x-rays or scans of the brain, liver, spleen, bones, etc. In addition, direct visual examination of other likely areas is performed during surgery along with removal of suspicious lymph nodes and biopsies of commonly involved organs such as liver, bones, etc. It may even require, in special circumstances, further and more extensive surgery. If more surgery is advised, it illustrates how critical and indispensable the staging process is to the complete surveillance of any cancer case. Many times the use of the x-rays, scans and blood tests are not enough to determine the stage of the disease without further biopsies.

Pathological staging means the taking of additional biopsies or samples of tissue from highly suspect areas to confirm or rule out the presence of spread. Since organs can be enlarged without being involved with the cancer makes additional biopsies necessary. Frequently the organ enlargement indicates the patient has other unrelated diseases in progress which are unrelated to the cancer but also need treatment. Since treatment can aggravate these other conditions investigating these other conditions is especially important. Also, if an area is presumed involved with cancer incorrectly the patient may receive an erroneously worse prognosis and the wrong choice of treatment. The chance for a cure could be lost, forever.

The need for further staging procedures, and whether they will require more surgery or not, depends on the original biopsy report. It also depends on the safety of the second surgery. The physician should explain the reasons for these choices. If the choices are not explained, ask for the explanation. You have the right to know.

Staging Designations: When both the clinical and pathological staging is completed it is customary to assign a simplified numerical designation to each cancer case. What follows is a description of these numerical staging systems.

The lack of universality and uniformity in the terms used in the staging system has caused much confusion in this area. In some cancers the stages are designated by Roman numerals I, II, III, etc. In other systems they are designated by capital letters A, B, C, D, etc. And still in other systems they are combined as IA, IIB and so on. Many times a particular system is used because it is traditional, and in others because it is easier for physicians around the world to understand. The practical reasons for using any staging system are, however, two fold. First, to allow for ease of research reporting of large groups of patients in different research centers with some consistency. These results can then be compared and combined in order to report, with some degree of uniformity, the end results to assess the effectiveness of various treatments.

Second, the staging system enables your physician to design a sensible treatment plan and present you with a reasonably accurate prognosis. In addition, the discussion between the physician and patient is made easier when there is a simple common language without use of technical terms.

The reader need not memorize or even know these staging designations to have the basic questions of prognosis, treatment and side effects answered clearly. However, every patient has the right to these terms, if they so desire. However, if the staging systems are misunderstood they can cause confusion or concern in your mind leading to errors in judgements and faulty decisions. Sometimes the prognosis and treatment choice between, say, a Stage IA or IIB, is so small as to be insignificant even though the extent of disease is different. Your physician should be willing to clarify these points for the reader.

Unfortunately, there are times when the cancer is so widespread that any further staging serves no real purpose. At other times the risk of further staging is too great because of other serious, concurrent complicating illnesses. Your doctor can explain these complicating circumstances and explain to you why the more prudent, conservative approach is best. When more extensive major, high-risk surgery is required to complete the staging process is a good example. At such times, often, other safer and simple tests, such as x-rays, scans, spinal taps and certain needle biopsies are still reasonable to perform.

On the other hand, the patient should never be dismissed offhandedly by the physician as—'a case of widespread cancer and nothing can be done'—without some simple staging tests being performed.

The specific details of staging depend on the individual case and on the precise type of cancer diagnosed by the biopsy. More particular information about the minimum amount of staging for each cancer type is discussed in more detail further on in this book.

The basic axioms used to decide on staging procedures are: perform only those tests which substantially alter the choice of therapy or significantly influence the prognosis; start with the safest and least costly; and choose those which have an acceptable degree of accuracy and reliability. Even if a testing procedure changes the stage, but does not change the treatment, it is not needed.

Chapter 10

"The Cancer Check-up"

A more accurate heading for this chapter would read, 'the so-called *cancer check up.*' Because there is, essentially, no such specific check up, just as there is (are) no specific *cancer test(s).*

Of course, someone can go to a physician with a specific concern about cancer in mind and the examination might focus on the areas of concern but this is a customized examination. It is not a general cancer examination. Even then the scope of the examination depends on the type of cancer under consideration since, as we have already learned, cancer consists of a group of diseases. Therefore, there is no standard battery of tests or x-rays which are performed under the title of, *The Cancer Check Up*.

There are groups of tests carried out—when indicated—to detect specific types of cancer in particularly high risk groups of the population. They will be discussed in detail later on. There are also groups of tests which are utilized to detect a nonspecific abnormality, and nothing more, with cancer as one of the more common possibilities. These are also discussed in detail below.

There is also a large group of unproven, unconventional tests done under the guise of *Cancer Tests* which have no proven value at all. These are not even accepted as proven general medical tests to anyone except the charlatans who profit from the sale of them.

Since there is no specific cancer checkup, a thorough medical examination is done beginning with a complete history of the present complaints, and past illnesses, and a basic survey of detectable physical changes in all parts of the body. An example of such a process is outlined as follows:

History of the Illness: Your physician begins with ascertaining your so called chief complaint or major symptom. That is, the primary symptom, physical change or health concern which prompted you, the reader, to seek an examination in the first place. Whether it is pain, weight loss, fever, fatigue, bleeding, or fear of illness the process follows the same general steps. The questions which follow are an attempt to obtain some of the characteristics of the symptom. They include such questions as; how long has it been present; is it a mild, moderate or severe change; what situations precipitate the symptom or make it better or make it worse? In other words, all the details about the chief complaint(s) should be touched upon to narrow the list of possible causes.

Then more pointed questions are asked to lead the physician to conclusions regarding the organ system most likely diseased. Let's say, for example, that abdominal pain is the chief complaint. Your doctor may ask if it is accompanied by nausea and vomiting, a change in bowel habits, caused by ingestion of specific foods or beverages. Is it relieved by a change in position, ingestion or administration of certain patent remedies? and so on. These questions are useful especially in problems in the abdominal cavity since there are so many different organs and systems located in this area.

Review of Systems: Several general questions are asked about all the other body systems if they were not already mentioned. The inquiry begins at the anatomical top of the body, namely the head, and runs down in an orderly fashion to the lower extremities, even to the feet.

Note that at this point your doctor has not yet placed an examining hand upon you, the patient, except, perhaps, in a greeting hand shake. And this is as it should be since it is your answers which direct your physician to the most likely diseased areas. The physical examination adds more information to the data bank later.

Past Health History: Questions regarding all past illnesses, even as early as childhood, are now asked. The questions are limited to only major illnesses which may now be producing residual or delayed symptoms.

Past Surgical History: Past surgical operations and major injuries are delved into at this point. These earlier events might reveal previous suspicions of cancer or other pre-cancerous conditions. In females, a history of difficult pregnancies, spontaneous abortions (miscarriages), menstrual abnormalities are all very important facts to uncover.

Personal Habits: The habitual use of tobacco, alcohol, and harmful drugs are recorded since some of these increase the risk of cancer and other diseases.

An **Occupational History** is very important to uncover facts about previous exposure to disease causing substances in the work environment. These include such things as asbestos, beryllium, uranium mining, benzene, and other less publicized substances.

Medication Use: Facts in relation to prescribed or over-the-counter medications are asked at this time since some medicines do increase the risk of diseases including, rarely, cancer.

Family Medical History: Herein lies one of the most useful—and most neglected—areas in diagnosing disease, especially in reference to cancer since some do have familial/inheritance tendencies. For example, a history of breast cancer in the mother, sisters, or daughters of a female patient is extremely important. A history of colon cancer in any first degree relative is also of significance.

The cause of death and the age at death of parents, siblings, or children is obtained. The presence of active diseases in living relatives is also important.

At this juncture the physician may not have even considered cancer as the cause of your medical problems, unless you had specifically mentioned it earlier in the history. And this is appropriate, since it is best for the doctor to keep an open mind to all possibilities until some concrete and highly suggestive evidence raises the possibility of cancer.

The Physical Examination: The physical examination consists of the very basic, simple maneuvers the physician carries out in his examining room using the simple instruments with which we are all familiar. The blood pressure cuff, stethoscope, ophthalmoscope, the thermometer, and other rudimentary tools are typical examples. Also included are the five senses of sight, sound, touch, even occasionally the sense of smell and taste.

Often, by the time the history of the present illness and the basic physical examination are completed the physician is 90% certain of the cause of the problem, or at least the organ system in which it originated.

The first pieces of data obtained are the subject's weight, height, blood pressure, pulse and temperature by a nurse or other assistant.

A well trained and alert physician begins the next step by simply observing the patient, looking at the face, the eyes, the way he walks into the room, takes a seat, sits in the chair, arises from it, and mounts the examining table. He looks at the texture of the skin, its color, or the lack of color. Simply stated, a keen eye for details, no matter how small or insignificant, is the mark of a thorough and meticulous physician.

The remainder of the examination proceeds as a systematic, anatomical scrutiny of all the parts of the body. Surface observations are usually made first. Eye inspection is made of the skin, hair, nails, eye lids, the outer covers of the eye including the whites of the eye (sclera) and pupils.

Then the examination begins with the head and neck, and proceeds through every organ down the body to the feet and toes. Of course, in females this always includes a thorough examination of the breasts.

Internal examinations then follow. Included are inspection of the internal structures of the eyes, ears, nose, mouth and throat. A pelvic examination is done in females to survey the reproductive organs— the uterus and its cervix, ovaries, tubes, vagina, etc.

In both sexes, the rectal examination is imperative. In males careful assessment of the size, texture and structure of the prostate gland must not be omitted. Chemically testing the stool for hidden (occult) blood is obligatory in all patients over 40 years of age.

Frequently, your physician has already formed a working diagnosis, and occasionally a conclusive one, by the time the history and physical examination is completed. Some easily visible and palpable (tangible) lesions on the skin, in the mouth, and in the breast certainly suggest cancer... but they still must be biopsied. Because a presumptive or suggestive diagnosis is never good enough.

Why do I bother to take the time and space to discuss such a elementary part of medical diagnosis as the *History and Physical Examination?* Why does it deserve such emphasis? Especially since it is not a recently developed, highly technological process? The reasons are essentially simple. First, there is so much misunderstanding about the *History and Physical Examination* that the public and physicians have a tendency to neglect it. The second reason is so the reader and any prospective patient knows what to look for to identify an ideal examination, as opposed to one which is cursory, inadequate, and, as result, of little value.

Now is when some basic laboratory tests and x-rays are performed to support the suspicions of your physician. Sometimes unusual tests are added early in the diagnostic investigation because the suspicions are so strong for cancer. Several tests and x-rays, however, are mandatory for general surveillance in all cases. These include blood cell counts, urine analysis, a general chemical survey of the internal organs' functions. This last test is known by many other titles, such as: a SMAC 12, Chemistry profile, Internal Organ survey, etc. Although the tests are named differently they essentially all measure the same thing, i.e., the function of several major organ systems; the liver, kidney, bones, pancreas, general mineral survey, circulatory system, cholesterol or other metabolic processes. It provides valuable clues to any structural dysfunction of the heart, brain, blood and lymph system, general nutrition, the lungs and many other organs.

Although there is some disagreement among physicians on this point, it is now generally believed that an electrocardiogram and chest x-ray are not routinely necessary unless there are specific symptoms or physical abnormalities to suggest the need. More will be said about these tests later in this work.

The 'Pap Test' (named after Dr. Papanicalou who developed it) is required for all females who have symptoms in this area; for all females who are sexually active, regardless of age; and for those women in the child bearing age group. Although significant debate exists regarding the frequency of the Pap test—annually versus every three years—and regarding the age groups which require regular periodic testing, the above guidelines are generally followed.

The author's personal preference is to perform the test: whenever any patient requests it; annually in women in their reproductive years and those who are sexually active; every six months in patients taking birth control medication; every three years in all females after menopause; and in all patients having gynecological symptoms—i.e., vaginal bleeding after menopause, painful menstrual periods, painful intercourse, vaginal discharge, etc.

The term *specific cancer tests* requires special attention. As already pointed out there is (are) no such test(s). There are several tests which have been found useful in; (1) highly suspicious clinical situations, (2) screening certain high risk groups for certain types of cancer, and, (3) as an aid in following the course of known cancers. But as far as a specific or highly sensitive test for screening the general population for the presence of *any and all* types of cancer, such a test doesn't exist. At least not yet.

Some of the more useful cancer screening tests are commented upon below.

The Pap Test: Although this is actually a sample of cells from the uterine cervix it only acts as a stepping stone. Even when highly suspicious, it is not diagnostic of cancer of the cervix, per se. Interpretations of the test are graded from Class I to V. Class V is highly suspicious for cancer but it only functions to alert the physician to proceed to a more conclusive examination... the biopsy.

The Pap test is also adaptable to other organs of the body from which cells can be easily scraped or from which cells are extruded spontaneously. The cells found in coughed up sputum, the urine, cells lining the stomach, esophagus, and other organs are examples. These, however, are not recommended for general routine surveillance use but are indicated only in specific cases where other clues point to these organs.

The Mammogram: Now that the level of radiation dose exposure has become acceptable this x-ray examination of the breasts has gained in popularity and prominence. However, it cannot be overemphasized that it does not replace but only complements the monthly self-examination of the breasts carried out by the reader and the periodic examination by a physician.

Nevertheless, the mammogram has added a much needed dimension to the early detection of breast cancer. Its greatest application is in the discovery of the breast lesions which are too small to be detected by palpation by the physician. The significance of the detection lies in the fact that the smaller the breast cancer at the time of discovery the higher the chances of cure.

In addition, it helps augment the physician's ability to decide if a biopsy is needed in a questionable lesion. Such a dilemma arises frequently in the patient who has had previous multiple biopsies which have been benign. Also, the physician frequently cannot judge by palpation if a lump is likely to be malignant or benign. Even in the rare instances where the mass is accompanied by the highly suggestive *dimpling* of the overlying skin, the so called *orange peel* appearance of the overlying skin, or the presence of enlarged lymph glands in the armpit on the same side, the biopsy is still required.

Because it is so important, this point must be emphasized. Regardless of how experienced, how expert, or how extensively trained any physician may be—even the specialist in breast diseases— it cannot be unequivocally stated whether a breast lump is benign or malignant. It may, on occasion, be decided to simply watch a 'benign' appearing mass for a few weeks after obtaining a normal mammogram of the area. And this is an acceptable choice as long as careful and frequent follow up examinations are carried out.

Proctoscopic, Sigmoidoscopic, Colonoscopic, Exami-

nation: In performing this examination an instrument is passed into the subject's anus to inspect the large bowel for colon or rectal cancer. Unfortunately, the examination has fostered much confusing debate and disagreement among physicians. At the present time there is no real consensus as to how often this test should be done as a screening procedure for the general population.

The relative high cost of the examination; the degree of discomfort and pain to the patient, and the real, although rare, occurrence of serious and even fatal complications have caused some of the disagreement. The experience of others has indicated the examination is not needed in all patients or in all age groups as a *routine* screening examination. If there are specific symptoms which suggest colon cancer or if the patient is a member of a group with high predisposing risk factors then the examination should be done.

The author's choice is to obtain: a thorough, specific history of bowel habits; a clear history and documentation of cancer of the colon or rectum in the family; a factual record of any previous colon polyps and colon cancer in the reader; and finally, a careful and thorough digital examination of the rectum with a chemical test on the feces sample for hidden blood. In most cases these steps appear to be adequate for screening purposes.

Prostate Digital Examination: Here is another step in the physical examination which fits into the same category as the pelvic examination and the Pap test in that it is simple, safe, inexpensive and valuable for screening large groups of the population. Also, for the same reasons, it is almost criminally negligent for the physician not to perform this examination especially in men over age 40.

As is the case with most tests and examinations, the digital prostate exam is not infallible. But it is a good threshold exam which leads to further testing, when indicated. It is a routine part of any examination of the male population. Whether symptoms of the urinary tract are reported or not, the examination is mandatory.

The physician palpates the prostate gland, through the rectal-digital route, for hardness, tenderness, or the presence of nodules which suggest cancer. If the findings are suspicious, more specific tests should follow, such as: a prostate related blood test—called the prostate specific antigen (PSA); or by a needle biopsy of the prostate gland via the rectum; or surgical biopsy of the gland if the suspicion of cancer cannot be settled by the simple steps elaborated.

Other so called screening blood tests are discussed later in this section but *the prostate blood test,* namely the prostate specific antigen (PSA) is elaborated upon here.

Although it seems logical to use the prostate specific antigen as a tool to screen large segments of the male population for prostate cancer, research has not proven this concept to be fruitful. The reasons this rationale fails are, as in most simple tests, there is a high incidence of *false positive* and *false negatives*. The term false positive refers to those cases who have a blood test value above the normal limit but who do not have cancer of the prostate; and the false negative refers to the cases which **do** have cancer of the prostate but have a normal prostate specific antigen. Both sets of circumstances are all too common in medical practice. But they have to be dealt with since they are presently unavoidable even in the light of our present advanced technology. Ergo, the profound observation, 'medicine is, at best, an inexact science.'

Research and population studies have shown the digital rectal examination coupled with the prostate specific antigen is much more useful and accurate as a means of screening for prostate cancer. Unfortunately, the general public finds it the least desirable because it is uncomfortable and requires an office visit to the physician. Be that as it may, the digital examination is still best.

The same general statements can be made regarding the older and less sensitive test called the serum acid phosphatase which was replaced by the PSA test.

The Screening Chest X-Ray: A simple and safe, but moderately expensive examination, it has been touted as a useful test for screening large segments of the population, especially smokers, for lung cancer. Epidemiological studies have also shown that this concept is not correct. More than one patient has stated, "I prefer to continue smoking and have a chest x-ray done every six months. Then, when lung cancer is found, I can have surgery and be cured."

Unfortunately, such an approach fails on several counts. First, the chest x-ray can only detect large cancers which often is synonymous with *advanced cancer*. That is to say, too late for any chance of cure. Research has demonstrated that only about 10% of lung cancers when large enough to be seen on x-ray are even approachable by surgery because they have already spread or are too extensive locally to be safely removed by surgical excision. It has been further demonstrated that less than 5% of the original number of people with lung cancers found by x-ray live beyond five years... even with successful surgical removal. These are quite dismal odds for those who choose to continue to smoke.

Second, it is recognized that a cancer seen on a chest x-ray reveals only 50%, or less, of the actual amount of cancer present. This technical reality explains why some smaller lung cancers are not even visible and those which are will be judged as operable erroneously.

Third, many lung cancers detected by the chest x-ray already have distant spread of the disease—to brain, bone, liver or the opposite lung—when first detected. This set of circumstances makes any chance for surgical cure extremely unlikely.

Fourth, using the annual-screening-chest x-ray-philosophy also results in many patients undergoing surgery needlessly. And since a certain amount of anesthetic deaths are unavoidable, a significant mortality rate will result from some unnecessary surgery, thereby, defeating the very purpose of screening examinations—namely, the saving of lives.

Lastly, the worst product of this philosophy is that cigarette smokers are given the false sense of security which encourages them to continue their disease producing habit; auto-pollution of the lungs.

Many other techniques have been studied in hopes of finding an ideal way of screening large numbers of the smoking population for lung cancer but to date none has proven useful, accurate or reliable. But, of course, research continues in this area.

Stool Examination for Blood: Theoretically, this is an ideal test for screening because; it can be done in the doctor's office, in the most basic of medical laboratories anywhere in the world, or even at home by the subject. It lacks, however, two basic requirements, i.e., specificity and accuracy.

It lacks specificity because the exam accomplishes only that which its name states—the detection of blood in the stool not visible (occult) to the naked eye. Here is where any degree of specificity is lost. Any abnormality producing small amounts of blood in the feces will give a positive result. The long list of abnormalities includes such common entities as; hemorrhoids, peptic ulcers, rectal fissures and fistulas, swallowing of coughed blood from nose bleeding or lung bleeding, swallowing of blood due to gum disease, etc. The list is almost endless. And, as is obvious, many of these conditions are not serious enough to warrant the major testing to which a positive result leads. These tests, of course, would include x-rays of the intestinal tract, proctoscopy, colonoscopy, and, occasionally, exploratory abdominal surgery.

In addition, the lack of accuracy of the stool test can have these same results. Many, if not all of the tests utilized, cannot detect minute amounts of blood which can be produced by serious disease. Also a positive reaction can occur in the presence of ingested red meat in the diet and by certain other types of foods.

What then is the purpose of the test as presently recommended by physicians? As is always the case, the results must be supported by and followed by other simple, logical steps before proceeding to the major tests mentioned previously. Which brings us full circle back to my original claim that the simple and basic process of a complete historical inquiry and a meticulous physical examination by a physician is still the best for screening purposes. Thereafter, the physician can—by the process of elimination—decide which individuals require the major tests to establish a diagnosis of cancer in the intestinal tract.

Therefore, it must be clearly understood that this *is a test for occult blood* in the stools in which cancer of the bowel is the *least* likely cause of a positive result. It is *not* a specific test for bowel cancer. Again, keeping the facts in proper perspective achieves a more desirable result than the fear of cancer produces.

Special Cancer Blood Tests: There are several tests which are specifically useful to either investigate suspected cancer or as a means of following the progress of a known cancer. It is emphasized, however, that these tests are generally not useful for screening the general population for cancer unless that population group has specific symptoms or specific findings on physical examination that suggest cancer. Another example would be in the case of high risk groups such as smokers or asbestos workers.

The 'Gold' Test derives its name from the physician who developed it. It has nothing to do with measuring the element—gold—in the blood, urine or body tissues. Carcino-embryonic antigen (CEA) is the complete scientific name of the test.

The CEA's greatest utility is in following the progress or response to treatment of an established case of cancer of the colon-rectal area. Although, it seems logical to use this test to screen the general population for colon cancer this has not been found to be the case. This is true, primarily, because the test is not specific enough, not sensitive enough and too costly.

The test can give a false-positive result in cigarette smokers without any evidence of cancer, in certain noncancerous liver diseases, in cancer of the ovary, lung, breast and other cancerous and noncancerous disorders.

The Sedimentation Rate (SED RATE, ESR) is a test widely used for a variety of purposes and was once used to screen subjects for cancer. But there are many infectious (pneumonia), inflammatory (Rheumatoid arthritis), and noncancerous conditions which can produce an abnormal result. In the light of present day knowledge the test has no validity for use in diagnosing cancer. It is included here only for the sake of completeness and not as an endorsement of its value in cancer screening. It can be used in following the course of certain kinds of cancer—such as Multiple Myeloma—but only as an adjunct since more specific tests are better suited for this purpose in that particular malignancy.

Other Cancer Tests: There is an ever increasing group of tests known as *Tumor Markers* which comprises a long list of tests with which the reader may be familiar. The alpha-fetoprotein, Human Chorionic Gonadotropin, CA 125, serum Acid Phosphatase, serum Alkaline Phosphatase, LDH, the Prostate Specific antigen, etc., are among some of the more familiar test names. These tests and many others not mentioned have specific uses for following the response to therapy or the recurrence patterns of some cancers but none is useful in screening the general population. These will be discussed in more detail later.

Screening X-Rays or Imaging Scans: It might appear justifiable to use the technology which has so greatly improved our accuracy to diagnose disease as a method to screen the population at large for early cancer but this has not always proven to be the case. The screening chest x-ray and the screening mammogram alluded to above illustrate both sides of the rationalization.

Other commonly known x-rays include: colon studies (barium enema), upper gastrointestinal x-rays; CAT (Computerized Axial Tomography) scans of various and sundry internal organs also have failed to stand up under the scrutiny of clinical study.

When entering into the area of using screening x-ray tests another dimension enters into consideration. There is the real, although small, risk of the damage that might result from large doses of radiation. In most situations individual x-ray studies carry a low risk from radiation exposure. Nevertheless, the frequency of the x-ray studies performed, and the risk versus benefit ratio must be monitored by a physician since the hazards are real.

The indiscriminate use of a multitude of x-rays to screen large groups of non-symptomatic subjects cannot be condoned or recommended. Aside from the radiation exposure hazard, especially in pregnant females, the cost of such a program does not justify the results in the number of lives saved. These facts have been verified by many large studies conducted by universities and medical centers around the world.

In summary, regarding the question of searching for the ideal cancer screening test, the essential characteristics of such a test(s) must include: ease of application; high degree of safety; low risk of complications or fatalities; acceptable cost; high degree of accuracy and specificity; relative ease in providing follow up and further diagnostic steps. There is still only one method that has all these characteristics—*THE COMPREHENSIVE HISTORY OF ILLNESS AND THE METICULOUS PHYSICAL EXAMINATION.*

Chapter 11

Unproven Cancer Tests

Although more specific details are given later about unproven methods of cancer *treatment* a general statement regarding the same category of unproven cancer *testing* seems appropriate here.

Most of the so called *cancer tests* which fit into this group are based on the same false or unproven premise upon which its treatment is based. Therefore, the testing itself has no basis in fact.

If a particular substance or chemical is given for the unproven treatment, very often the *cancer test* applied is used to measure a deficiency of the same substance in the blood. A typical example is the case of Laetrile (also known as amygdalin or vitamin B 16) where a test is used to demonstrate a deficiency of Laetrile in the blood of a patient. Also, the same test is used to screen an otherwise healthy group of subjects for an unproven 'predisposition toward cancer', or to follow the course and progress of a patient being given injections of the substance for the treatment of cancer.

Another recently touted, unproven method was to measure the subjects general immunity to determine if a deficiency in these functions exists. It is supposed to test for a tendency toward cancer development. If found deficient, the subject was given substances which supposedly stimulate his natural immune defenses.

All of these unproven methods essentially fail in the same areas which are discussed in more detail later. Briefly, however, they all fail to demonstrate that the therapy or the testing method is truly effective by generally accepted and proven systems of scientific medical research.

These unproven methods are frequently accepted on blind faith or for political reasons by a frightened, and paranoid segment of the population desperate for a cure.

Part Three

Cancer Therapy

Chapter 12

Definitions

Introduction

Cancer therapy is simply defined as any treatment or series of treatments administered for the purpose of specifically removing or killing all viable cancer cells in the body. The primary aim is the prolongation of the life of the patient and relief of any and all symptoms produced by the cancer.

However, stated in a more scientific way it is a treatment which when completed has removed all objective evidence of the cancer when tested by conventionally accepted medical research methods.

What it does *not* mean is that the treatment only makes the patients feel better or causes them to *believe* they are *cured*. Although relief of all symptoms is one of the ultimate goals of therapy it cannot be used as a means of concluding that the patient is cured or the treatment is effective. The major reason these are not used as end points is that the therapist has at his disposal many methods of improving the sense of well being of the subject or relieving his symptoms—let's say, pain—without really altering the status of the cancer. Therefore, the patient and therapist can be easily fooled into thinking the treatment has effected the cancer growth without objective evidence of having done so. Herein lies the trap many unproven therapies use to lure patients into their obscure web.

The concept of *objective regression* of cancer growth is a very important one to grasp. This is especially true in light of the many misconceptions about cancer therapy and cure.

One of the major advances in cancer research and management has been the general acceptance by the medical profession of the principle that cancer is a *systemic disease* and not a localized process. The phrase, *systemic disease*, indicates that although the major manifestations of the condition may appear localized—such as a lump in the breast, a tumor on a chest x-ray, etc., —the disease is already often disseminated beyond its *apparent* confines when first discovered. The significance of this systemic disease principle has spawned to the idea that cancer, therefore, requires therapy applied systemically and not only applied locally. Consequently, surgical excision or localized radiation therapy are frequently not curative in themselves and other systemic therapy is required to increase survival rates and, it is hoped, to improve cure rates.

As simple and as logical as the concept might appear it has taken many decades for physicians to embrace it. Many still have not accepted this concept and still refuse to consider any systemic therapy for some cases of cancer. The general public's acceptance of the notion has been even slower. Herein lies one of the reasons many readers believe surgery alone is the ultimate and final answer in the treatment of all cancers. If nothing else is learned from this portion of this work except that the reader appreciates that cancer is a *systemic* (not a localized) *disease* the writing of it has been worthwhile.

The appreciation of this principle helps the reader to understand that after the initial localized therapy (surgery or radiation) for some cancers, further systemic therapy is required. It also becomes obvious that future follow up examinations and tests for both local *and* systemic recurrences by the physician are mandatory.

It is the realization and appreciation of these philosophical points which has led to the development of contemporary forms of therapy which have produced cures for cancers previously considered hopeless.

Since the ultimate goal of cancer treatment is the total eradication of the cancer and the prolongation of survival of the victim an understanding of the terms used to identify the end-results of these goals is needed.

Definitions

Cure: Because of the ambiguity and non-specificity this is an almost meaningless term. There are probably as many, and varied definitions of the term, as their are physicians.

One popular laymen's dictionary defines cure as, 'a remedy, a healing or a system of treatment that restores one's good health.'

Even the definition obtained from a commonly used medical dictionary is unclear. It reads; a successful treatment for an illness or wound; or a special treatment for a malady or injury.

When discussing cancer treatment the definition becomes even more nonspecific or more vague depending who is expounding on it. However, since it is a universally accepted term, and probably irreplaceable, it's best to reach a consensus agreement on a definition of the term-*cure*.

Therefore, the following is the author's simplified definition of the term cure as it applies primarily to cancer.

"Cure": is defined as a treatment, a series of treatments, or a combination of treatments which prevents the recurrence or spread of the original cancer with the end result of preventing the death of the subject from the disease.

The greatest difficulty arises in identifying this end point because detecting the recurrence of cancer can be as difficult as detecting any cancer at any stage. The only meaningful measure of the endpoint or a cure is duration of survival of the patient which requires years of observation of individual cases, as well as, large groups of cases.

The following is a list of the terms commonly accepted by physicians and scientists to describe the end results of cancer treatment; such as remission, control, no evidence of disease (NED), five and ten year survivals, palliation.

I now submit my definition of these terms and their practical utility.

Remission: In the practical sense, this is a more useful and meaningful word to use to identify the immediate results of cancer treatment. Simply defined it means that all the evidence of the original cancer has been removed or is now undetectable by scientifically accepted means of such detection.

Remissions are further subdivided into complete and partial remissions.

Partial Remission: signifies that after examination by objective, clinical measurement—such as x-ray pictures or physical examination— at least 50% of the original cancer has been destroyed. Rephrased in another manner, it means the original cancer mass has been reduced to at least 50% or less of its original size by actual measurement.

Complete Remission: Means eradication of *all* of the original cancer by the treatment modality used. However, the term is not synonymous with cure. Since it may takes months or years for the disease to recur or spread it takes months or years of observing the patient before such an end point can be identified. It is generally accepted, however, that the likelihood of cure is greater if complete remission is achieved but it is not a guarantee of cure.

The physician in charge of your treatment program should discuss your case in terms of remissions, complete or partial, or in the terms of duration of survival. Rarely, is the term 'cure' used.

The quantification of duration of survival known as; 5 YEAR SURVIVAL RATES, 10 YEAR SURVIVAL RATES, TWO YEAR SURVIVAL RATES, are also important for the reader to understand.

These terms were originally intended for the use of the scientific community in reporting end-results of treatment to other medical scientists. The terms were designed to avoid misleading and conflicting reporting of end-results of treatments under study.

It has been known for many years that in some forms of cancer the subject can survive for two, five and more years even without any treatment. These are known as spontaneous remissions or 'cures.'

Therefore, even though a particular form of therapy appears to eradicate a cancer or bring about its complete remission, the survival of the patient might not actually be prolonged as compared to that of the untreated patient. This is one of the reasons it takes so many years for cancer research to produce meaningful results which clearly show prolongation survival or production of cures.

It is most important that the reader understand this concept of 'years of survival' so it is not assumed to be synonymous with cure and he neglect returning to the physician for regular follow up examinations. The physician must discuss this concept of *regular, periodic* follow up examinations with the patient in order to avoid this pitfall.

The number of years the physician tacks on to the beginning of the designation of survival—such as FIVE OR TWO YEARS—should not be a matter of his personal choice or a reflection of his optimistic or pessimistic attitude. It should be a scientific designation chosen by a consensus of the scientific community based on the natural history of the cancer in question. For example, until recently survival in lung cancer seldom exceeded two years regardless of the kind of treatment given. Therefore, the reporting of new treatment programs for lung cancer are given in terms of *TWO YEAR SURVIVAL* rates. Whereas, breast cancer patients commonly survived for five years or more and thus, the treatment results are reported in terms of *FIVE YEAR SURVIVAL* rates.

Again, it must not be assumed a cure has been achieved when one reaches the five year survival point. If there is any misunderstanding about this point you must ask your physician about it if he has not already voluntarily offered an explanation.

Control of Disease: Cure may not be the only aim of treatment. Holding the cancer in check for a unspecified but significant period of time can also be a desirable aim of treatment. Some therapeutic modalities do not produce any reduction in the size of the cancer but clearly prohibit the cancer from enlarging or spreading. Although this is not the ideal situation one cannot deny it is a worthwhile goal of treatment especially if it alleviates pain or other uncomfortable symptoms of the disease and prolongs the life of the patient.

Such an achievement can have very special meaning for the subject who wishes to remain active and functional for whatever length of survival can be accomplished. Who is to say that six months of disease control, without reduction in cancer size, is not important to a person who wants to survive to see a child married, or see someone graduate college, or see a first grandchild born? As long as the physician is honest with the patient and doesn't mislead them into a false impression of cure or remission. Only the patient can then decide if this is a worthy goal.

Palliative Therapy: The purpose of this goal in therapy is solely and primarily to relieve any of the discomforting symptoms of the disease. Even if given the knowledge that the cancer growth itself is *not* effected this can be a useful tool for the therapist, and most important the patient.

Palliative therapy differs from *control therapy* in that the cancer itself is not expected to decrease in size or severity. Of course, the physician must make the patient and the family aware of this fact. It is also your physician's obligation to keep the cost of such palliative therapy to the barest minimum. He must also stop the treatment when no further benefit is accomplished. And there is no doubt this can be accomplished in many cases, even in terminal cancer, by very simple, inexpensive, low risk medications and other maneuvers.

However, reader beware the charlatan who claims to have produced a *"partial or total cure"* because the symptoms have been alleviated. And there are too many such unscrupulous individuals who would not hesitate to make such claims. False and unproven methods of cancer therapy are discussed in more detail in another section of this book.

Chapter 13

Types of Cancer Therapy

There are basically only five general types of cancer treatment currently recognized. They are surgery, chemotherapy, radiation therapy, and biological response modifier therapy (formerly known as Immunotherapy) and any combination of two or more of these. But because each can be combined with one or all of the others, in sequence or concurrently, a larger total number of treatment approaches are possible.

Surgery or Surgical Therapy: In this form of therapy an attempt is made to physically remove (excise) the visible cancer from either the surface of the body or from some internal organ. There are now other methods besides the obvious excision by a sharp instrument which have been added through new technologies. Such modalities include laser surgery, ligature, freezing, and the like. But these are still essentially another form of excision and are discussed below under another heading.

However, the reader must understand that not all surgical procedures are necessarily done with the intentions of a therapeutic end point or a cure. In other words surgery is sometimes required to obtain a biopsy for diagnosis. In doing so, either a small portion of a mass may be removed or the entire mass itself, depending on the clinical situation. Therefore, most, if not all, cancer cases may have some type of surgery performed without any therapy being accomplished. This should be obvious since as previously defined therapy is given with the ultimate aim of eliminating *"all the cancer."*

Thus, cancer surgery falls into one of five categories. (1) Biopsy surgery, (2) Surgical Staging, (3) Exploratory Surgery, (4) Emergency Surgery, and (5) Therapeutic or Curative Surgery.

Biopsy Surgery has been defined as a means of obtaining tissue for diagnosis.

Surgical Staging. Surgical staging is simply a means of determining if the cancer has spread and how extensive it has become. Sometimes this requires extensive surgery to achieve naked-eye-examination of internal organs and the biopsy of those organs which look suspicious. Occasionally actual removal of those entire organs is necessary for microscopic examination.

In other situations, such as Hodgkin's Disease, it amounts to major surgery even after a diagnosis has been established by some other simpler biopsy technique. Using Hodgkin's Disease further as an example, after a lymph node is biopsied, say, in the neck it may then be necessary to examine the abdominal organs. At the same time surgical removal of the spleen, and several other lymph nodes is carried out and there is visual examination of the liver and several biopsies are taken of the liver. The ultimate aim here, again, is not to treat the disease but to determine the extent (stage) of the disease.

Exploratory Surgery. Implicit in this term is the impression that your physician is fairly certain—from other findings from blood tests, x-rays, etc.—that a cancer is present but it cannot be proven without surgery. Consequently, a body cavity or other part of the body is *'explored'* surgically to pinpoint the sight of disease and obtain the necessary biopsy or remove the cancer, if possible.

Almost any part of the body may require exploration, but the more common ones are the abdominal cavity, the chest cavity, or the internal confines of the skull. Remember, that at the time of exploratory surgery it may or may not be possible to cure the cancer. Only the surgeon can determine this after he has entered the explored cavity and examined the situation. Of course, the surgeon along with your primary physician discuss the findings with the patient and family after the surgery is performed. If this is not done the reader has the right to ask for such information.

Curative or Therapeutic Surgery: In many, although not all, circumstances the intent of surgery is to effect a cure of the cancer. When such a situation exists the surgeon usually knows prior to surgery that a cure is possible depending on the type of cancer being attacked. Most times, however, the surgeon does not know if cure is possible until the surgery is performed. Only after the other neighboring organs are examined with the naked eye and biopsied, where indicated, is the possibility of compete excision and cure considered.

As always, these options and possibilities are discussed with the patient before any surgery is planned or carried out. Except in dire emergencies, when a life or a limb is at risk, there is always enough time to discuss the proposed surgery, safely.

Emergency Cancer Surgery: In a few relatively uncommon circumstances surgery is performed on an urgent basis in order to save the patient's life even when cancer is not suspected. In these cases time is of the utmost importance so that only brief discussion may be possible. But even then some brief discussion is mandatory between physician, patient and the family.

A common example is the case in which a cancer of the colon has caused obstruction of the intestinal flow. The result is shock, life threatening infection (peritonitis or blood stream infection) and death if surgery is not performed immediately. The surgeon recognizes the immediate threat to the subjects life but may not suspect the presence of cancer. Such a dilemma is not rare since some of the tests ordinarily required to diagnose colon cancer are too time consuming and can cause delay which is not acceptable in such an emergency.

Often in these situations two surgical procedures are required. First, the emergency surgery is performed to relieve the intestinal blockage and to save the patient's life. Then, perhaps weeks later, the curative surgery can be more safely performed to remove all of the cancer, whenever possible.

What exactly constitutes a so called *'life threatening emergency'?* It exists when the current circumstances pose an immediate threat to the subject's life. *Immediate threat* applies only to clinical situations in which the death of the patient is imminent—within hours or days—if some definitive, aggressive step is not taken. The point is emphasized to distinguish it from the patient's fear based on the unfounded beliefs about cancer. A typical example is the case where the family feels the cancer is spreading by the minute or hour, or at the very least by the day. There is no shock, peritonitis or intestinal obstruction but they demand immediate surgery to remove the cancer when immediate surgery is not indicated. As a result the patient or family often may refuse needed, and even mandatory, testing before undertaking high risk surgery.

It has never been demonstrated, and few if any physicians believe, that waiting even several weeks for surgery or other treatment has altered the long term prognosis or the chance for cure of any cancer. However, this unwarranted concern cannot be allowed to shorten the required time to insure maximum accuracy in diagnosis and absolute safety for the patient before embarking on any high risk surgical approach. Although one can understand the sense of urgency and concern that is felt for a loved one, logic and constraint must prevail. It is your doctor's obligation to inform and reassure the patient and the family.

Discussion Before Surgery: It behooves the patient and the family to discuss the planned surgery before undertaking it so they can clearly understand the reasons the surgery is indicated. It also helps to alleviate often exaggerated and unfounded fears. The following is a list of questions suggested the reader ask before agreeing to surgery unless a dire emergency exists.

(1) What is the precise purpose of the surgery anticipated? Is it done for the purpose of diagnosis by biopsy? Is it indicated for the purpose of accomplishing cure, staging, palliation or relief of a life threatening emergency? Is it an exploratory procedure to solve an undiagnosed problem and establish a diagnosis? The patient or their designated spokesman must have these questions answered before agreeing to any surgery. None of the answers to these questions should be taken for granted.

Although it may seem logical to the reader that surgery is only done for curative purposes this is often not the case. This principle applies to all kinds of surgery, not just cancer surgery, and should be strictly followed.

(2) Exactly what structures and organs will be removed or what anatomic alterations will be made? One does not need to know all the jargon and technical descriptions to comprehend your physician's response to the questions. A simple diagram with some plain-language-explanation by the surgeon can clarify any confusion. It is astounding that a large number of patients who have had major surgery have no idea of what organ(s) was removed; what disease or condition was being treated; or what change was accomplished. Everyone has the right to know this information before or after surgery.

In certain special situations the surgeon may truly not know exactly which organs will be removed prior to the surgery. But they should have an approximate idea or at least have a list of the options and possibilities. These special situations arise not because of a physician's incompetence. They happen to the best physicians because of the limitations of medical scientific technology and the unavoidable inaccuracy of diagnostic methods.

(3) What kind of risks are involved? What is the general risk of death or other major, permanent complications from the surgical procedure chosen? This question should first be asked in reference to national or at least regional experience. Finally, the reader should ask about the personal experience of the hospital, the staff, the support facilities and the surgical team for this type of operation. In other words, is it a procedure that is seldom or frequently performed at this locality?

Next, the question should be asked in a specific sense as it applies to the current patient. The answer to the question, as it applies to the current case, may be influenced by the age, the general overall health and preexisting medical conditions of the patient. The risks of surgery can also be influenced by the type of cancer present.

(4) Complications: If there are any complications, which are the most likely and what kind of disability, if any, could remain after re-

covery? Can the complications be corrected later; is comfortable survival possible with the residuals; what kind of quality of life is possible if the complications do occur? In other words, it must be known if the cure is going to be worse than the disease, as the saying goes.

(5) Is there any evidence of spread of the cancer before surgery? This is a very important question to ask before surgery. Because, if spread or dissemination is already apparent, what is the purpose of the surgery?

This doesn't mean to imply that there are not often very good reasons to go ahead with surgery because very often there are. These reasons to proceed may include; confirming diagnosis, confirming suspected dissemination, staging of the cancer, relief of disabling symptoms, improving the chances of cure with additional types of therapy. There are many such good reasons but the patient has the right to know what those reasons are and if dissemination is already noted prior to surgery.

(6) Less important, but equally reasonable questions, include the anticipated cost of the surgery; the duration of hospital stay; the length of recovery time at home; ability to remain active, or even employed, during and after recovery. These are essentially quality-of-life questions and will be addressed in detail later.

(7) What are the chances of being *'cured'*—in accordance with the definition of cure given earlier—by the surgery or its combination with other therapy?

Evasive Terminology: Beware some the evasive phrases which have mislead patients and families because they are, unfortunately, still utilized today by some physicians when discussing the results of surgery.

"I THINK I GOT IT ALL" - this is one of the more popular and most meaningless phrases ever uttered after surgery. In light of contemporary knowledge this statement never suffices as an answer to question number seven above. The reason this is a meaningless proclamation is that cancer is a microscopic disease which requires several millions to billions of cells to make a cancer large enough to see or feel. Therefore, there are often, if not always, some microscopic cells

left behind no matter who performs the surgery—except perhaps God. Thus, if a few cells or a few hundred cells, or a few thousand invisible, undetectable cells are left behind no one can ever say, honestly, "I think I got it all."

How, the reader may ask, can the surgeon or any other physician give the patient any idea of his prognosis and chances for cure? The doctor can obtain published percentages and average figures for cure, five year survival, etc., from the medical literature based on the national or international experience of cancer centers and cancer physicians. These figures are readily available to all physicians through there local medical library, cancer society, or cancer specialists.

While it is true that the figures are constantly changing, the changes are small over a one year period and the new figures are published each year by the American Cancer Society. Not only are the percentages available for almost all groups of cancers but they are even available for the various subgroups of cancers based on the stage, the age, and race of the subject.

Consequently, after surgery a statement can be made—or at least searched out by the physician—in regards to the prognosis of as long as the stage and type of cancer are known, along with the other factors of age, race, etc.

The following list includes more of the other infamous, *meaningless* phrases used by physicians when discussing the outcome of surgery or any form of treatment for that matter. And it is most certainly an incomplete listing.

To wit; *"The operation was a success"*; *"Everything went fine, or well, or came out good"*; *"I think she'll make it"*; *"I don't anticipate any problems"*; *"I think it has been arrested."* The greatest fallacy of these nonspecific vagaries is they seem to imply prognosis or long term cure. Which they, of course, do not.

The patient and the anxious family are awaiting some sign or gesture or even facial expression from the surgeon which even implies hope. Therefore, they are easily mislead even by well meaning attempts at reassurance. They will readily expand these small statements beyond their true meaning. Much more information must be given to the reader than that which can be implied in a single positive statement.

The sad result, which is usually seen later in the course of the illness, is an unexpected and ignored recurrence because the patient was sure they were *'cured.'* And this results from all the false assumptions made by the patient because of those statements. These false assumptions included; *"I don't have to back to the doctor again unless I have trouble," "I can continue to smoke," "I don't have to have any regular checkups or tests," "I do not need any other kind of treatment," etc.*

Thus, except in the rare case of one hundred percent complete cure the patient should always be advised—after completion of all therapy—about the need for frequent and regular periodic follow up visits and examinations by the physician.

Old Witches Tales and Myths: The outside world abounds with these kinds of statements as they refer to cancer surgery and its hazards. As stated previously no surgery is without its risks but they are seldom the ones which we hear about from neighbors and relatives. Among the more common ones are: *"If they operate they will spread the cancer all over the place"; "nobody ever survives cancer surgery"; "why operate when everybody knows there is no cure for cancer"; "you should hold off on surgery until it's the last resort."* All of these statements have been made based either on a lack of understanding and knowledge about cancer; or anecdotal evidence experienced by friends, relatives and neighbors. Which brings us back to exactly the reasons it was decided to write this book—to dispel the myths, half-truths, misunderstandings, incomplete information and total lack of knowledge about cancer that is rampant among our citizens.

Radiation Therapy: This modality is also known as irradiation therapy, cobalt therapy, x-ray therapy, radiotherapy, linear accelerator therapy, radioactive therapy, cyclotron therapy, radium therapy, and many others. These are basically all the same type of treatment methods. They differ primarily in the type of equipment used, number and types of unwanted side effects, how quickly each therapy session can be given, the number of patients treated per day or hour, the cost, the safety, etc. All of these differences are of course worthwhile and useful but they do not necessarily change the *cure rates or remission rates* of cancers.

Radiation therapy was one of the first methods which specifically attempted to destroy the cancer cells while they resided in or on the body. Such an approach is in contrast to surgical techniques which attempt the gross physical removal of the cancer cells by excision or extirpation.

The precise scientific and biological way in which radiation therapy accomplishes the destruction of cancer cells is very complex and beyond the scope of this book. Suffice it for our purposes to summarize by saying, the cancer cells ability to grow and reproduce itself is altered by radiation so it can then be removed by the bodies natural defense and other natural healing mechanisms.

As in the case of any cancer treatment method, the same type of questions must be answered by the radiotherapist (also called the Radiation Oncologist) before embarking on the radiation treatment program. Also, the same goals and objectives apply to radiotherapy as they to do to surgical therapy. These goals are; curative intent, remission induction, palliative intent, and so on, as detailed above under the discussion of surgical therapy. And, therefore, the same questions must be asked by the reader and received. You have the right to these answers before therapy is begun.

There are, nevertheless, some special differences between surgical therapy and radiation therapy which are unique and must be addressed. Each of these types of therapy do have in common the same objective of eradication of all the cancer, whenever possible, albeit via different mechanisms.

Means of Administration: Radiotherapy is administered via an external source of radiation and on occasion via a temporary internal source. Thus the radiation beam penetrates the skin to a calculated and anticipated depth to reach the cancer cells to eradicate them. The subject is placed in the path of the radiation beam for a very brief period of time which varies with the radiation source and type. The subject feels no discomfort—except perhaps some anxiety in the beginning—or only the mild discomfort of warmth while the radiation is being administered. It is a quite painless and easy process for the subject at least. This is not to say there are no side effects. But these side effects usually occur later as the radiation doses accumulate. Side effects are discussed in detail below.

The brief periods of radiation beam exposure occur on a daily basis with a rest period on the weekend, both Saturday and Sunday. This rest period allows the damaged normal tissue and the total body systems time to recover.

The number of radiation treatments given in this sequential manner varies from as few as 7 to 10 up to as many as 35 or 45. The precise number of treatments is determined by your radiation oncologist and calculated in terms of total tumor dose called *rads or Gy.* These are technical details the reader can have, if they wish, but are not really needed to prepare you for the program.

After the initial series of treatments have been administered to a specific limited area further treatments cannot be given again to the same area. At least this is not ordinarily done because of the very high risk of serious and permanent damage to normal structures. Even death can rarely occur from excessive radiation therapy. This is another way in which it differs from surgery which can be repeated on the same organ if needed.

Onset of Effects: Generally speaking, radiation therapy has little perceptible effect on the cancer in the early phases of therapy. But as the series of treatments and the total radiation doses begin to accumulate changes become apparent. Naturally, relief of symptoms may take a little time to occur as well. This delay in response is part of the reason other forms of treatment and alternate means of pain relief are administered until the radiotherapy takes effect.

Consequently, the duration of the therapeutic effects of radiotherapy can be longer lasting, even to the extent of total cure, long after the treatments are completed. Unfortunately, the same is true for the side effects. But, eventually, both side effects and therapeutic effects disappear.

Side Effects: The undesirable side effects of radiotherapy are unique to this mode of treatment and must be considered before the patient and physician decide to administer the course of treatments. Although fatal side effects are extremely uncommon, severe and debilitating discomfort is fairly common. However, almost all of these debilitating side effects are temporary and reversible over time. But some of the minor side effects are irreversible. The permanent side effects occur because there is always some *unavoidable* amount of damage caused by the radiation to the surrounding normal tissue and the damage is irreversible.

The expertise of the radiation oncologist is a major factor in minimizing this damage. He calculates and predetermines the extent and severity the expected damage as well as the therapeutic benefit. Then the therapist decides if the amount of therapeutic benefit outweighs the permanent tissue damage—this is known as the therapeutic/toxic ratio. As a matter of fact, all forms of therapy must be considered in the light of this ratio whether it is in the form of medication, drugs, surgery, etc. The same principle should apply to therapy for all diseases not just cancer therapy.

There are basically two kinds of side effects which can be anticipated from radiotherapy based on when they occur. They are divided into the immediate and the long term. The manifestations of these side effects varies with the location of the body radiated and the organs which fall in the path of the beam. Therefore, the topic of side effects can only be discussed in general terms along with some specific examples.

For example, let's say the subject is receiving radiation therapy for a brain cancer. Not only will the cancer tissue be effected but the surrounding normal brain tissue suffers some damage. This damage can result in: nausea and vomiting; loss of hair in the area which falls into the beam's path; fatigue and decrease in appetite with resultant temporary weight loss; irritation and burning of the skin surface exposed to the beam. These are some of the immediate side effects.

Long term side effects, for instance, include impairment of the motor and sensory functions of that portion of the brain radiated producing such side effects as weakness of a hand or foot, numbness or loss of pain sensation in the same extremity, etc.

Another common example is the patient who is treated for a lung cancer with radiotherapy. The immediate side effects may include cough, shortness of breath, difficulty and pain on swallowing. A second example occurs when the path of the beam falls over the heart this organ can suffer damage but this is usually one of the long term, delayed side effects.

On the surface, the side effects appear terrible and hardly worth the risks. And before the era of modern radiation therapy technology the dangers were often too great to administer radiation therapy. However, with the advent of the newer, more sophisticated equipment utilized to administer radiotherapy, and the methods used to shield the normal tissues the curative effects of radiotherapy can be outstanding.

General Side Effects: There are some general side effects which occur with radiotherapy regardless of the area being treated. These include: mental depression and fatigue; loss of appetite; bronzing of the skin area treated; a decrease in the normal red blood count and the white blood count with increased risk of infection. A careful therapist, however, regularly checks for these changes during the course of therapy and, either lowers the dose of radiation or allows a longer rest period to minimize these problems.

Fatalities: As mentioned earlier, death from radiotherapy is such an uncommon occurrence it is barely worth mentioning. But for the sake of completeness it is touched upon here. However, when a patient actually dies during a course of radiotherapy it is more often caused by some other preexisting disease unrelated to the cancer or by the rapid progress of the cancer itself. Some examples include; the patient with severe heart disease who cannot tolerate even the smallest amount of damage to that organ caused by radiation; or the patient with severe lung disease who cannot tolerate the minor damage caused to even a small amount of surrounding normal lung tissue; and lastly and least likely, the patient who suffers severe depression of the blood count and encounters a fatal infection or severe hemorrhage.

Because of the multitude of types and locations of cancers which are treated with radiation therapy more details are given later under the discussion of each of the cancers in another section of this book.

To summarize, a well trained and meticulous radiotherapist, in conjunction with the general physician or medical oncologist, assesses all these dangers and hazards before recommending this form of therapy. But, as always, they must discuss these factors first with the subject before starting therapy. If this information is not volunteered to the reader you should request it. No, you should demand it.

Side effects notwithstanding, there is no doubt that radiotherapy is an indispensable part of the treatment of many cancers and in some cases it is the *only* modality capable of producing cure or complete remission of the disease. However it is not a universal panacea. That is, it is not indicated or even useful in *all* cancers. Only the oncologist and family physician can determine which cancers are amenable to treatment with radiation therapy. In many cases the best approach is a combination of radiation with either surgery or chemotherapy, or sometimes all three are required either concurrently or in sequence.

Evasive Terms: With regard to radiation therapy here are a wide variety of words and phrases used to evade the real issue, which is, the statistical chances of cure or remission of the cancer.

Such phrases as; "Your cancer is all gone," "it has been all burned away," "you have had a good result," and the like, do not indicate the likelihood of recurrence or spread of the disease. True cure rates, remission rates, and recurrence rates are generally known or written somewhere to help the physician give the patient an accurate assessment of his prognosis. The reader must ask for these figures if they are not offered by your physician.

Myths About Radiotherapy: There are many 'old witches tales' and other misconceptions regarding radiotherapy. Some of the more common ones are listed here.

Permanent Radioactivity: There is a mistaken idea that the individual treated remains radioactive for the rest of his life and poses a danger to his family and those around him. The notion is totally incorrect because the source of the radiation used in therapy exists outside the body only. The radioactive particles emitted from it pass through and into the body but then they dissipate and the energy produced is gone in a short time and forever. The only practical exception is the occasion where a radioactive substance (i.e., radium implants and seeds) is placed inside one of the body cavities for therapeutic effect and then later removed. Even in these circumstances the radioactive material is eventually removed and so is all the radioactivity. Therefore, any danger to the surrounding environs only exists temporarily. The therapist takes all the necessary precautions, including radioactive warning logos, while this short-term hazard exists. The scientific guidelines are very clear and strict in this area of radiation therapeutics.

"Everyone loses there hair and never gets it back; everyone will vomit and be sick; the rays make the disease spread; you never completely recovery from the damage to your insides;" etc. These are all statements of generalization which have very little or no validity. The risks and side effects of radiation therapy vary according to the area treated and the duration of treatment. These are not the same for all cancers and may not even be the same for any one group of cancers in all patients. The radiotherapist discusses these particular factors with the patient before beginning therapy.

When the reader considers that all human beings do not react to the same forces or events in the same way it becomes obvious that such generalizations are meaningless. Therefore, it is best not to draw parallels between one cancer case and another in regards to side effects or therapeutic benefit. Even the therapist can give only estimates of risks and benefits. Just because nausea or vomiting is discussed as a possible side effect does not mean all patients must experience it in the course of their therapy.

As far as therapeutic results are concerned there is no physician on earth who can look at, say , one hundred patients and pick the 75 who will be cured and the remaining 25 who will not. He can only make the statement that 75% of subjects with this type and stage of cancer will be cured and the remaining 25% will not. This is all he can say with any degree of honesty and accuracy. He may have a "gut reaction," or a "good or bad feeling" about a particular patient but this is not concrete evidence by any stretch of the imagination.

Cancer Chemotherapy: The most popular definitions of this modality of cancer therapy are variable, vague, and sometimes confusing at best. But some background information and discussion should clarify the definition the author has chosen. I have chosen the definition of *cancer chemotherapy* I have found most understandable by my patients over the years.

Practical Definition: Stated simply as possible chemotherapy is the term utilized to describe a method of treatment in which chemical agents or drugs are administered to the patient, either by injection or orally as tablets, which attacks the cancer cell and destroy it in a variety of complex ways.

The term chemotherapy is derived by contracting the two words, chemical and therapy. Therefore, literally interpreted any therapy applied by administering chemicals— antibiotics, blood pressure medicines, etc.,—could be called chemotherapy. However, the present day use of the term, 'chemotherapy,' is applied primarily to cancer chemotherapy.

Mechanisms of Action of Chemotherapy: The mechanisms of action of chemotherapy drugs are scientifically complex and can be confusing to the layman. Suffice it here to plainly state that the drugs work by preventing the rapid growth and reproduction of cancer cells. The cancer cells then undergo a natural demise and then the bodies natural defenses remove the dead or injured cells and excrete the by-products.

One of the first anticancer drugs ever tested was a direct result of observing the toxic and fatal effects of the mustard gas used against allied troops in World War I. It was noted that the gas damaged or destroyed the most rapidly dividing and growing cells in the body. These cells included the bone marrow and other blood forming organs, the gastrointestinal tract, and the skin and its appendages, namely the hair and nails.

It was known to scientists at that time that cancer cells were also rapidly dividing and growing cells. Thus, the research which followed involved developing chemicals similar to mustard gas but different enough to allow the normal cells to recovery and the cancer cells to be killed. Consequently, the first chemotherapy agent developed was called Nitrogen Mustard. It is still used today.

Once this compound was perfected it then became the research scientists' long and complicated task of screening all newly discovered chemicals and drugs for anticancer activity. The screening process is done by testing the chemical agents in experimental animal cancer models.

As a result of these research efforts there are now more than seventy-five anticancer drugs available for use by the general medical community. In addition to these seventy-five single agents available there are an infinite number of combinations which can be devised using two, three, four and even more dissimilar drugs together or in sequence. Furthermore, there are now hundreds of new compounds still under study and development.

The reader might wonder, why is there a need for more than one chemotherapy drug? The answer is because not all cancers are successfully eliminated by the same drugs. Also, since some drugs can only produce a partial or temporary remission it became obvious that more than one agent might be needed to reproduce a subsequent remission and possibly a cure.

One of the most important and unheralded discoveries about chemotherapy is the fact that a much better therapeutic result—even occasionally a cure—could be achieved by using several drugs simultaneously (combination chemotherapy) or in sequence. This discovery was a major step forward since until that point most chemotherapy agents were used alone. Then, when it was no longer effective it was replaced by a new single agent. When the use of single chemotherapy agents was common there were few, if any, true cures achieved.

Another momentous development was the observation that when chemotherapy was combined (combination modality therapy) with either radiation therapy or surgery, and sometimes both, previously incurable cancers could now be cured.

Therefore, the reader might ask, what is the best chemotherapy drug(s) for the treatment of cancer. There is no single best therapy for *all* cancers. Remember, as we discussed earlier, there are over 250 types of cancer worldwide and at least 100 types known in the western hemisphere. And each of these types has a different therapeutic program for the best treatment results. There are also several stages and substages within each of these cancer types which may be treated completely differently as the stage of disease changes.

Stated another way, there is no single *'magic bullet'* for cancer and there probably never will be. The reader should not be discouraged by this statement, however. It has been a scientific fact throughout medical history that most diseases, even those that are curable, have not had a single, best curative treatment. As a result, there are dozens of antibiotics available to treat several kinds of infections. There are dozens of medicines used to treat high blood pressure, diabetes, heart disease, and now, cancer.

When people ask, "when are we going to have a cure for cancer?" The author's usual answer, "we already do have several cures but it depends on what kind of cancer is being treated." Most people are amazed by this answer and it does open the door nicely for the presentation of the scientific facts.

How is the best treatment plan chosen by the physician? The answer is that the physician, either alone or with the help of an oncologist, chooses the best therapy according to the research reports disseminated by cancer researcher centers. They then tailor the therapy plan to the type of cancer, the stage of the cancer, the general health of the subject, the age and sex of the subject, the side effects of the therapy, and in accordance with the choices of the subject.

Therefore, it is not wise for the reader to compare his therapy plan with a treatment plan from newspaper or television reports; the results of treatment of a relative or friend, or anecdotal reports given by acquaintances. Even if those reports are for the same type of cancer as the reader they still may not apply because the stage of your cancer, along with all the other factors listed above, may alter the choice and the results of the chosen therapy.

For example, let's suppose Mr. Jones and Mrs. Smith each have lung cancer. Yet Mr. Jones is treated with surgery and his cancer is cured. Mrs. Smith, on the other hand, has limited surgery, radiation therapy and combination chemotherapy for her lung cancer, and she is cured.

Mr. Jones may have had a small, localized, non-disseminated type of lung cancer; he may have been young enough and healthy enough to survive extensive surgery; and his type of cancer may have been known to be insensitive to radiation therapy or chemotherapy.

Mrs. Smith, on the other hand: may have been much older and in poor general health for extensive surgery; her cancer may have been at a more advanced stage or had even spread to another organ; her type of cancer may have been one known to her oncologist to be sensitive to radiation or chemotherapy alone.

And these case scenarios sited are not at all unusual in the practice of oncology. As a matter of fact they are very common sets of circumstances. This is precisely the reason each individual patient has their therapy plan tailored to their situation and cannot be administered in a *cook book* fashion by just any physician who decides to do so.

Methods of Administration of Chemotherapy: Since cancer chemotherapy entails the use of a drug or a combination of drugs it can be given by mouth as a tablet, capsule or liquid; by injection through a vein (intravenously), deep into the muscle (intramuscularly), or under the skin (subcutaneously). Under more special circumstances it can be infused into an artery (intra-arterial) very close to the cancerous growth; or into the spinal canal (intrathecal); into the abdominal cavity (intraperitoneal); or into the chest cavity (intrapleural). The intravenous and oral are the most common routes of administration.

In most cases the patient does not require hospitalization but can receive the chemotherapy in the doctor's office, in the hospital outpatient department, and, on occasion, by the patient himself or a family member at home. The physician in charge makes this choice after discussing the options with the patient. However, there are circumstances in which a drug can only be administered safely in the hospital under the careful, close supervision of a physician or nurse. The way in which these choices apply to any individual cancers, and cancer drugs, is discussed more in detail in later pages of this book.

The degree of discomfort experienced by the patient during administration of chemotherapy is usually minimal and tolerated quite well. The tablet form, of course, is painless as is the liquid form. Some patients report mild nausea or a burning sensation in the abdomen after ingestion of the medications. Often these complaints can be prevented if the drugs are taken with food.

The amount of discomfort experienced with the intramuscular and subcutaneous forms of injection is similar to the degree of pain experienced when receiving a 'flu shot,' which is usually a minor discomfort.

The intravenous injection form of administration is like the discomfort experienced when the reader has blood taken for laboratory tests or when one donates blood. There is a sensation of coolness in the arm as the drugs, which are usually at room temperature, flow into the vein and up the arm. Some drugs cause a mild burning or stinging sensation as they flow into the vein. If there is any actual pain or discomfort experienced it should be reported to the physician or nurse.

Synonyms: As a group, chemotherapy drugs are known by many other names. Some of these are; Cytotoxic drugs, Radiomimetic drugs, Alkylating agents, Antimetabolites, Vinca Alkaloids, Anticancer antibiotics, Anthracyclines and there are many more.

In some cases these designations are actually 'classes of drugs' used in cancer treatment. In other cases the names indicate the mode of action of the drugs.

Side Effects of Chemotherapy: Unfortunately many patients still refuse life saving curative chemotherapy because of a misunderstanding about, and an inordinate amount of fear of the side effects of chemotherapy. Perhaps a definition of the phrase side effect can clarify these misconceptions and fears.

The term, ***side effect*** is best defined as the *undesirable and unwanted* changes or symptoms caused by the administration of a drug or treatment. The term does not mean that these side effects have to be dangerous, serious, lethal or permanent. And, indeed, most of them are not. It also does not mean that every patient must suffer these side effects and, indeed, many patients never experience any side effects during the course of treatment.

It is your physician's duty to discuss these side effects before proceeding with chemotherapy. She can also estimate the likelihood of each of these side effects occurring; the symptoms you might experience and their severity; if the effects are permanent or temporary and approximately how long they will last; if the effects are serious or minor; the degree of suffering from each and if any chance of fatality exists from the side effects; what organs might be involved in the side effects and if the organ will recover. Also, she should discuss the ways in which these side effects may be prevented or reversed.

Ordinarily the side effects of a chemotherapy drug are known well in advance of their clinical use on humans through prior research and experience. Your physician must then determine if the risk and type of side effect are acceptable for your particular case. The effectiveness of chemotherapy pivots upon the fact that the normal tissue and organs eventually recover from the effects of therapy whereas the cancer tissue does not. Also, it is not necessary for a patient to experience side effects in order to achieve a therapeutic benefit. The ill effects are discussed with you with the understanding that they only *might* occur. There are many occasions when a patient does not experience any of these side effects but still experiences a cure or remission of the cancer.

Also there is no relationship between the rate of occurrence of side effects and the rate of successful results of the therapy. Conversely, if the side effects do occur it does indicate that any therapeutic effect has also occurred.

The most common side effects experienced are nausea and vomiting; hair loss (alopecia); fatigue; loss of taste for food, loss of appetite and loss of weight; increased risk of infection; decrease in the blood count including red blood cells, white blood cells and platelets (cells needed for the clotting of blood). These are in general the side effects most often experienced with most chemotherapy drugs whether used alone as single agents or used in combination.

In some cases there are some side effects which are unique to one chemotherapy drug or one class of drugs. The chemotherapy physician must discuss with reader these specific side effects and the other risks in relation to the agent(s) used in the therapy program chosen. These special side effects are discussed under each of the drugs to which they apply in a later section of this book.

During the course of the therapy program the physician must monitor the patient for both therapeutic benefits and side effects through the use of questions about symptoms, physical examination, laboratory tests, x-rays and scans.

Onset of Therapeutic Effects: Frequently, the reader is disappointed with their therapy program because they don't experience immediate relief of the symptoms of their cancer. It is normal and to be expected that there not be any improvement in symptoms until at least six to twelve weeks of therapy are administered. Also, in the majority of cases, the objective signs of improvement as measured by physical examination or testing do not occur for as long as three months after starting chemotherapy. This lag period is not an indication the therapy will not eventually be effective. A certain amount of delay in therapeutic response is to be expected. The reader must not become discouraged because of this delay in response. The chemotherapist physician should point this out to the reader early in the patient-physician relationship so there will be no surprises or realistic expectations. If the expected onset of improvement is not discussed the reader must ask the question regarding time to expected improvement before embarking on the therapy program.

Prevention and Treatment of Side Effects: Because of the contemporary developments in medicinal science there are now available several agents which are helpful in either preventing or reversing the undesirable side effects of chemotherapy.

Nausea and Vomiting: Without a doubt these are the most common and the most troublesome side effects of chemotherapy. However, with the discovery of several new anti-vomiting drugs it is now possible to prevent, or at least modify the severity of these side effects. Unfortunately, their prevention cannot be accomplished in all individuals nor can it be done even in the same person each and every time therapy is administered.

In most circumstances the vomiting doesn't last more than 24 to 48 hours after the administration of chemotherapy. Also, depending on the specific drugs and the sequence of their administration the vomiting may occur only on the first day of therapy even if several more doses of drugs are given later in the sequence. Contemporary chemotherapy programs begin with a large dose of one drug or a combination of drugs given on the first day of a series of treatments, these series are called cycles, and then a cycle is repeated 4 to 6 weeks later. During the rest interval between cycles the normal tissues are allowed time to recover and the patient is allowed a respite much like the interruption of therapy which takes place during radiotherapy.

In addition to using medicines for preventing vomiting it is now possible to successfully treat it when it does occur. Several drugs are given in prevention before starting the chemotherapy injections. Among the many are; metapropamide (Reglan®), chlorpromizine (Compazine®), Ondansetron (Zofran®), dexamethasone, nabilone (a marijuana derivative), and a few others of similar chemical structure.

In addition, alteration of the method of giving chemotherapy agents can, in itself, reduce or prevent vomiting. One of the alternate methods of the therapy is to give it in cycles with interspersed rest periods. Such changes in the methods of administration is another of the unheralded advances in cancer chemotherapy. The recognition of the benefit of giving more than one agent at a time and giving large doses on a single day has turned many previously ineffective and highly toxic forms of therapy into ones which achieve much better results.

Incidentally, readers often ask if it is advisable to eat anything just before receiving chemotherapy. This author's clinical experience suggests that whether the patient eats or not just before chemotherapy seems to have no influence on the occurrence of vomiting. Actually, it becomes a philosophical question more than a medical question. Since the author's philosophy is that the patient try to continue their usual life-style in the same manner as before chemotherapy, and since maintaining good nutrition is important, patients are advised to try to eat a normal meal whether they are scheduled to receive chemotherapy or not. If, and when, vomiting does occur taking large amounts of clear fluids only until the side effect passes is recommended.

Many patients and families are concerned about malnutrition or starvation during this short period of no food intake. They need not be concerned. The effects of undernutrition take at least several consecutive weeks of decreased caloric intake to cause any serious consequences, as long as fluid intake is maintained. The nutritional aspects of cancer therapy are discussed in more detail in later pages.

Preventing Hair Loss (Alopecia): Many methods have been advocated for the prevention of the hair loss caused by chemotherapy. Unfortunately, none of these methods have been shown to be useful. At least in this therapist's experience they have not proven to be effective. The methods used have included; placing a tourniquet around the crown of the skull just below the hair line; application of ice packs or other forms of cooling devices over the skull during and before therapy; ingestion of large doses of vitamin E, avoiding application of shampoos and other chemicals to the hair, etc. My personal observation has not shown that any of these methods are effective. However, since they are harmless and relatively inexpensive there is no reasonable objection to prescribing these if the reader requests them.

Alopecia is one of the most feared side effects of cancer therapy. Therefore, the physician must discuss the possibility of hair loss with the patient, especially female patients and children. The topic acquires even more significance because *not all* chemotherapy drugs can be expected to produce this side effect. Your doctor must also point out that the hair loss is *usually* temporary and full regrowth of hair *usually* occurs. It may take several months but it will happen. Equally important information is that the hair loss may be total or partial but the quantity of loss does not alter the chances of the hair growth returning. As stated earlier, the therapeutic effectiveness of the chemotherapy drugs has no relation to degree or occurrence rate of hair loss. The therapy can still produce remission or cure even if hair loss does not occur, a parallel many patients erroneously take for granted.

The subject must be advised before starting therapy that they may need to wear a wig. They are advised to cut off a lock of hair that most represents the color they would prefer for the hair piece to save for later, if needed. They are also advised not to purchase a wig until the hair loss occurs since it may not happen.

Fatigue: Patients often characterize this symptom as weakness, listlessness, a worn out feeling. Fatigue is one of the more troublesome side effects and one with which the patients desperately need help. They are informed of its possible occurrence so they might prepare for it. It seems to be handled better if they are advised to expect it and to be prepared. However, they are encouraged to maintain normal activity when fatigue does occur. The author's personal clinical experience has been that bed rest is not helpful in subduing the fatigue caused by the chemotherapy. On the contrary, it is probably worsened. But remaining active and fully involved, unless a serious disability exists, appears more beneficial in combating the side effect of fatigue. The patient is informed that their life-style need not change because of chemotherapy. The more they remain in their usual groove, so to speak, the better they feel.

Occasionally, medications are helpful in combating the problem of weakness and fatigue. The medications which are used include the classes of drugs called mood elevators, antidepressants, etc. However, psychological counseling, encouragement and a great deal of support from the physician, the nursing staff, family and friends, ministers and priests and support groups are more desirable than drugs. If used properly, these support systems can reduce the patient's already deep concern regarding side effects of medication.

The majority of patients are not physically hindered by their chemotherapy regimen and many go to work immediately after receiving their therapy. Normal activity is the best tonic for this side effect. Patients are advised to maintain this philosophical attitude before starting chemotherapy.

Nevertheless, this philosophical approach should not become a form of nagging or badgering the subject. The result of such pressure by your physician is only loss of confidence and patient resentment. As it is, there is always enough patient resentment over having acquired the disease in the first place. But gentle, firm encouragement and assistance by your physician can be of significant benefit to the patient.

Loss of Appetite: Most often these side effects are the result of the effects of the chemotherapy drugs on the taste buds on the tongue and the appetite center in the brain. On occasion the loss of taste is a result of a fungus infection on the tongue and in the mouth (oral thrush). Your physician can treat or prevent this fungus with the appropriate antifungal drugs. A large part of the problem is a result of the depression that patients experience. The management of depression has been touched upon in earlier sections of this book.

However, in addition to encouragement and support your physician can do a great deal to improve the eating habits of the reader. Normal caloric intake is so extremely important because good nutritional status is so vital to a good response to chemotherapy. A well balanced diet which contains all of the four basic food groups must be maintained. However, the problem needs to be handled in a realistic manner. If the patient has never been one to ingest fruits or green vegetables, or even animal flesh-meats it is not likely they can be converted. Instead, the important nutrients can be supplied in other more palatable ways to the patient. For example, protein can be supplied to the vegetarian from dairy products, eggs, gelatin desserts, nutritional supplements and the like.

If the subject has a particular taste preference for certain flavors this can be utilized to blend that flavor with other food substances to encourage their intake. Eating several small meals a day rather than the traditional three larger meals can be effective in some subjects. A dietician or nutritionist can be helpful in the area of nutritional support, as will be discussed in later pages.

There are many readers who have the mistaken impression that special, exotic diets *alone* can cure or prevent cancer. Careful scientific research has not demonstrated that a dietary program can, by itself, combat cancer. While there is no question good nutrition is important in aiding the body's natural healing powers remission and cure can only be accomplished with other concurrent, conventional therapies. For that matter, good nutritional status is important for all forms of cancer therapy whether it be surgery, radiation therapy, chemotherapy, or any combination thereof. The same statement is applicable to the prevention of cancer by diet alone. That having been said, there is a substantial body of evidence that a high fiber diet may be useful in preventing cancer of the colon. There has been no substantial and reliable evidence presented to date supporting the claim that large or standard doses of vitamins are effective to treat or to prevent cancer.

There are many other specific ways to prevent some of the special and unique side effects peculiar to certain chemotherapy drugs and classes of drugs. These specific methods are discussed in the section which gives more details about each cancer chemotherapy drug.

Hormonal Therapy: Technically known as hormonal manipulation, this modality of treatment eliminates the cancer cells by altering the hormone balance of the patient by administering drugs which alters this balance. The hormonal drug agents are usually given in tablet form. In some cases the choice of hormone is a logical one, such as administering male hormones (androgens) to a female patient with breast cancer. In other instances the therapeutic effect may have been a chance observation without much scientific rationale. An example is the use of hormonal cortisone drugs to treat certain leukemias and other non-leukemic types of cancer.

The primary difference between hormonal therapy and chemotherapy is that the normal cells are usually not damaged or killed by the hormonal drugs. However, this is not to say there are no side effects from hormonal therapy. Side effects do occur with this type of treatment but not through cell destruction or damage.

Each hormonal drug agent has its own unique group of side effects and is discussed in detail with each agent presented in future pages. Some of these side effects are purely cosmetic and some can be fatal. Your physician should discuss these side effects with the reader before beginning therapy.

Anti-hormone drug therapy is included in the class called hormonal treatment because it is a form of hormonal manipulation used in certain types of cancer. Examples of these anti-hormones include tamoxifen and flutamide.

New and Evolving Therapies: Because of the vast amount of research presently in progress discussion of this topic could very well produce an endless and on-going list. Thus, only those therapies that are included here are those which have just recently come on the scene or those which are just about to appear over the horizon.

Biological Response Modifiers: Biological response modifiers are defined as a group of agents which either stimulate or modify the bodies natural immune defense systems in order to achieve cancer cell death and then the cancer cells removal. This therapeutic end point can now be accomplished by several new agents which operate by several mechanisms. Immunotherapy is another name for the use of this group of therapeutic agents.

Included in the group are the Interferons, Interleukins, BCG vaccine, levamisole and some others discussed below.

Suffice it here to state that these agents are just beginning to be fully developed and they are not a panacea—*a cure-all*—for all cancers. As a matter of fact, there are very few cancers which are effectively treated with these agents at the present time.

It should also be understood that although this type of therapy sounds wholesome and pure, it is not without its major and minor side effects. It is hoped that further research and development can help to eliminate or reduce these side effects and improve cure rates. The entire area of biological response modifiers is still very experimental and not generally applicable to cancer therapy.

Experimental Cancer Therapies: Since this term has come up at this point its meaning needs defining and clarification. The first step is to define what this experimental therapy *is not*.

Experimental treatment modalities are not those which are exclusively available to a select few people based on their; political connections, wealth, social status, race, religion, or any other such mundane qualifications. And, clearly, there are many readers who labor under such false notions.

The selection of any patient as part of any experimental therapy program is a purely scientific and clinical choice. Patients are chosen based on their meeting a specific set of scientific and clinical requirements, such as; cancer type, location of the cancer, and lack of response to standard forms of therapy. Also, patients are chosen based on previous research which has clearly demonstrated that this particular type of cancer has had some response to the experimental therapy under study. The experimental therapy must also have been shown to have relatively low toxicity and acceptable safety standards.

For example, in some programs the patients are screened out on the basis of age and not because the program director or the doctors involved in the study are only interested in saving the lives of the young. Such a screening and selection process is necessary because many forms of experimental therapy have an extremely high risk of serious side effects and a high fatality rate among subjects over the age of fifty or in some cases even over the age of forty.

The major point to be made is that a scientific project, in order to yield some meaningful results must be designed in such a way wherein all the variables are known and reduced to the smallest possible number.

In most cases the patients in an experimental program are divided into two groups which are matched by cancer type and stage; by age, sex, race and the general health of each subject chosen; by those who have or have not received prior therapy; and by many other factors which alter the response of the cancer to treatment or by the toxicity of the therapeutic agent for the patient. Then, the results are matched against either the previous known effective therapy or no therapy at all, if that applies to this cancer type.

Therefore, when your physician or the program director states you are not eligible for an experimental form of therapy they mean that your case does not meet the scientific qualifications for that particular program. The decision to exclude a case is not a financial, personal, racial, or political one. For these reasons I believe that the government, the politicians, the news media, the social agencies, or any other group not involved in the scientific design of the program should not be involved in the decision making process when choosing patients for an experimental therapy study. Otherwise, the end result yields no scientifically useful information and might actually hinder the research effort.

Of course, the medical community would like to cure everyone, now, but the scientific process is a slow, tedious one and must be conducted under strict guidelines and principles. If these principles are not followed valuable time and resources are wasted and new therapies are placed further out of our reach.

Supportive Therapy: Support therapy programs are extremely vital to the care of cancer patients, even to the point of calling them indispensable. Without these support systems any cancer therapy program is doomed, if not to failure at least to a very poor success rate. Patient therapy support program is a concept which consists of a large team of specially trained professionals including; dieticians, clergymen, nurses, physical therapists, psychiatrists or psychologists, social workers, and, most importantly, the physicians. The physician members of the group should include the medical specialists, as well as, the family physicians and other primary care physicians.

Performance Status: It has been demonstrated in many research studies that performance status is a strong determinant in the patient's positive response to any kind of cancer therapy. Performance status is defined simply as the subjects ability to perform ordinary every day tasks in the manner and to the degree which they were able prior to receiving cancer therapy. It is clear the remission rate and cure rate are directly effected by this variable. For this reason it is important to encourage the patients to try to maintain their usual life style. Supportive therapy programs are designed primarily to achieve this end. Thus, the subjects physical, emotional, and spiritual needs are to be normalized as much as possible.

Dietary Status: The importance of good dietary support in cancer therapy support cannot be over emphasized. A well balanced nutritional status must be achieved. Encourage good nutritional status is not to say the subject must be made to over eat or to gain weight beyond their healthy, normal weight. However, if the patient has lost weight every effort must be made to regain the lost weight in the form of healthy flesh and muscle, not in the form of fat. Encouragement, support and education of the subject and the person who provides their food is absolutely necessary. The dietician or nutritionist are very useful in providing helpful tips in accomplishing this goal. A dietary plan is organized to provide the four basic food groups for the individual but an effort must be made to keep the plan within any specific ethnic or social taste to which the subject is accustomed. They must not be forced to eat in a taste-fashion not attractive to them as long as the menus have a good balance.

Physical Activity: Maintaining normal physical activity is another vital area which needs emphasis if the subject is to respond well to therapy. Clinical experience has shown me that well meaning family members and friends often unintentionally hinder this process. Of course, it is not intentional. But in their effort to demonstrate their love and concern for the patient they tend to wait on the subject hand and foot. Or they encourage the patient to rest more and nap frequently during the day. Thus, the recommended physical activity and exercise is not forthcoming. The patient's emotional welfare is also injured by this attitude. The patient often feels more like an invalid than their condition warrants. They sometimes become suspicious and doubtful of the honesty of the therapy team and feel they are not being told all the details of their prognosis. They often suspect the physician is keeping some important and damning information from them but the family has been given the 'bad news.'

Apparently, the outdated idea of excessive, forced bed rest was fostered by the approach used to treat many illnesses in the past. All illnesses do not necessarily respond faster to treatment if the patient is made to rest excessively. On the contrary, clinical research has shown that excessive bed rest—such as after childbirth or surgery—increases the complication rate. And the mortality rate has been shown to be higher with prolonged bed rest.

The skeleton muscles of a cancer patient need as much exercise and use to maintain their integrity as is required by a healthy person.

Of course, excessively vigorous athletic training programs are not necessary but regular, normal paced walking and maintaining the upright, out-of-bed position is beneficial. The physical and recreational therapy teams are indispensable in achieving this goal. Moreover, the physician can add credence to the team effort by encouraging the patient and assuring them that activity is not harmful to their general well being. Your doctor must also reassure you and your family members that normal physical activity does not cause more rapid spread of their cancer nor does it hinder the therapy effort. Support, encouragement and realistic reassurance are the major ingredients provided by the physician. The therapy team can devise an ideal activity program to suite the taste and needs of the subject.

Nursing Support: A supportive nursing staff is an invaluable part of the therapy team. There are nursing school teaching programs which now provide specialty-nurses training in oncology care. The oncology nurse can provide instruction and support for the patient which the physician cannot provide. Included in this education area, but not limited to it, are the instructions concerning: the administration, dosage, safety of medications; maintenance of personal hygiene; feeding and bathing techniques for the handicapped; and just plain moral and emotional support. All of these factors are important for the continued normal life style of the patient.

The specialized area addressing the care of contemporary injection devices and vein access devices is provided by the oncology nursing specialist. In addition, they supplement and augment the information given by the physicians, nutritionist, etc. Sometimes, just knowing they are there and that they do care gives the patient a much needed bolstering of morale.

Emotional and Spiritual Support: The patient need not be a religious individual to require emotional and spiritual support. Of course, they must not be forced into religious counseling if it is not their desire. Ministers, rabbis and priests, however, can provide valuable assistance in these areas but it is not limited to the clergy as providers. The needed counseling can also be provided by trained social workers, psychologists or psychiatrists who have an interest in this kind of program. Peace of mind and peace of soul are extremely important if any therapy program is to succeed.

Of course, the family members and friends are an irreplaceable part of the entire team effort. The love provided by these individuals cannot be replaced by newly found supporters. They must be involved as soon as possible in the therapy plan when it is still being formulated in order for the plan to be effective.

The physicians must also be a part of the support group effort. If a physician's wishes are only to provide the technical and professional skills of the therapy program he is derelict in his duty in my opinion. Physicians must demonstrate their interest and faith in the support of the team concept in order for it to be effective.

Part Four

Prognosis

Chapter 14

Prognosis of Cancer

The formulation of a prognosis is a process which is frequently misunderstood by the cancer patient and their family. There is some misconception that the physician has some magic formula for calculating the exact minute, hour, day, month and year the patient's life will come to an end. There is also a mistaken idea that the physician has the ability to predict the manner in which death will occur. Immediately, it must be understand that there is no such magic formula for making these predictions.

Definitions: The definitions below are offered as working interpretations of the term— prognosis. The first definition is from a well known medical dictionary and the second from a layman's dictionary. A third definition, derived from my personal clinical experience, is a variation on these interpretations.

Medical Definition: Prognosis is a prediction of the duration, course and termination of a disease, based on all information available in the individual case and knowledge of how the disease behaves *generally.*

Layman's Definition: Prognosis is a forecasting–especially in medicine–a judgement in advance concerning the probable course of a disease and the chances of recovery.

Author's Definition: The prognosis is an approximation of the duration of survival which the patient can expect after a specific course therapy. It must be modified to each particular type of cancer based on the clinical stage of the disease, and the age, race, sex and general overall health of the individual affected by the disorder.

Reader please make note that in all three of these definitions the use of vague, imprecise and generalized terms. These generalizations and ambiguities are used not in an attempt to hide information or avoid the issue of life expectancy. They are used because there are no precise factors which can be utilized—with any degree of honesty—in predicting the outcome of any illness. Regardless of the competency, ability, training or experience of the physician involved he can never forecast the precise outcome for any single patient or even for a group of patients with any type of cancer.

The best your physician can offer is the *likelihood* of response, expressed as a *percentage*, and an *estimate* of the duration of survival. For example there may be a 30 to 60 percent chance of five-year survival, two-year survival, complete remission, or partial remission based on your physician's general knowledge of the type of cancer involved.

Those numbers are **not** based on the individual physician's personal success or failure rate. Nor are they based on his own particular skills and end-results unless he is a research physician as well as a practitioner in the field of cancer therapy. Even then his estimations are based on the results of other researchers who have duplicated and verified his results. These calculations are derived from nationwide or even worldwide end-results of a particular therapy program for a particular type and stage of the cancer in question. Herein, arises the major reason a universally agreed upon and utilized group of terms and definitions are used by cancer research scientists around the world.

There is no way any physician anywhere in the world can line up a thousand, or even a hundred cancer patients and predict which 50 percent will survive and which 50 percent will not survive. He is also not capable of, if he is honest, calculating a specific number for Mrs. Smith or Mr. Jones because he has been their physician for many years. Having knowledge of the general health status and the lifelong habits of the patient does lend some useful data in providing medical care but it does not give the physician extrasensory magical ability to make predictions regarding the therapeutic outcome any better than the known national statistics.

In an attempt to clarify the definition of the term prognosis it must be pointed out what the term *does not imply* and what *it cannot do*.

It is not a precise, accurate statement indicating how long an individual patient will live; or how they will respond to therapy; or how likely they are to have any side effects from therapy; or what their quality of life will be like during a specific therapy program.

The prognosis statement is a rough estimation of the possibility of the patient's length of survival based on the type of cancer and its likelihood to respond to therapy based on general, worldwide results of that particular therapy. It is an approximation also based on the clinical stage, type and grade of cancer, and on the sex, age, general health and compliance of the patient to a particular program of therapy.

There are not, nor can there ever be, any guarantees of how the subject will fare under the effects of therapy. This is the honest, current situation not because physicians are inept, uncaring or incompetent; or because medical science has not made the research effort . It is so because of the variability of the biological responses of the human species to a variety of clinical circumstances. Each and every individual is capable of responding in a totally unpredictable and previously unexperienced manner. Many years of clinical experience has demonstrated to physicians that anything is possible when it comes to the responses the human body can arouse to any of our therapeutic manipulations. It is exactly for these reasons that imprecise qualitative and quantitative terms are used so often in the practice of clinical medicine. Terms such as; probable, most likely, on the average, in general, five-year survival, unavoidable complications, percentages, ranges, etc. are an indispensable part of the vocabulary of physicians.

Part Five

Choosing a Physician

Introduction

Choosing a Physician to Manage Your Cancer

In this section I have attempted to provide the reader with some guidance as to the way in which an individual goes about choosing the type of physician—based on their specialty and training—who is most likely capable of treating and managing the readers particular cancer related problem. The discussion is divided into two distinct areas. The first portion discusses the situation of the reader who has nonspecific symptoms but who is looking for answers to the cause of his symptoms, especially if his major concern is whether or not he has cancer. The second portion discusses the possible choices and some recommendations when a reader is *definitely known* to have cancer which has been diagnosed by a biopsy.

However, there are no hard and fast rules, nor is their any mandatory way in which a physician should be chosen. This freedom of choice is one of the many blessings of living in a free democracy such as the United States. You, as a free, adult individual, therefore, can choose any type of physician you wish and you are even free to choose *not to be treated* at all. No one can forcibly deny you these rights. It is my hope, however, that after reading this book the reader will see the rationale and plausible arguments for and against my points of view. However, the final choice is always up to the individual reader as long as they are mentally competent and able to speak for themselves.

Chapter 15

The Undiagnosed Patient

Many readers automatically think of seeking out a medical specialist when they have a medical problem. And there are those who hold with the idea of the family physician as the guardian of their health. Either approach is acceptable. However, the claim that the family physician is more likely to think of the patient as a whole person rather than a specific part and the specialist is not likely to do so is a narrow minded generalization. Considering the patient as a whole person is an individual and personal human trait based on the physician's character, morality, ethics and his philosophy of approach to medical care. There is no inherent guarantee that any type of medical training—specialist or generalist—will result in either type of approach.

Nevertheless, speaking strictly from the point of view of economy and preservation of financial resources the primary care physician *is* perfectly capable of diagnosing or ruling out cancer. A medical specialist, oncologist or otherwise, is not required to arrive at the diagnosis.

There may be some confusion in the reader's mind as to what constitutes a *primary care physician,* therefore, a simple definition is offered. The medical profession's concept is that the primary physician constitutes the *'first line of defense'* in providing medical care. They may or may not be specialists, such as in the case of those who are pediatricians and internists. They are called generalists. That is, they manage the patient's general medical problems rather than focus their attention on a specific organ or limited group of diseases such as, a pediatric oncologist (children's cancer), pediatric surgeon, pediatric cardiologist (children's heart diseases), etc. Ordinarily, primary care physicians include; the family physician or general practitioner, the general internist, the gynecologist-obstetrician, the general surgeon and the pediatrician. Each of these groups of primary care providers is perfectly capable and adequately trained to either, establish a diagnosis of cancer or, at least, to direct the patient to the specialists—namely the secondary care physician—who is able to establish the diagnosis.

Eventually, the primary physician will need the help of other specialists to confirm the diagnosis of cancer. A radiologist helps him read and interpret the x-rays needed; a surgeon performs the surgery necessary to obtain a biopsy specimen; a pathologist or hematologist helps him interpret the biopsied material. The therapy program is provided by a medical oncologist, a surgical oncologist or a radiation oncologist or a team of these experts. Even within these specialties other more specific medical specialists (or subspecialists) may be consulted. The subspecialists might include; a neurosurgeon to perform brain surgery, a thoracic surgeon for chest surgery, and so on.

Initially, if the reader is not yet certain of the cause of their symptoms or even the organ system involved they need not seek the aid of a specialist. However, that is the reader's right if they so choose. The only exceptions might include choosing a dermatologist for a skin lesion; a pediatrician for children; and a gynecologist for obvious problems in the area of female reproductive organs, i. e. vaginal bleeding. The public impression that only a specialist thinks in terms of *'serious diseases'* and the primary care physician only thinks in terms of minor diseases is erroneous. All physicians are trained under the axiom, *always look for the worst but hope for the best.* Additionally, all doctors are trained to suspect cancer as a possibility to explain any symptom and all symptoms and to pursue this specific line of investigation when warranted.

On the other hand, it is a mistake for the reader to believe that the specialist or subspecialist can only think exclusively in terms of serious diseases. He may refer the patient back to the primary care physician once he has ruled out disease within his area of expertise rather than treat it himself. His decision will be based on practicality and cost effectiveness.

In the final analysis, the management of any medical case should be a team effort with the universal goal of establishing the diagnosis as quickly, safely and economically as possible with as little discomfort and apprehension to the patient as possible. The emphasis is vigorously placed on the phrase, *team effort*. None of the physicians involved in the case should think of the patient in question as his personal property. But they should, instead, think of the patient as a whole human being in need of help with the ultimate goal being cure, if possible, and to return the patient to their normal life style as soon as practicably possible.

Chapter 16

Guidelines for the Patient with Known Cancer

The following is a practical guide to aid the cancer patient in choosing the proper course once a diagnosis of cancer has been clearly established. Understand, however, there are no hard and fast rules or laws on how one must proceed. The ideal arrangement is an organized, cooperative team effort in the management of any particular patient. In an another section of this book is listed each type of cancer and within this framework I list the type of physician I believe is best to serve as the *"quarterback,"* if you will, of the cancer treatment team. There must be an organizer to call the signals if the team is to function effectively.

In most circumstances the primary care physician—the general practitioner, the internist, the gynecologist, etc.— initially directs the team until the appropriate course of therapy is chosen. Very often the team leader will change as the treatment of the cancer proceeds because of the technology involved and the special expertise required. For example, the primary care physician may feel radiotherapy is the best choice of therapy but the radiotherapist might disagree and suggest surgery or chemotherapy.

At this point the team members will hold a joint discussion of the case to determine a consensus recommendation as to the best therapeutic approach. Once a course of action is chosen it is seldom possible, if ever, for the primary care physician to administer the chosen therapy because his training in primary care medicine doesn't include cancer therapy. The highly technical knowledge and skill of a radiation oncologist, or a neurosurgeon requires someone specifically trained and experienced in those areas.

The team must function in a way which makes the patient feel comfortable in knowing there is a team leader. Knowing who the team leader is and what is his function adds to the patient's confidence in the team. The patient should also know which member of the team to contact should complications or problems arise during the course of therapy. The immense amount of security experienced by the subject with this arrangement is a major factor which allows the therapy program to proceed smoothly. The physician members of the team or the designated team leader will discuss these points with the patient and a family member as early in the process as possible.

Of course, the patient is always free to request a second opinion or to request the involvement of another type of specialist at any time. However, this request should be done with full knowledge of the team or team leader and should be discussed before making the request. If the team leading physician is a mature, wise and experienced practitioner he will not object. He may, and is obligated to, advise the patient regarding their choice to be certain the appropriate specialist is requested and to insure there is no undue delay in the treatment program. My personal practical experience has taught me that the reader should not undertake this step without professional advise.

Frequently, because of misunderstanding and inadequate knowledge about cancer the reader seeks a second opinion from an inappropriate type of physician. For example, there are clearly situations in which a medical oncologist is *not* appropriate for the proper management of certain kinds of cancer. The same can be said for radiation oncologists, surgical oncologists etc. Also, there are clearly situations in which highly specialized physicians who do not primarily treat cancer must be involved in the case, such as, neurosurgeons, thoracic surgeons, cardiac surgeons, etc. Such choices will be discussed in more detail in the section of this book which considers each specific cancer and its management.

The confusion may arise in the reader's mind because of the failure of the language of medicine to convey the appropriate function of many medical specialties. For example, it might be logically concluded that a dermatologist is necessary for all cases of skin cancer. But this is clearly not the case. In many situations a general surgeon or a plastic surgeon is required. It is advisable for the reader to discuss these points with the primary care physician before making any choice.

In my opinion the patient should not begin the process by seeking a specialist without the guidance of the primary care physician, although they do have the freedom to make any choice they wish. However, there are definitely situations in which the involvement of a specialist is mandatory. Radiotherapy, for instance, can only be given by a trained radiation oncologist; chemotherapy should be given only by a trained medical oncologist or chemotherapist; neurosurgery should be performed only by a trained neurosurgeon, etc. The only exception is the occasional situation in which a dire emergency exists and to save the life of the patient immediate action is undertaken by the most immediately available physician. However, with the high degree of development of contemporary communication systems available today the advice and guidance of a specialized physician can always be obtained by telephone if necessary.

Below I have listed the surgical specialists, the medical oncology subspecialists and the circumstances under which I believe they should be involved in the cancer treatment team effort.

Radiation Oncologist: In all cases in which radiation therapy is considered part of the therapy program requires a qualified radiation oncologist. The actual list of cancers and the sets of clinical circumstances needing radiotherapy is too long and complex to be given here. The sets of circumstances vary with the stage of the cancer, the general medical health of the subject and the treatment choices the patient has made as to whether or not radiotherapy is needed. Nevertheless, there are situations in which the advice of these various specialists is valuable even if radiotherapy is not administered. Their early involvement can only be a positive attribute in any case of cancer management.

Medical Oncologist: The medical oncologist's expertise is needed in any case in which chemotherapy, in any form, is administered in treatment of a cancer case. In view of the highly complex and sophisticated nature of contemporary chemotherapy agents only a clinician highly trained and experienced in their administration can give these agents safely and effectively. Obviously it is difficult, if not impossible, to make such a statement without being prejudiced and influenced by my own background in this subspecialty field. Nevertheless, I make this statement in good conscience based on my years of clinical experience with the many hazards involved in chemotherapy administration. As stated above, there can only be benefit incurred in involving a medical oncologist in the choice of treatment even if chemotherapy is not finally chosen as a treatment modality in the therapy program.

Surgical Oncologist and Gynecologic Surgical Oncologist: Unfortunately these subspecialists are few and far between but wherever they are available their involvement is strongly recommended. However, their involvement is not mandatory since adequately trained general gynecologists and general surgeons are perfectly capable of handling the majority of these cancer cases.

General Surgeon: In the case of cancers of the abdominal organs, of the breast, the extremities, the neck etc., a general surgeon is most often the best choice. However, when special organs within the abdomen, chest or brain are involved the general surgeon ordinarily seeks the assistance of the appropriate subspecialists. For example he may call on: a urologist for a kidney cancer; a gynecologist for a pelvic cancer; a neurosurgeon for a cancer close to the spinal cord, etc. As the reader can see the choice of the appropriate subspecialists is not always clear cut even to the physician, let alone the patient or their family. The complexity of these choices are some of the reasons the treatment plan must be customized for the individual case. There is no single best way to approach any case.

As far as learning of the qualifications of the physician you have chosen these can be obtained simply by asking the physician if he is Board Certified or Board Eligible. Also, the documentation of these qualifications can be requested. Board Certification or Eligibility are the minimum requirements your choice of physician should meet. Since there is some confusion as to what these requirements signify I shall try to clarify some of them.

Board Eligible indicates that after graduating medical school the physician has studied his specialty as part of an *approved* specialty program and at an *approved* institution of postgraduate medical training. The approval of these training programs is administered by the American Medical Association under strict guidelines. The Board Eligible physician has in his possession, and sometimes appropriately displayed, certificates which document his successful completion of the required specialty training program.

Board Certified or Qualified means that in addition to having completed the specialty training program the physician has taken and passed a written—and in some specialties a practical—examination given by the Board of Examiners for that particular specialty. The successful completion of these requirements is also documented by an appropriate, official certificate of Board Certification.

However, the reader should understand that there is no state, federal or local law requiring a physician to have these qualifications to practice any particular specialty or subspecialty. The law only requires the physician have a valid state medical license to practice medicine and surgery. I consider this a major flaw in our current licensing system. Usually, however, the hospitals are the guardians of these training and certification requirements. They should be continually monitoring all physician's qualifications and his standards of professional behavior.

If any reader is not familiar with the medical specialties available in their area the information can be obtained from the state and county medical societies. These are listed in your local phone book. In this contemporary age of marketing and advertising of medical services the listings of the physicians by specialty can be found in the yellow pages of the phone book. The reader should exercise caution here since simply listing oneself as a "Medical Oncologist" does not indicate the physician listed is officially *"certified."* The previously described documentation is still required.

Second Opinions: The second opinion is a very popular and fashionable concept today especially since it has been fostered and encouraged by the government and medical insurance companies. In some cases the patient has no choice in the matter. They are required to obtain a second opinion before the insurance provider agrees to pay for the medical services provided. A major difficulty which arises in the mind of the public as to when to obtain a second opinion if it is not required by the insurer. Sometimes, because it is trendy or fashionable, second opinions are requested by the patient or family for the wrong reasons. The decision to obtain a second opinion comes down to two basic questions in my view. First, when the diagnosis of cancer cannot be clearly established; second, whenever the optimal treatment modality indicated is not locally available or not clear, then a second opinion is usually recommended.

In the final analysis it is up to the patient to decide if and when they would feel more comfortable and more secure with a second opinion. However, if the patient is comfortable with the diagnosis, the recommended treatment program, and their physician, a second opinion may not be necessary. The essential ingredients should be trust and confidence in your physician. If the patient has confidence in their physician and trusts their judgement a second opinion may not be needed. If the physician in charge of your case is sincere and competent he will be the first to admit when a case is beyond his capabilities and will recommend a second opinion with the appropriate specialists. Nevertheless the reader should know that there is no legal obligation that another opinion must be obtained by your physician unless it is required by the insurance carrier.

Would I advise the reader to go to a large and famous medical center? The answer to this question is not always clear. Sometimes the limits of the patient's financial resources and geographic traveling distance precludes this possibility. If such a choice is made it should not be based on the notoriety of the referral center alone. Certainly it should not be misconstrued that special treatments for cancer are available exclusively at the famous medical centers. When the concept is examined carefully it is not the institution which provides the medical care. It is the individual physicians stationed at the medical center and the local hospitals who provide the care. In addition, it is the personality traits, the moral principles and the ethical characteristics of the individuals which determine the quality of care, not the buildings, equipment or furnishings. If the physicians are Board Eligible or Board Certified they most likely have had their training at a large university or an approved medical center. These desirable medical qualifications and character traits do not fade with movement to a different geographic location. Indeed, if this were the case then many rural areas in our country would not have access to contemporary medical care. And this is just not the case.

By all means, the reader is always free to discuss these options with their physician and they should be discussed. If your physician is truly interested in your welfare he will readily admit the need for having your case judged by a large medical center. However, it is best to follow your physician's recommendation regarding the choice of the medical center best qualified to examine your case. It is a common error for patients to assume that *all* large and famous medical centers are expert in *all* areas of cancer medicine. And this just isn't true, either.

Your doctor should be more familiar with the well known and competent physicians in a particular field and where they are located. In many cases it is the type of cancer in question which determines the best choice of consultant-type. There are many physician-researchers who have devoted their entire careers to the understanding and management of a single type of cancer for which they are world renowned. The physician or oncologist in charge of your case should know who these individual consultants are and how to make contact with them regarding a second opinion consultation.

Also, there is sometimes confusion about the availability of special treatment modalities offered away from the large medical centers. In this modern era of sophisticated communication and rapid transportation it is seldom, if ever, true that a particular form of cancer therapy cannot be provided outside of the referral centers. Many local and rural specialists maintain a liaison with a large cancer center primarily in order to be able to provide the latest and even the experimental modalities which might be recommended in your particular cancer.

There are now available many sophisticated means of communication between physicians and researchers around the world. One of the major purposes of published medical journals is to serve as an outlet for the reporting of new discoveries to physicians outside of the research centers. Their ultimate goal is to keep other physicians apprised of the latest in developments in the diagnosis and treatment of all diseases. In addition, all medical centers conduct regular, periodic educational seminars and work shops to add to the growing fund of knowledge in all fields of medical science and practice. Your physician only needs to maintain contact with the current medical literature and attend seminars to sustain and enrich his knowledge and skills in the field of cancer. These efforts toward remaining current are part of the moral, ethical and conscientious makeup of the dedicated physician.

Because of these contemporary means of communication and transportation it is never correct to assume any treatment modality is an exclusive or secret possession of any medical center. The antiquated notion which says—'there is only one physician in the world who can perform this operation'—is a melodramatic throwback from the motion picture shows of the 1930s. The same can be said for any new drug, chemical or dietary treatment of cancer. This is one of the reasons quack cures and quack physicians in any field cannot substantiate their outlandish claims of *"secret cures"* they alone possess.

In the final analysis the decision whether or not to visit a major medical center is the free choice of the patient and their family. For whatever reasons they decide to obtain a second opinion from these medical centers no one can prevent them from doing so, including their personal physician. Our legal system prevents the physician or anyone else from impeding the second-opinion-process by refusing to provide medical records, x-rays and other test results to aid the medical center in its evaluation of your case. The law does not allow such impediments since upon written request, after signing a legal release and request of your medical record, the physician must comply.

Depending on the state and local laws the physician may not be required to provide a copy of the records directly to the patient but he must supply it to any other physician making such a request. Also, there is no means by which physicians can penalize a patient for seeking another opinion. It is not possible for them to prevent the provision of medical services in the local community when the patient returns for continued care. The local physician does, of course, have the choice of not providing the care himself but he cannot prevent the local hospitals or other physicians in the community from providing medical care. The only damage which can occur is the injury to the physician's ego which should never be placed above the welfare of the patient. If it is apparent to the patient that medical services are being unjustly denied, I would advise that they seek another physician whose personal glory does not take precedent over his medical judgement. No physician is indispensable and no talent or skill is so unique as to be the exclusive possession of a single individual physician regardless of how outstanding his reputation may be.

The main purpose in my discussing this choice in seeking a second opinion from a large medical center is to remove the glamour from the kind of treatment result which can be unrealistically expected when making this choice. For example, it is unrealistic to expect a mystical revelation from the medical center physicians that they have a magical drug or a fabulous surgical procedure previously unknown to the medical world which will cure your cancer.

It is also unrealistic to expect that an error was made in the diagnosis of your cancer case and there is no cancer after all. However, there are occasional rare instances in which the diagnosis is initially not clear and when the medical center does further testing and biopsies it may decide that a cancer is not present. If your local physician is candid and has not withheld any information from you, he should have made you aware of this diagnostic dilemma before he referred your case to a medical center. In fact, this is precisely the situation in which physician should suggest another opinion from a medical center.

There are rare situations in which a clear cut case is sent to a center because of great expense, technical complexity, the small size of a community in which a special test, unusual form of treatment, or piece of equipment is available only at a university medical center. But every state in the United States contains within its boundaries a medical center which has these special modalities available or at least has the ability to obtain them. In fact, there is available a list of designated regional cancer research centers provided by the National Cancer Institute for the use of physicians and the general public.

In summary, any reasonable, caring physician realizes that the emotional well being of all cancer patients is an important, inseparable part of the complete care they require. Therefore, if for no other reason than the peace of mind of the patient he will be willing to assist you in obtaining the second opinion you desire.

Chapter 17

Philosophical Approaches to Cancer Management

The principles of practice style, bedside manner, patient advocacy, reflects the concepts which are discussed under this subheading. Unavoidably, the only way a patient can determine the style in which a physician practices medicine—whether he is an oncologist or not—is to actually meet several times with that physician. My experience suggests when readers follow the advice and observations of a relative or friend alone in choosing a physician they more often disagree, than agree with the recommendation. This is much the same as reading a critics review of a book or a film. You, the individual reader, still has to actually read the book or see the film to make your own decision.

In my view, there are essentially three practice styles a physician may choose in the management of cancer patients. However, it is probably not even a conscious choice the physician made through any special effort on their part. It is more often a slowly developed philosophical approach to the practicing medicine they gradually build by following their intuition, instincts and inherent personality traits. First, there is the traditional style which follows the philosophical line—tell the patient very little or no more than they actually need to know about the diagnosis or the treatment of their cancer. And, if the reader asks no questions about their disease, the doctor does not volunteer any information. Happily, this is a fading, uncommon style of practice. But unfortunately, it still does exist.

The second style is the more contemporary and reasonable approach which believes it is best to inform the patient as much as possible about their diagnosis, treatment and prognosis. More importantly, the physician must impart this information in an understandable, unslanted way. In other words, the patient must be educated in a lucid, unpretentious manner.

In the third style, there is a combination of the first and second methods of management. Usually, this approach surfaces only after the cancer patient or his family asks some pointed questions. The questions may be the result of undesirable side effects from the chosen therapeutic regimen or it may follow the observation of the patient's lack of improvement. The third practice philosophy is discussed first since it is, the most common type encountered.

The fourth system—which is not systematic at all and is therefore a misnomer—is an episodic, haphazard stopgap manner of cancer management which more often fails than succeeds. It often ends in medical malpractice suits simply because there is no rapport established between the physician and the patient or family. And, as a result, that which is implied or presumed to be understood by the patient is more often misunderstood. The patient may assume from the phrase *'you have been given the available or preferred treatment'* that imminent cure or at least a high rate of therapeutic success can be expected. The patient's anticipation of immediate improvement results in unrealistic expectations but not through any fault of their own. This false assumption actually results from the physician's failure to communicate information to the reader before beginning the therapeutic program.

The same dissatisfaction with the therapeutic result also occurs because of misinformation about the side effects of the therapy. The patient and family are left with either hearsay information; anecdotal experiences of friends and acquaintances; or partially true facts from the mass media. Again, the fault lies with the physician in failing to convey the appropriate information before starting the treatment program. However, it is the author's impression this does not come about because of the physician's deliberate attempt to deceive. Instead, it is simply a reflection of his personality and character structure. In all fairness, nevertheless, part of the fault does reside with the patient. It is much too easy for your physician to assume the patient has no questions because none are asked. By the same token, it is easy for the reader to assume there are no problems or side effects from the treatment because no information is offered. It is human nature to choose the path of least resistance and both the physician and the patient are human. Each of these situations of mutual mutism is correctable and avoidable. The only question remaining is with whom does the responsibility lie for avoiding and correcting this mutism? Tradition and logic dictates it is the physician's duty to undertake the task of informing and educating the patient.

Frequently, the patient is so emotionally involved in dealing with the psychologically devastating burden of their cancer that their rational thinking is impaired. When coupled with the general public's poor understanding and misconceptions about cancer even the most educated and cool headed reader cannot be expected to automatically ask the appropriate questions. Any physician with even the smallest amount of experience is aware of this impairment. It is his duty to guide the subject into the correct path of questioning. Your physician must be certain that you obtain the necessary information required to make an informed decision about treatment choices.

The second practice style of telling nothing, even when questions are asked, is indefensible. While it is true many physicians are extremely busy and distracted by the flood of trivia now imparted by government regulations and overbearing bureaucrats they *must* find the time to discuss the diagnosis, prognosis and therapy plan with the patient. The simple expedient of stating, *"I am the physician and I decide what is best for you,"* is simply not appropriate or acceptable in this day and age. The concept of omniscience and omnipotence previously claimed by the 'old school' of physicians is not justifiable today.

The third philosophical style is to tell all which is within reason and practically significant to the cancer patient. As you can see, even the *'tell-all-concept'* has to be quantified and qualified. These modifiers are necessary simply because of the overreaction to the concept which has been fostered by the public press and the government. If the reader examines any popular public text or technical text on the *possible* side effects of medications, radiation therapy and surgery they would immediately be overwhelmed beyond comprehension. As a result, all patients would probably refuse all therapy. The ubiquitous threat of medical malpractice suits is one of the reasons for this overreaction. In reporting clinical studies and investigations on drugs and treatments the manufacturers are required to state ***all*** side effects reported by the test subjects no matter how rare or harmless they may be. When one considers the known fact that some deaths are reported each year with even simple, common remedies such as aspirin, acetaminophen, penicillin, cough syrups, nasal sprays, diet pills and other over-the-counter proprietary remedies the list will obviously become endless.

None of the laymen's texts report the frequency of these side effects or if the side effects are inconsequential or reversible. The mildness and temporary nature of these side effects is the concept referred to previously in this book as the therapeutic/toxic ratio. It is a principle physicians must consider in choosing any therapy for any disease, in any set of circumstances. If adequately trained in their field physicians will have the information necessary to judge the therapeutic/toxic ratio. If the information is not immediately at hand they at least know where to find the information quickly and how to use it before making a judgement.

For these and many more reasons complex, contemporary rational medical care requires more than the possession of a textbook and the ability to read it. The insight and judgement required to make these judgements can only come from the experience and exposure of an adequately trained individual in the basics of clinical medicine. In other words your physician must decide if the treatment is worse than the disease itself. Even then, he must discuss the decision with the patient and offer you all the other legitimate and reasonable options available.

If necessary your physician must find the time to have several discussion sessions with you and a responsible spokesman about the diagnosis, prognosis and treatment and give them time to reach a decision unless a dire emergency exists. Explanations and definitions must be put forth in clear, simple, intelligible language in which all technical terms and jargon are avoided. For example, the physician must tell the patient that the chemotherapy may cause the white blood cell count to be suppressed which could result in serious life threatening infection. They should not state, *"the drugs may produce severe leukopenia and granulocytopenia through bone marrow suppression and result in fatal septicemia, meningitis, pneumonitis, etc."* Such is the language one uses to impress and befuddle an adversary not to counsel a patient.

Usually more than one counseling session is required to convey all the data and its explanatory notes to the reader unless you are a physician or a nurse. However, it cannot be assumed that even a physician or other trained medical persons can easily grasp the concepts put forth. As human beings even they are as effected by the emotional upheaval of the diagnosis of cancer as anyone else, and are often as befuddled and confused as any lay person.

Most cancer patients are so overwhelmed by the simple fact they have the dreaded disease in the first place that they cannot absorb all the necessary information heaped on them in the first patient-physician contact. The same can be said for the family members because they are as emotionally labile as the patient. It is best in the initial meetings to discuss—in broad terms only—the meaning of the diagnosis, the staging and the treatment. Then later, after sufficient time has passed and rapport is established, more details can be added. The patient and family must be given all the reliable and useful printed literature available in reference to their cancer. They are instructed to read them over carefully and underline or mark any areas or terms which are not clear and to ask questions which will help to clarify the facts.

It is good practice for the physician to introduce the words cancer, chemotherapy, radiation therapy, side effects, staging and chances for cure versus remission, as early as possible into the discussion. It is also useful to define what is meant by an 'oncologist,' and what purposes they serve and objectives they seek in reference to the patient's case. This initial discussion session helps to eliminate barriers, relieve apprehension and establish an effective, communicative relationship. This initial discussion often takes place before the physician carries out the comprehensive history and physical examination so that pertinent questions can be answered more clearly by a patient who is more at ease.

The counseling process is different only when the precise diagnosis of cancer has not yet been clearly established. In this case the testing procedures planned in making the diagnosis are explained; why they are chosen over others; and why they are chosen in the sequence planned. The reader is informed that a cancer is *suspected* in their situation but it is far from confirmed.

Establishing the diagnosis and completing the staging process ordinarily allows enough time for your doctor to better introduce the reader to the particular background information regarding the diagnosis, stage, prognosis and cancer therapy plan. By the time this plateau is reached the patient and family should have developed some confidence in the physician's competence and you will have observed his style of practice. If you do not have confidence in your physician by this time the reader should seek another physician or another opinion—if that option has not already come up.

In the final analysis, it is you, the patient, who must be comfortable with and have confidence in your physician regardless of the way anyone—be it family or friend—else involved with the patient may feel about his abilities. It is improper and futile for a friend, spouse or other relatives to force the patient into accepting any physician, institution or management plan if they are not comfortable with the choice.

Chapter 18

The Patient's Right 'To know' or 'To not know'

Certainly it is quite clear and obvious to the reader at this point that this writer's personal choice is to divulge all necessary information—and even unnecessary information, if requested—about a subject's cancer. At the same time, however, the physician must respect any person's right to choose *'not to know all about their cancer.'* Because this statement appears contradictory on the surface, it needs some elaboration.

Let's analyze what is the purpose of, and who is served by this principle of total disclosure? I believe it is safe to assume that everyone has the same worthy motives in advocating such a philosophy. When professional care-givers are serving the needs of a patient, who may soon lose his life to cancer, the following is a list of my primary reasons for advocating such a policy of total disclosure.

First, knowing what lies ahead and what the future holds is a dream which mankind has dreamed for centuries. In other words, what is the prognosis for recovery from cancer or any illness? The purposes for wanting this information varies from individual to individual. But, presuming the noblest of purposes, each person must be allowed to choose their own reasons. These reasons might include; preparing the soul for death and in achieving readiness to meet your God; to prepare family and loved ones for the person's departure, both spiritually and financially; endeavoring to enjoy life and treat themselves to all the earthly pleasures possible before death; to see and to do things they have always wanted to do but could not before their demise; and on, and on. If these are the individual's desires, and it can only occur after full disclosure, so be it.

My second reason is the fundamental, undeniable right of every living human being. That is, the right to choose the type of treatment they feel most suitable to their needs and desires. Included in these options, of course, is the right to receive *no treatment* at all but instead to allow nature to take its own course. Even to the extent, although I deplore it, of your choosing *unfounded* and *unproven 'quack'* treatment.

As you can easily see the two groups of reasons given ultimately serve the end which makes the individual reader feel most comfortable physically, emotionally, and spiritually.

The following reasons, which are certainly the least important, are those which make the rest of us—the care givers—feel comfortable. This includes those of us who are the reader's physicians, nurses, therapists, moralists, social workers, the lawmakers, politicians and protectors of the subject's rights; the relatives, friends and other loved ones who are left behind to endure the grief; the medical and other professional associations assigned to monitor our behavior; the intellectuals; the priests, ministers, rabbis and other spiritual leaders; and the contemporary thinkers who feel that the fashionable principles of man's behavior must prevail. All are great and noble ideals, of course. However, in the end they are not really intended for the patient's comfort but for our own. Therefore, they must take a secondary place when compared to the patient's comfort. It is doubtful that many people would take exception to this statement.

Now, to examine the first premise—the comfort of the afflicted individual. One of human nature's most prevalent mechanisms for avoiding discomfort is psychological denial of the unpleasant facts. Of course, everyone including the counselors, the psychoanalysts, the psychologist and the psychiatrists know these mechanisms are unrealistic, unsophisticated and immature. True enough in most circumstances, but is it applicable in the face of what might be inevitable death, if that is the individual patient's final outcome?

After my many years of first hand experience it is obvious to me that it is unwise and unreasonable to expect myself to be able to force another human being to face that which he chooses not to face. Many patients have been driven to mental breakdowns and psychotic behavior because someone insisted the patient *'must'* face up to the fact of imminent and impending death.

The better approach is to discuss the possibility of shortened survival and failure of therapy with the patient on at least three separate, carefully conducted private sessions. This number of meetings should allow enough time, for those who need more time, to absorb and digest the information which has been placed before them. If the reader still appears not to understand, assuming they are mentally competent, it is often because they have chosen the defense mechanism of denial. It is seldom possible to force someone to accept their fate once they have utilized the denial mechanism. Approximately fifty percent of people choose the denial mechanism. Certainly, unless someone has faced the situation of having cancer, we cannot imagine how these people must feel. Therefore, it is not the place of the care-givers to condemn or criticize the patient for using this mechanism.

One can even see, after careful examination, that this mechanism may be a good thing if our real aim is to promote the comfort of the patient when we can offer no other assistance. Perhaps this is the very reason the powers that be have allowed such a mechanism to exist. Who are we to chastise and judge? Especially if we have never faced certain death long before it actually occurred.

Thus, one can defend the patient's right—*'to not know'*—as long as reasonable and gentle attempts have been made to advise them of their life threatening situation.

It is the physician's obligation to take the initiative in offering the basic information about their cancer to the reader. They must not assume the individual reader has chosen the denial defense mechanism because no questions are asked by him or their family. The physicians must try to put themselves in the patient's place and imagine facing the devastation of the diagnosis of cancer. They must try to realize that the impact of the diagnosis might stun the readers and prevent them from asking the appropriate questions.

It is our duty to pursue the proper areas carefully and give the patient time to fathom the seriousness of the situation. Care-givers must cautiously and charitably lead them into the proper territory of questioning. If three sincere attempts do not appear adequate the physicians must modify their approach to suit the circumstances and the patient's personality. Once it appears the individual reader cannot abandon the denial defense mechanism the physician must make certain that a responsible family member is apprised of the situation.

Chapter 19

Physician Attitude

There can be no doubt the attitude and posture of the physician can effect the outcome of the therapeutic plan just as it can be effected by the patient's attitude.

The doctor's general demeanor and style should impart a definitive sense of control and understanding so he can transfer the same attitude to the patient. The physician must exude confidence and competence which is the only way the reader can acquire them.

The physicians' attitude toward their profession, their specialty and themselves are equally important. Nothing is more disconcerting to a patient than a physician who is cavalier and careless about his style of approaching the cancer victim.

In presenting information about the organized plan for approaching the diagnosis and staging of the disease the physician must be assertive, and yet, it must not sound like a sales pitch for a used car. An honest, candid attitude toward the prognosis outlined is very influential in having the reader consider the future with hope. But the doctor must not portray unrealistic expectations and unattainable goals. If the treatment can only offer some prolongation of life it must be stated as such. And yet, the patient must be assured that every effort will be made to preserve a good quality of life along with the survival time offered. A promise of cure, in the true sense of the word, should never be uttered or even implied if it cannot be delivered. The physician might even have to go so far as to state the treatment is not a 'cure' since so many times the lay person equates, incorrectly, the terms 'treatment' or *'therapy'* with *'cure.'*

If true *'cure'* is possible or within reach, the doctor must define the word 'cure' and state, to the best of his honest, culpable knowledge what the average chances for achieving it are. And yet, the doctor must not exaggerate the statistics or his enthusiasm for the statistics.

When cure is not possible it must be stated in a way which does not portray hopelessness or doom. If significant *remission* is attainable it must be defined within the confines of reality and in thc simplest, most understandable language possible without appearing to talk down to the reader. The meaning of *'five year survival,'* or whatever term applies, must be described and explained in detail so there can be no misunderstanding what a remission can provide, as well as, what it cannot provide.

When the physician can only offer *'comfort therapy'* it must not be presented as a last resort, even if that is all it can be. It must be offered with reassurance, and compassionately, and with sincere interest in the quality of time the patient might experience.

In outlining the side effects and dangers of the therapy plan the physician must not hide any of the major risks involved. And yet, the doctor cannot instill an exaggerated dread of the risks in the patient's mind. The reader must be reassured that the risks are worth the possible benefits if that is the fact. The definition of the toxic/therapeutic risk must be discussed with clarity and simplicity. When the physician has no confidence in the chosen therapy plan the patient senses it and transfers the no-confidence perception to himself. Even a therapeutic plan with a high success rate is doomed to failure when the confidence of the patient has been eroded.

Even when a positive attitude has been accomplished in the early days of the physician-patient relationship it must be reinforced periodically during the course of the management program. If any changes are made in the therapy plan the patient must be informed beforehand and the reasons for the change in the plan must be explained. The patient must be reexamined frequently to reassure them the physician is monitoring the situation and watching for improvement or worsening of the disease process. This 'laying on of hands,' or 'touching' is very important for instilling confidence and a sense of concern.

The ultimate aim of the physician and the management team must be the physical, emotional and spiritual well-being of the patient.

Part Six

The Gathering and Interpretation of Cancer Information

Introduction

The Gathering and Interpretation of Cancer Information

As stated at the outset, one of the major purposes of this book is to improve the understanding and knowledge of the reader regarding the diagnosis, treatment, and prevention of cancer. The need for such an endeavor was brought home to me not only by a glaring lack of information but also by the superabundance of misleading and distorted information which abounds. For these reasons the sources of information utilized by the reader must be scrutinized very carefully. Given the choice, I would prefer to start with an uninformed reader rather than with one who has been adulterated by the surplus of misinformation now available. My preference is especially applicable to the cancer patient because they are so vulnerable and desperate for easy answers and quick cures. This extreme vulnerability and sense of desperation is incurred by the social stigma of having cancer caused by the widespread false impressions of this group of diseases and the publicity it receives.

The patient, with the help of the physician and his management team, must seek out only authoritative sources of information for the particular facts about their cancer. The key word here is— *"Authoritative."* The readers are advised first to use common, ordinary, everyday horse sense. If a problem exists with the plumbing in your house you don't call the electrician. And more importantly, don't ask a neighbor or relative, unless of course they happen to be a plumber, electrician, or a physician. There is no doubt the advice of friends and relatives is offered out of sincere concern and love for the patient. But if several unauthoritative sources of information are mixed with the facts gleaned from the authoritative sources the end-result is simply a confused patient who is already being torn in several directions at one time. The confusion of mixed messages only complicates matters and the result can be an unnecessary delay in starting the treatment program.

The most authoritative source of medical information is your local physician whether he is a primary care person or a specialist in oncology. Your doctor can also provide the reader with multiple secondary sources of reading material and cancer support groups. These printed materials are readily available through the local chapter of the American Cancer Society and its main branch in Washington, D.C. The National Cancer Institute and the National Institutes of Health, both branches of the U.S. Department of Health and Human Services, offer a wide variety of printed matter on the treatment, diagnosis and detection of all types of cancer. Often this same printed material is available at your local pharmacy, hospital, nurses association and medical association offices.

There are also regular periodic cancer seminars and support group's lectures available in many communities. These are usually publicized in the local newspaper, on radio and television. In general these are reliable sources of information.

However, the reader must be alerted to the wide variety of misleading information published in a free-speech society such as ours. Many of these sources are the product of misguided reactionaries but some are more bent on luring the public into their financial trap. Beware the individual or group which claims to have the *'secret cure'* or *'magic remedy'* which no one else possesses.

Chapter 20

The Public Press and the Mass Media

The mass media and public lay-press do a fairly good job of disseminating useful information regarding cancer and other diseases. However, it could and should do much better. There is, unfortunately, a tendency toward overdramatizing and sensationalism in cancer news reporting. The reasons for this tendency is not for me to judge or discuss here. But the sensationalization of the facts only leads to false impressions and improper reactions by the public.

Much of the sensationalism apparently results from the phraseology used by the mass media. The overuse of words and phrases such as; 'major break through,' 'new hope for cure,' 'a new cure discovered,' and the like, are usually exaggerations of the facts or are partial truths. If the reader examines the scientific publications which are quoted or summarized by the news reports he does not find these terms used by the authors of the scientific articles.

The reasons for avoiding these sensational phrases are many and are dependent often on the character and personality of the researcher investigators. Certainly, it is not because they do not hope their work and reporting will lead to a true improvement in cure rates. Also, it is not for the purpose of hiding the facts. The primary reason for avoiding these terms is they know that the uncovering of one scientific fact is only a single building block, if it is found to be valid, in the foundation of constructing a huge pyramid of facts leading to a complicated solution. They are aware, as are most researchers and practicing physicians, that it requires many years and the work of hundreds or even thousands of other researchers to lead to a solution for any complex scientific problem. History and experience have taught there is seldom, if ever, a single event or revelation which has resulted in a new scientific advance by itself. Even if a single new fact is startling and momentous scientists know the work must be duplicated several times by many other independent researchers before the new fact can be accepted as valid. And even if it is found to be valid it has to be tested and applied to the treatment of human disease before it can be considered useful and meaningful. Research workers realize that such is nature and the way of human biological research.

It is the lack of this wisdom and knowledge which has lead to so many false prophets into the error of proclaiming they possess *'the secret cure'* or other so called *'unproven remedies'* and *'quack cures'* for cancer and so many other diseases.

Sadly, it is this kind of sensationalism which sells newspaper, magazines, and high television viewing ratings. Therefore, the temptation to report in this manner is very strong and almost irresistible. I doubt the sensationalism is a result of deliberate planning on anyone's part. However, regardless of the intention and motives of the reporter the result is the same. It causes much undesirable, damaging confusion, and nurtures misconceptions and unrealistic hope for a group of desperate, frustrated cancer patients and their families.

Some of the other drawbacks of using the public press for medical information includes the lack of depth in reporting and the absence of clear, complete interpretation of scientific data. The absence of depth in many popular publications results in a brief, superficial report of an apparent new advance with only sketchy details. There is very little to be gained from this kind of reporting other than boosting newspaper sales and television ratings.

The concept of medical reporting should provide a more comprehensive amount of information regarding such medical advancements so the public can properly apply the knowledge to their own problem. Ambiguous promises of 'things to come' simply result in unrealistic expectations. The physician can help in this area by filling in the details for the individual patient. Therefore, the reader should feel free to raise any questions about so called 'new advances' reported in the mass media. Better yet, they can bring in the newspaper clipping itself to physician so that he can explain the significance of the report before the person makes any judgements about its validity or applicability. The public must be made aware that so called 'new discoveries' are often not really new, or that so called 'promising advances' are merely a first step in the very long journey leading to meaningful scientific developments and truly new treatments.

The second drawback of the medical reporting system in the public press is the of lack of expert interpretation of the reported information. It is a common error for reporters to assume that the reader knows the meaning inferred by the phrasing of a report. As I have stated earlier, there are so many misconceptions of what cancer actually is and is not, let alone a clear understanding of new advances. Although it is the primary responsibility of the medical profession and its associations to educate the public, the public press and mass media has not been as helpful as it could be in meeting this responsibility.

Medical encyclopedias and medical advice books have also failed in this public education effort. Again, too much is taken for granted by the publication as evidenced by the use of highly technical terms and medical jargon without any clear definition of these terms.

The books and pamphlets provided by the American Cancer Society and the National Cancer Institute have taken the most practical and simplified approach. Each pamphlet is limited to discussing each of the more common forms of cancer on an individual basis so the patient is not overwhelmed by a mass of data presented but is limited to data which applies to their cancer. The various kinds of therapy programs available are also presented in the pamphlets in a simplified manner and is limited to one kind of therapy in each pamphlet. The reader is given only the literature which applies to their cancer, unless of course they request others. The physician must encourage the patient and family to read over the appropriate literature. Then they can bring it back on the next visit to their physician to discuss any portions which are not clearly understood.

The publications provided by these two organizations need improvement in only one respect—more widespread distribution and greater awareness through increased publicity. It is my hope that these defects will be remedied through a more concerted effort. It is also my hope that this book will help to increase and stimulate a greater level of public awareness, at least in small measure.

Chapter 21

The False Prophets

The reader might ask, if the mass media and public press is not an authoritative source of cancer information where can one turn for guidance and hope? Unfortunately, for many the answer to this question is gladly provided by the numerous disciples of the *'false prophets.'* The number of followers of these groups has increased because of the general loss of faith and trust of the public in the physician, the medical profession, and the system of traditional medical research. The exaggerated reports of some dishonest health dealers and unethical physicians has lead to the distrust of the public for all of the health professionals. I believe it is the duty of these professionals, as individuals and as groups, to help restore the faith of the public. Unfortunately, too many physicians and their professional associations have failed to fulfill their duty by not exerting enough effort in public education.

Much more effort is needed by health care professionals to demonstrate and explain to the public that the traditional and time tested scientific methods of research are not to be abandoned because of the desperation, frustration and slowness of medical advances. It should be pointed out to the readers that it is unreasonable to abandon the system which has lead to the discovery and development of so many outstanding medical advances, such as; penicillin, cortisone, vaccines and other forms of immunization, anti-tuberculous drugs, anti-hypertensive drugs, diagnostic and therapeutic x-ray, curative surgical procedures, organ transplant, cosmetic surgery, artificial organs and limbs, effective screening tests, and so on. It is the traditional system which has lead to the almost complete worldwide eradication of small pox, poliomyelitis, typhoid fever, whooping cough, rheumatic fever. This same system also has resulted in significant reduction of other killers such as syphilis, gonorrhea, meningitis, malaria, pneumonia, and many others too numerous to list here.

The disciples of the 'false prophets' defend their support for unproven remedies in a variety of ways.

An example typical defensive statement: "But this article was written by or the claim was made by a doctor who is an M. D." However, with today's high degree of specialization and in view of the massive volumes of information available there can be no M. D.'s who are omniscient or infallible simply because they possess a degree in medicine. Such a statement is not meant to degrade the generalists, such as family physicians, general surgeons, internists, specialists or subspecialists. It is merely meant to point out that with the very specialized knowledge and training required to perform medical research and reporting the results of that research requires more than a medical degree.

As an obvious and exaggerated example, because a physician has a medical degree and a license does not mean they are capable of performing open heart surgery, neurosurgery or are able to administer radiotherapy or chemotherapy. The specialty training programs provide us with the certified and experienced physicians in these specialty ar eas. The hospitals also help to screen their staffs to be certain all physicians are adequately trained and experienced in these special areas. Unfortunately, the hospital's limitations are that they cannot control the quality of care delivered in a doctor's office or anywhere else outside the hospital. This is not to imply the hospitals should have control outside of the institution but some quality control mechanism is needed.

For a second example: "But this treatment was discovered by a famous and world renown researcher." The same principle applies to this statement as it did to the preceding one. There are areas of specialization in research as there are in medical practice. An award winning researcher in the area of, let's say, virus research is not necessarily capable of research in organ transplant or clinical cancer research. The degree of his fame and notoriety also does not have any influence on his ability to perform research in all divisions of the field. There are even subdivisions within the already narrowing areas of cancer research. For instance, one scientist might be expert in the screening and development of cancer chemotherapy drugs but he may have no training or experience in actually prescribing these drugs to human patients. The clinical research—the actually treatment of patients—is usually left to the clinical oncology researcher who applies the new agents in an actual clinical situation.

In summary, expertise and excellence in one area of medical practice or research does not necessarily indicate ability in all or even the majority of these areas. When judging the validity of any report the reader needs more information about the reporter than his degrees or the number of awards previously received. Again, the patient's physicians can provide some guidance because of their training in this area. If your physician cannot personally provide guidance and information he can at least get the information from a colleague or from an authoritative reference source.

Another commonly used defense for 'unfounded remedies' is the anecdotal report. "My sister-in-law had this special treatment and now she is living and well." Prior to the days of refined and controlled research systems physicians and scientists made the same mistakes by reacting to single case reports or an individual experience. The sad result was the propagation of many worthless remedies, sometimes with damaging results. The recognition of this erroneous approach lead to development of the contemporary research tool called *'controlled research study.'* This phrase does not imply *political or government* control of the research. It means that the variables in the research are 'controlled' to reduce error as much as possible. A controlled study means that patients with the same type of cancer; in the same age group; of the same race; with the same general health status; of the same sex; with the same treatment are selected for the research project. The size of the group of patients studied in the research is also controlled so that adequate numbers of patients are studied to avoid errors caused by the study of small numbers of cancer cases.

Thus, unless an individual happens to have two hundred sisters-in-law who can be matched in all these parameters and then divide them in half and treat each group differently, the anecdotal report has no validity regardless of who the reporter may be. The same requirements for controlled standards in study trials applies even to highly qualified and credentialed physicians, scientists, and researchers.

Testimonials provided by famous and well known persons is another way in which false claims are supported. The principle of personal testimonials and endorsement may work in advertising and marketing breakfast foods and soft drinks but it has no place in promoting medical remedies. As much as we may adore our professional athletes, movie stars and TV stars, their ability in their respective fields of endeavor in no way lends credibility to their judgement of medical remedies. Just as a physician's training in medicine does not make him an expert in football or book reviews, the reverse is also true.

Chapter 22

Interpretation of Information

I believe that just simply supplying the public with pertinent health information is also not enough. Some explanation and interpretation is necessary because medical information is difficult and complex. Also because the patient's ability to rationally interpret and decipher the facts is impaired by the emotional upheaval caused by their illness. The physician should not assume anything. Even the simplest concept may not be clear in the subjects mind no matter how sophisticated and educated the reader might be.

All applied words and phrases must be defined and explained by the physician from the very beginning when contact is first made with the patient. Arrangements should be made to have a second responsible party present to help record and store the information since there is so much to be handled in the beginning. The purpose of the second individual—and perhaps even a third person—is to avoid overwhelming the patient with reams of data at the outset.

The physicians must explain the character and extent of the patient's illness; the nature and the type of treatment planned along with the character and severity of its side effects; the expectations of what the treatment program is intended to accomplish and what it might not accomplish. They must discuss the support systems available to help with emotional, spiritual, nutritional, financial, nursing and all other forms of aid needed to make your treatment program as comfortable and as effective as possible.

These areas of discussion may have to be handled in small doses over several contact sessions with the patient. The information may have to be repeated several times over for the sake of achieving clarity. But it must all be done, eventually.

The readers and their spokesmen should be encouraged to ask questions, express doubts, concerns and fears; admit to any questionable or unclear ideas and clarify them; and reveal any needs or desires they have. When these questions are not forthcoming the physicians must not assume that the patient's silence is synonymous with understanding or acceptance. Some gentle prompting and coaxing may be required.

When your physician is reasonably convinced that the patient is clealyr and completely informed in regards to your cancer then, and only then, the process of cancer management can begin in earnest.

Part Seven

Synopses of Cancers

Introduction

Synopses of Cancers by Location and Type

By way of introduction to this portion of this book allow me to explain the arrangement of the facts and what each is intended to accomplish. Also, again it is important to understand that these details are not needed by the reader to make rational decisions. But the information is yours to utilize if you are so inclined. As a matter of fact, you are encouraged to keep the decision making process as simple and clear as possible. Therefore, you can retain and use whatever information you desire and discard the rest.

It should also be pointed out that the information which follows is not a magic or infallible formula for success. No such formula exists. The following information is a compilation of facts and concepts gleaned from many years of personal, practical experience in dealing with cancer patients. It is, nevertheless, a matter of personal opinion and choice. It is not the *only* way.

Each **type of cancer** is listed and named according to the more common names used in the lay press. Each is also listed by the more common and accepted method according to the organ or organ system in which the primary cancer arises. The listings are not arranged alphabetically but, instead, are arranged by their frequency of occurrence with the most common cancers given first and progressing to the least common. Any useful and simple synonyms are given but complex scientific designations are not given to avoid unnecessary clutter and confusion.

The **incidence or occurrence rate** of each cancer is listed according to the most current and reliable statistical sources. The average fatality rates for each cancer type are given. Wherever sex and racial differences exist they are pointed out and expanded upon where appropriate.

The **causes or risk factors,** when they are known appear under each type of cancer. If the causative agent(s) is only suspected it is designated as such.

The most common **signs and symptoms** encountered by the patients are given in as simple terms as possible with the understanding that they are not the only possible clues, and they are not exclusive or specific. A reader could still have one of the specific cancers discussed even without having any signs or symptoms. In fact, the individual may not feel ill at all.

The best **screening procedures** which are most commonly and widely recommended are listed and discussed briefly.

The means of establishing the **diagnosis** of each cancer type is listed and discussed briefly. The various ways the diagnosis may be obtained are listed in systematic order beginning with the simplest and safest methods. The listing of the various diagnostic methods starts with the easiest and progresses to the most difficult methods.

The **staging** procedures and tests considered most useful and most accurate for determining the extent of the disease are listed and discussed briefly.

The **prognosis** of each general, broad type of cancer is given in terms of the overall results for all subtypes and stages listed under the general heading of the specific cancer type. Some subtypes are listed and discussed in more detail when the difference in prognosis is significant and meaningful. The prognosis for each type of cancer is given in terms of cure rate, remission rate and duration of survival when applicable. However, it must be understood that the figures given are only averages, medians or means and are not absolute numbers. Some patients do better than the averages, some do worse. And a small number of people defy the figures all together. It must be accepted that these exceptions are one of the many quirks of the natural sciences, and completely unexplainable.

The kinds and locations of cancer spread—the **metastases**—that are most likely to occur and which most often alter prognosis or survival rates are given.

The **types of therapy** recommended for each cancer group will be listed in accordance with this author's judgement of the most useful and most reasonable choices—in most cases. Therapy choices by subtypes and stages are discussed only when appropriate. Again, these are not magic formulas for guaranteed success. Because of the rapid advances being made in the field of cancer research they may even be outdated by the time this book is read. You should discuss these treatment choices with your physician as to their current accuracy and general acceptance. And, it must be kept in mind that the choice of therapy is 'custom tailored,' if you will, for each case depending on the clinical circumstances.

The more common and most troublesome **side effects** of each type of treatment are listed and discussed in limited detail. But because of biological variability it is not possible to list all the conceivable adverse effects. These adverse effects are discussed in the broadest sense because the number of combinations and variations of the treatment programs are as numerous as the possible combinations of side effects. It must be stressed that a patient does not necessarily have to experience any of the listed side effects in order to have a therapeutic effect. Wherever possible, an approximate percentage of the risk of experiencing the side effects is given. Also, the risk of fatal side effects and their types are given.

The recommended composition of the **management team** is presented along with a designated coordinator of the team. Here again, it is often a matter of individual physician opinion and varies with the geographic locale and the availability of certain physician specialists. There is no 'super team,' as it were, which produces a guaranteed successful program for any type of cancer in every instance. The team recommended in each case is that which, in the judgement of the author, is most likely to produce the best results.

Synopses of Cancers

Most of the statistics quoted are compiled from data published by the American Cancer Society or the National Cancer Institute.

Chapter 23

Lung Cancer

Lung Cancer: Lung caner is in reality a group of cancers, and is defined as, and limited to, cancers which have started in the lung, and does not include those which have spread to the lungs. It also does not include cancers which begin in those structures or organs within the chest cavity but are not basically respiratory organs. Excluded are organs such as the esophagus, heart, lymph nodes, thyroid, fat, muscle, bone, etc. And, as we have already learned, the organ of origin of any cancer is of primary importance in outlining treatment and estimating prognosis. Primary lung cancer is the cause of the greatest number of deaths due to cancer in all races, sexes and socioeconomic groups. Alarmingly, the death rate from this cancer has been steadily increasing for several decades. The increasing death rate parallels the increasing number of cigarette smokers in the United States.

Synonyms: Some of the more common names used to designate this group include carcinoma of the lung, cancer of the lung, bronchogenic carcinoma, lung tumor, pulmonary cancer, etc.

Two large subtypes of lung cancer are worthy of mention because of the vast difference in survival and treatability between the two. The two distinct types of lung cancer are called small cell lung cancer (SCLC) and large cell lung cancer (also called non-small cell lung cancer-NSCLC). The first type (SCLC) has a higher degree of treatability and remission as compared to the second which has a very poor response rate to any form of therapy.

Incidence: According to statistical estimates for 1995 lung cancer will account for 18% of all cancers in men and 12% of all cancers in women. It will cause 34% of cancer deaths in men and 22% of all cancer deaths in women. The most disconcerting figures are those which indicate the occurence rate of lung cancer in woman is fast catching up to the incidence rates in men. The increase is apparently related to the increasing number of women who smoke cigarettes. There will be 168,000 lung cancer cases and 146,000 lung cancer deaths in 1995.

Causes and Risk Factors: Smoking tobacco is unquestionably the number one cause of lung cancer. The risk increases with the number of cigarettes smoked per day. The generally used number is 40 pack-years. The number is derived by multiplying the number of years of cigarette smoking by the number of packs smoked per day. For example, two packs per day for twenty years equals 40 pack-years. The same general risk is also associated with smoking pipes and cigars if the smoke is inhaled. There also may be a relationship to the brand of cigarette smoked and whether it is filtered or non-filtered but this point is less clear. Quitting smoking does reduce the risk of lung cancer in previous long time smokers. However, at least six years must transpire before there is an appreciable decline in the cancer risk in those who quit. More recently, so called 'passive smoking' has been implicated in causing cancer and other diseases. I believe that the passive smoking issue is not settled as of this writing.

Asbestos exposure is associated with an increase in lung cancer especially if the subject is also a tobacco smoker.

Other environmental factors which have been implicated in the causation of lung cancer have included: atmospheric pollution; radioactive ore (uranium) in miners; high industrial exposure to metals such as nickel, chromium, silver, cadmium, beryllium, cobalt, selenium, and steel.

Chemical products such as chloromethyl ethers have also been implicated.

The readers should make no mistake about it, however, tobacco smoking is by far the number one cause of the vast majority of lung cancers.

Signs and Symptoms: Unfortunately these signs and symptoms are all nonspecific and are extremely common of many other noncancerous diseases and they often appear too late in lung cancer.

The most common symptoms can be grouped under the heading 'a change in the quality of or the appearance of new respiratory symptoms.' Such changes in symptoms include increasing cough, chest pain, increase in sputum production, rust colored or bloody sputum, and increasing shortness of breath. There are many symptoms and signs in lung cancer which can occur away from the chest cavity but they are too numerous and diverse to be of use to the laymen although they are valuable to the physician. The best advice I can give to tobacco smokers and those exposed to agents in their occupation is to seek medical attention when symptoms occur, have regular periodic examinations, and do not smoke.

Screening: Unfortunately, methods of screening high risk groups for lung cancer have not been found reliable or practical. Regular and periodic chest x-rays, and examinations of the sputum for cancer cells (cytology) have limited utility. As previously pointed out I believe a comprehensive history (inquiry of symptoms) and a meticulous physical examination are indispensable for screening and probably gives the highest yield of useful clues.

Diagnosis: As always, obtaining a sample of tissue is the only reliable way of establishing an accurate diagnosis of lung cancer. The actual sample may be obtained in variety of ways. These include, bronchoscopy; examination of sputum obtained either from spontaneous or induced coughing or through the bronchoscope; a needle biopsy obtained via a needle inserted through the chest wall; a tissue specimen obtained via minor chest surgery for biopsy or, major surgery by removal of a portion (lobe) of the lung or removal of a single suspicious nodule; removal of abnormal collections of (pleural) fluids in the lung; removal and biopsy of lymph nodes in the neck; and mediastinoscopy (biopsy obtained through a tube inserted in the space between the lungs).

Staging: Staging is defined as the procedure used to determine the extent of the spread of the disease within and beyond the chest cavity, if any. Chest x-rays and CAT scans of the chest are done to determine if the tumor has extended locally into surrounding organs. Scans of the brain, liver and bones are also performed. Bone marrow biopsy, especially in cases of small cell lung cancer, are mandatory. Blood tests such as CEA, complete blood count, blood tests which evaluate the function of the liver, kidneys and other distant organs are included.

Prognosis: The best that can be hoped for in lung cancer is an increase in the five year survival rates. True and lasting cures are extremely uncommon. A ten to twelve percent 5 year survival rate is the average outcome which can be achieved with any and all forms of treatment. These are rather dismal statistics for so common a form of cancer especially since it could all be avoided by abstinence from the tobacco habit in the first place.

Approximately 85% percent of cases which cannot be treated with surgery have a short remission with a combination of chemotherapy and radiation therapy but practically no cures result. The average length of survival for the vast majority of lung cancer cases is approximately 12 months with any and all treatments.

Sites of Recurrences and Localities of Spread: It is possible for this cancer to recur almost anywhere in the body but the more common sites are, the same lung as the original tumor; the opposite lung; the bones; the brain; the liver; and the lymph nodes in the chest cavity and the neck area.

Treatments: The choice of therapeutic modalities or combinations, thereof, chosen are dependent of the cell type of the lung cancer, the extent or stage of the disease. The other factors which influence the choices of treatment include; age, status of general health, and the presence of specific life threatening and discomfort producing symptoms. The various combinations and permutations of treatment modalities available to the physician are constantly changing as research and understanding of the disease progresses.

Surgical Therapy: The use of surgery as the primary treatment is only indicated for very small and localized lung cancers. I believe the presence of distant spread is a contra-indication for the use of surgery except to relieve discomfort or establish diagnosis. Only a small number of patients, approximately 10%, have cancers which are amenable to surgical therapy. And, very often, when the surgeon opens the chest cavity he finds locally extensive disease which mitigates against complete removal of all the lung cancer—this is known as an 'unresectable lung cancer.' At this point the surgeon cannot remove any of the cancer at all or only a small specimen is obtained for biopsy.

The remaining 90% of lung cancer cases require either chemotherapy, radiation therapy or a combination of these if the physician and patient so choose.

Special Comment: The lung cancer cell-type called, *'small cell lung carcinoma'*, has the greatest response rate to these nonsurgical modalities but with only a small number of true cures resulting. The most commonly used drugs are given either alone or in combination, they can include—cyclophosphamide, doxorubicin, methotrexate, procarbazine, 5-fluorouracil, mitomycin-C, Cisplatinum, carboplatin, CCNU, vincristine, etoposide. Each of these drugs are discussed in more detail in a later section of this book. Suffice it, here, to say that the drugs chosen are determined by the medical oncologist involved in your case after discussing the choices with the patient and family.

The side effects of this chemotherapy may include nausea and vomiting, loss of hair from the head (alopecia), fatigue, a decrease in the blood cells counts, diminished immunity to infections, liver damage and heart damage and peripheral nerve damage (neuropathy). The only life threatening side effects involve serious infections, heart and liver damage, and hemorrhage due to lowering of blood cells—called the platelets—which aid in the clotting of the blood. Most of these side effects have an acceptably low incident rate and many are reversible or preventable. Nevertheless, the medical oncologist should discuss all these risks with the patient before embarking on the program.

The side effects of radiation therapy depend on the local structures which are irradiated and also should be discussed before starting treatment.

Management Team: Besides the usual combination of physical therapist, nutritionists, nurses, psychologist the kinds of physicians involved depend on the stage of the cancer and the treatment chosen. If only surgery is required then the thoracic surgeon is the team coordinator along with the primary care physician, if one was involved in your cancer in the beginning. When radiation is the only modality utilized the radiation oncologist coordinates the team effort until the course of radiotherapy is completed then the primary care physician can take over. When chemotherapy is administered the medical oncologist is the team leader, at least until the chemotherapy is completed.

However, in the early phases of the management program all of the above named team members confer on the treatment plan and come to a consensus agreement as to the best therapy program advised for the patient. The paramedical members of the team remain involved for as long as the patient requests their services, which may be indefinitely, or for as long as the patient needs support and rehabilitation.

Chapter 24

Breast Cancer

B**reast cancer** is the most frequent and the most feared malignancy of women. It is most frequent in the prime of a woman's life with most cases occurring in the 55 to 74 year age group. It will cause approximately 46,300 deaths in 1995, it is slowly increasing in frequency, and there is no clear cut known cause and no known method of prevention. There are, however, effective methods of early detection. And although the 5 year survival rate and remission rates have been slowly increasing there is no fail-proof method of cure. Since the female breast is perceived as a sexually important organ the emotional and physical impact of the disease can be devastating to women and their sex partners.

Incidence Rates: Breast cancer is the most common kind of cancer in American females constituting 32% of all cancers in women and it is responsible for 19% of cancer deaths in this group. However, it still ranks second behind lung cancer which is responsible for 22% of the cancer deaths in females. The disease is not limited to females but it is rare in males. Most of the information which follows refers to the disease in both sexes. Overall, it will strike one of every 9 American females sometime in their life times. In any given year their will be 100 new cases of breast cancer for every 100,000 American females. It is more common in the left breast rather than the right breast and is more frequent in the upper outer 1/4 of the breast. Ten percent of all breast cancer patients will have the disease occur in both breasts.

Causes or Risk Factors: Breast cancer has no known single cause. It is five times more common in females with a family history of breast cancer, and it is more common in women who have no children or whose first child is born after the age of 30-35.

Genetic and hormonal factors play some role in some patients. Viral and immunological processes can also be potentially contributing factors.

Low dose radiation exposure has been implicated in atomic bomb survivors, in patients who were treated for mastitis with radiation in the past, and in those exposed to multiple fluoroscopic examinations of the lungs in cases of tuberculosis. The last two causes are now outdated and rarely, if ever, encountered today.

Ingestion of excessive dietary fat has been implicated as a possible major environmental factor in the cause of breast cancer. Although not definitely proven as a cause, a decrease in dietary fat ingestion seems prudent.

Unopposed and uninterrupted estrogen stimulation has also been implicated primarily in adolescent and premenopausal females. However, as of this date, the use of oral contraceptives has not been definitely shown to increase the occurrence of breast cancer.

Signs and Symptoms: Breast cancer is most often discovered by the patient, either accidentally or during intentional self-examination of the breast, or by the physician during routine physical examination. The breast lumps are usually painless and, therefore, the patient's attention is seldom drawn to the mass by discomfort. In a few instances more obvious changes call the persons attention to the breast, they are; dimpling of the skin over the mass, nipple retraction, bleeding from the nipple, reddening of the skin and an 'orange peel' appearance to the skin over the lump, ulceration of the mass, enlargement of lymph nodes in the armpit (axilla).

Screening Methods for Detection of Symptom-Free Breast Cancer: There are essentially only three screening procedures presently available for the detection of early, symptom-free breast cancer. And all three of the procedures are of equal importance and utility. These procedures are: regular, periodic self-examination of the breast; periodic examination by a physician; and periodic mammography of the breasts. The primary observation leading to recommending these screening techniques is based on one premise, that is, that breast cancer detected early has a markedly increased chance of total cure. The cure rate of early breast cancer is in the range of 80 % to 95%. Whereas, when discovered later survival rates drop to 50%.

The first of these screening procedures, self-examination of the breast, cannot be overemphasized nor can it be overdone. The reasons for this statement are obvious. Self-examination is simple and safe, it is inexpensive, it is readily available and only requires a minimal amount of instruction to master the technique. Equally desirable is the fact that the patient can perform the examination on a monthly, weekly or even daily basis, if she so desires. But at least monthly self-examination is the general recommendation.

However, many women shy away from this procedure because they feel they are uneducated, untrained and do not want to "play doctor." But extensive higher education and medical training are not required to perform the examination properly. You are simply asked to 'memorize' the construction and texture of your own breasts and then to examine them regularly for gross changes in that configuration. You are not expected to make a diagnosis or to decide if a lump is serious or important. All that is required is that you watch for changes and when they occur to see your physician who will decide the significance of the changes. Less emphasized is that each patient has only two breast configurations to commit to memory, whereas, the physician can only make a poor attempt at memorizing many. It has been estimated that approximately 98% of all breast cancers diagnosed each year are originally detected by the patient herself by accidental or intentional palpation of the breast.

Periodic examination of the breast by a physician is the second screening technique utilized. At the least a yearly examination by a physician is recommended. And your doctor need not be a specialist in oncology or surgery. As a matter of fact, the general family physician is as capable as anyone to perform the breast examination. Since they are greater in number and more widely accessible in almost all communities the primary care physicians are the first line of defense against all diseases and they should be utilized as such. In some situations your physician may advise more frequent examinations than yearly because of some special circumstances. These special cases include; recent breast cancer in the other breast; a strong family history of breast cancer; a new and suspicious change in the breast indicating more frequent surveillance before deciding if biopsy is indicated; and for the peace of mind of a concerned patient.

The last of these points is not to be minimized or frowned upon since the emotional health of the patient is a part of your physician's responsibility. On the other hand the physician must not use the patient's fear for any ulterior motive, be it financial or otherwise. This is the place where trust and confidence in the physician is applied. If it is unclear to you why there is a need for more frequent examinations you should discuss the points with your physician.

Mammography, or specialized x-ray of the breasts, on a regular and periodic basis is strongly recommended by most experts in the field as a screening procedure for individual cases and on a mass population scale.

In the individual case the physician uses the technique to help him decide if a biopsy is indicated or to see if another cancer is present in the other breast.

In mass screening this examination is most useful for detecting breast cancers which are too small to be felt by the patient or the examining physician. Over 95% of the breast cancers detected in this way are still localized and have not yet spread to the lymph nodes. For each 1000 women screened by mammography approximately 3 breast cancers will be detected. The accuracy of the procedure exceeds 90%. The 10 year survival rate of patients with cancers detected solely by mammography is in the range of 90-95% as compared to an overall 5 year survival of 50-60% for all breast cancers treated each year.

Some other screening methods which are sometimes used but of less value and utility include; thermography, ultra sound, CT scans of the breast, needle aspiration of cysts or solid lumps. These are occasionally of value in support of and in conjunction with other screening methods but are generally not recommended for use alone for mass screening.

Diagnosis: As in the case of all types of cancer a definite diagnosis can only be established with some form of biopsy of any suspicious masses. The biopsy can be accomplished in a variety of ways but it cannot be avoided. This fact is especially significant since the vast majority of masses or lumps which can be felt by examination will be benign.

The most common method of obtaining biopsy material is the excisional biopsy. Excision implies the complete removal of the mass to be sent for processing and examination by a pathologist. In former days it was standard procedure to plan the mastectomy at the same time as the biopsy to avoid a repeat risk of general anesthesia. But since most lumps can be removed under local anesthesia this approach is seldom necessary today. The mastectomy can be planned at a later date when the diagnosis is confirmed without any danger of the cancer spreading in the two or three week waiting period.

Occasionally, when specific indications exist suspicious breast tissue can be obtained by needle aspiration of the mass in the breast. In this procedure a needle is inserted through the skin of the breast into the mass and some liquid and/or solid material is aspirated. In the case of very small masses the procedure can be done under fluoroscopy to aid the accuracy of the placement of the needle. Unfortunately, the procedure is not always accurate and an excisional biopsy still may be required.

The major point to be made, nevertheless, is that a diagnosis of breast cancer cannot be surmised or assumed without a biopsy. There is no other reliable method. As a matter of fact, on some occasions even the biopsy is questionable and may have to be repeated or further slices of the mass will have to be examined by a qualified pathologist.

Staging of Breast Cancers: In simple terms the staging of breast cancer is based on a measurement of the size of the primary breast mass (given in centimeters), and the extent of spread beyond the breast to such areas as; lymph nodes in the armpit (axilla), the nipple, the other breast, the overlying skin, and more distant sites such as neck lymph nodes, bones, lung, liver, etc.

In the majority of cases the most significant information is obtained from microscopic examination of the lymph nodes in the armpit since most cases will have not extended beyond this point at the time of first diagnosis. Regardless of the type of surgery for the breast tumor that is chosen the status of the armpit lymph nodes must be determined. In this way, and this way alone, can an appropriate therapy plan be devised and the most accurate prognostication be made. In addition, and probably without exception, the testing of the ability of the cancerous tissue to take up two hormones—estrogen and progesterone—is very useful information which must be obtained whenever practical.

Staging Terminology: The most frequently used nomenclature for the staging of breast cancer is the Stage I, II, IIIa, IIIb, and IV system. The complex definitions of these various stages is not of practical use to the patient—as it is to the physician— therefore, the reader will not be burdened with the excess details. However, you should feel free to ask your physician for this information if you so desire. More importantly you should understand how and why these stages are used to determine the treatment plan and the prognosis of your cancer.

Thus, comprehensive staging of breast cancer involves the following procedures in addition to mastectomy and removal of armpit (axillary) lymph nodes: complete history and physical examination; especially of the apparently normal opposite breast; chest x-ray, blood count; blood chemistry to screen for involvement of bones, liver and other distant organs. These are essentially routine but mandatory tests for screening of other organs frequently involved with breast cancer. Other specialized tests are chosen according to the results of the above mentioned surveillance tests and the judgement of your physician. These specialized tests might include: a bone scan to survey the skeletal system; x-rays and scans of the liver, brain, and biopsy of other lymph nodes might be required.

Because of the 10% chance of concurrent involvement of the other breast many physicians advise blind biopsy of this breast even if the physical examination and mammogram are normal. The need for the procedure is an arguable point but it is a safe and simple procedure.

Prognosis: The prognosis of breast cancer varies according to the many factors discussed below. Nonetheless, some general statements can be made about the overall cure rate, 5 and 10 year survival, and remission rates of breast cancer. The reader must remember that these figures are averages and medians for general prognosis for a large number of cases and not specific information for each individual breast cancer case. Each individual patient's prognosis must be discussed, in no uncertain terms, by your physician(s) involved in the management of your cancer.

Therefore, in broad terms, the 5 year survival rate for all breast cancer patients, including all stages and all age groups, is approximately 64%, and the 10 year survival is approximately 45%. These figures are a modest improvement over the period prior to earlier screening procedures and new treatment modalities such as chemotherapy. True cures, in the purist sense as previously define, probably don't occur in significant numbers. Of course, if a female develops breast cancer at, let's say, age 75 and then dies at age 78 from an unrelated cause, such as heart disease or stroke who can say if the cancer would have recurred if she had lived to age 90.

For the reason of this unpredictability the target of 'true cure' cannot be the only goal to strive toward in this group of cancers where long-term survivals are not unusual. But if treatment has prevented some of the pain, discomfort, anxiety and the cost of chronic debilitating disease it is generally worthwhile.

When divided into the two major subgroups—premenopausal and postmenopausal age, and stage of disease—there are distinct differences in survival rates. For example, in Stage I disease—the smallest lump and least amount of spread—the 5 year survival rate is roughly 85%. Whereas, is Stage IV disease—with the largest breast mass and the most distant spread—the 5 year survival rate drops to 10%.

In the premenopausal age group, arbitrarily defined as below age 50, the mortality rate is one-third that of the age group over age 50.

Again these are averages and medians and they may not tell the individual patient what will happen in the course of their disease.

Readers should not be discouraged by these facts and figures. There is no physician, anywhere, who can take a group of patients in the same age group and stage of disease and predict who will be in the high survival rate category and who will not. They can only quote the above numbers, do their best to achieve the best results and leave the rest in the hands of a greater power than themselves.

Equally as important as prolonged survival is the issue of quality of survival attainable with therapy. And, of course, the patient must discuss this point with the physician before embarking on any therapy program. The most difficult task for all concerned is defining the phrase "good quality survival" because it is subject to individual desires, variable tastes and personal values. Some patients state, quite frankly, they would rather die than live without one or both breasts, or without their hair, or live with the medicines side effects. Yet other patients say they want to have every minute of life they can get regardless of the quality of those minutes, days or months. As a result, it is not possible for your physician to mandate a universal definition of 'quality survival time' which suits all people. Each individual patient must be free to decide and define that for themselves as long as their expectations are not unrealistic.

Sites of Spread or Recurrence (Metastases): The distant spread of breast cancer has been known to appear in every conceivable location from the retina of the eye to kidneys and intestinal tract. However, both of these examples are distinctly rare. However, there are several more common locations of spread which the physician must check regularly with symptom-questions, physical examination, x-rays, scans and laboratory tests.

Among the more common locations checked by history and physical examination are: the skin overlying the chest wall from which the original breast was removed; the remaining opposite breast; the lymph nodes in the armpit and the neck; the bones, most often in the back and hips; the lungs; the liver; and the brain. However, meaningful, good quality survival is still possible even with spread to these areas because of recent advances in therapy even when it is not possible for your physician to prolong your survival.

Confusion apparently exists in the minds of readers regarding the spread of breast cancer to the other reproductive organs such as the uterus, ovaries and vagina. It might be that the confusion arose from the fact that removal of the ovaries (called Oophorectomy) has been used to treat recurrent and metastatic breast cancer. However, the ovaries are removed in these cases, even when they are normal, simply to attempt to cut off the production of female hormones (estrogen) by the ovaries which are known to encourage the growth of breast wherever it exists in the body.

Although it is true that breast cancer does frequently spread to the ovaries these ovarian metastases rarely, if ever, produce symptoms. Therefore, your physician does not suspect they are involved before the ovaries are removed but it is usually found coincidentally at surgery. As far as spread to the other reproductive organs, the uterus and the vagina, I have never seen this occur in my 20 years of practice and, therefore, it must be very rare.

And, finally, the breasts are not part of the same organ system as the ovaries, uterus and vagina. The last three named structures are true 'reproductive organs' and are necessary for reproduction of the human species but the breasts are not. The breasts may very well be utilized as 'sex organs' but they simply add to the pleasurable side of sex but they do not influence reproduction as such. It is these same misconceptions which cause women to fear being impaired sexually after mastectomy. Of course, the female breasts may be used for nourishing the infant by breast feeding but many women choose not to breast feed and the infant is provided other forms of nourishment quite effectively.

Therapeutic Approaches to Breast Cancer: The four major therapeutic approaches to breast cancer are surgery, radiation therapy, chemotherapy and hormonal manipulation. Often these modalities are used effectively in combination either simultaneously or sequentially. The research being conducted in breast cancer is very brisk and continuous. Therefore, the variety and combinations of therapy utilized are continually changing. There is no single 'magic therapeutic formula' which is used for or recommended for all breast cancer patients regardless of type, stage or age. However, there are some, more or less, standard general therapeutic principles which are applied.

Surgery: There is no doubt that surgery is still the primary mode of therapy for patients with breast cancer. However, some debate and controversy does exist as to how much surgery and what type of surgical procedure is best. But removal of the entire primary breast tumor is mandatory except is those patients who are already terminal at the time of discovery of the disease. Fortunately, through education and public awareness this situation of late presentation in the terminal state is becoming much more uncommon.

The original breast cancer operation described by Dr. Halsted many years ago was called the 'radical mastectomy.' At the time of its original appearance the mastectomy was considered by many physicians as an excessively aggressive approach but it unquestionably revolutionized the thinking of the medical community about the treatment of breast cancer. The 5 year survival rate was improved from a dismal 10% without mastectomy to a surprising 50% following mastectomy. The adjective 'radical' referred to the extensive removal of the muscles of the chest wall beneath the involved breast and all the lymph nodes in the armpit in addition to the entire breast.

Today most surgeons prefer a less extensive procedure called the 'modified radical mastectomy.' This procedure is less extensive in that none of the muscles of the chest wall are removed and a smaller number of lymph nodes in the armpit are removed. However, it is still advisable to remove the lymph nodes in order to access the extent of involvement since the degree of lymph nodes involvement is crucial in choosing the proper treatment plan and to determine prognosis. Except in those breast cancer cases which present with already widespread disease, or in patients who cannot tolerate major surgery because of poor general health, removal of the primary cancer mass and lymph nodes is standard therapy.

Considerable controversy and debate does exist among the medical community between the alternative of operative procedure known as "lumpectomy, teliectomy or quadrantectomy" versus mastectomy.

These lesser procedures try to preserve most of the breast, for cosmetic reasons, by simple removal of the main tumor mass and a limited number of armpit (axillary) lymph nodes. It is this author's carefully considered opinion that this lesser operation has not yet been shown to be as effective as modified radical mastectomy. However, when the patient is profoundly concerned about her physical appearance she must still given the option of choosing this less extensive procedure. But I would advise that it should always be followed by radiation therapy to the remaining breast tissue, axillary lymph nodes and followed by at least six months of chemotherapy.

Radiation Therapy: It was at one time standard procedure to apply radiation therapy to the chest wall and all the lymph nodes areas in the neck and axilla after mastectomy. However, it subsequently been shown that the addition of radiation therapy does not increase survival rates or prevent distant spread of the disease. It does, however, reduce the incidence of local chest wall recurrences. In addition, it can be used in treating chest wall, skin and axillary lymph nodes recurrences after they appear. However, some controversy does exist among physicians and researchers as to the need for radiation therapy in the prophylactic setting. In treating disseminated and locally recurrent disease, nonetheless, there is a major role for the application of radiation therapy. It is unequaled in the relief of pain from bone involvement by disseminated breast cancer and in many other situations too numerous to list here.

Chemotherapy: The use of cancer killing drugs can be applied in at least two ways in dealing with breast cancer. One way is in the case of distant and local recurrence of the disease; another use is in the so called 'adjuvant' i.e., the prophylactic setting.

Adjuvant or prophylactic treatment setting: In this clinical situation chemotherapy is given for 6 months after mastectomy—with or without radiation therapy—in order to reduce recurrences, prolong survival or improve the quality of survival for patients who achieve longer disease-free survival. Its use is based on several more or less valid assumptions. Number one, most, if not all, patients already have some microscopic spread (micro-metastases) of breast cancer at the time of presentation. However, these metastases, which are too few and to small, are undetectable by presently available testing procedures. Number two, these disseminated, but younger and smaller cancer cells, are more sensitive to the killing effects of chemotherapy. Number three, the side effects of the doses of adjuvant chemotherapy used are more tolerable and acceptable to the patient; and they have a low to nonexistent fatality rate. Number four; the duration and quality of the survivals, and the survival rate are significantly improved by its administration. Granted, these are all assumptions but several years of studies seemed to have borne out the validity of most of them.

There is little doubt that adjuvant chemotherapy has improved the outlook and survival for premenopausal patients with breast cancer. The degree of severity of side effects are tolerable and reversible, and the fatality rate from the chemotherapy is minuscule if given carefully under the diligent eye of an experienced chemotherapist. Some debate and controversy does exist over whether or not postmenopausal patients receive as great a benefit from adjuvant chemotherapy. Many physicians feel these patients do benefit from adjuvant chemotherapy but they must admit this is a 'personal impression' and the statistical proof for this assumption is not yet available. I believe the majority of medical oncologists would recommend adjuvant chemotherapy to postmenopausal patients with a high risk of recurrence because they have involved lymph nodes at the time of surgery and other high risk factors. These therapy choices and options should always be discussed by your physician with you before undertaking this major step. Even if the risks of therapy are small, tolerable and reversible the patient should still be made aware of their possibility. Thereby, the patient's choice is an informed and reasonable one.

The number of chemotherapy agents which have been found effective in treating breast cancer increases almost on a daily basis. And, of course, as the number of effective single chemotherapy agents increases so does the number and varieties of combinations which are possible. The following is a partial list of the more commonly utilized of these effective agents to treat breast cancer: cyclophosphamide (Cytoxan®); methotrexate; 5-fluorouracil; vincristine (Oncovin®);

doxorubicin (Adriamycin®); mitomycin C; vinblastine (Velban®); prednisone; L-phenylalanine mustard (Alkeran®); chlorambucil (Leukeran®); Thiotepa; BCNU; cis-platinum, and so on. The list of newer and developing agents is even longer and more impressive. The possible combinations and permeations are too numerous to even be attempted here.

Hormonal Manipulations: Defined in the broadest sense this form of therapy refers to altering the hormonal composition of the patient in order to discourage further growth of the breast cancer or to completely obliterate obvious recurrences. Also this modality can be used to treat known breast cancer relapse or to prevent it.

In former days this change in hormone composition was achieved through some kind of surgical procedure such as: removal of the ovaries in a premenopausal subject; removal of the adrenal glands (adrenalectomy) or; removal of the pituitary gland. All of these procedures tended to eliminate the source of natural female hormones—estrogens. And they were, indeed, effective means of producing and relieving symptoms but, unfortunately, no cures were achieved. These methods of hormonal manipulation had several disadvantages. They were found most effective in premenopausal patients; they were associated with significant surgical mortality and other serious side effects; they were slow in producing detectable benefits for the breast cancer patient.

In contemporary settings, however, the surgical means of hormonal manipulation are seldom utilized. It is now possible in nearly every situation to achieve the same result with drugs which are administered with minimal and tolerable side effects. There is almost no significant increase in mortality to produce the same therapeutic effects. These agents include tamoxifen—an anti-estrogen agent; megesterol—a progestational agent; and less commonly, aminoglutethamide—which suppresses estrogen production by the adrenal glands. Some other less common agents include androgenic hormones—such as fluoxymesterone (Halotestin®) and others; estrogenic hormones—such as Stilbestrol® and others. The side effects of the last two types of agents has precluded their use in modern breast cancer therapy programs. The number of ways in which these agents can be administered have increased by combining them with chemotherapy and/or radiation therapy.

Indeed, preliminary evidence is accumulating to indicate that administering anti-estrogens and chemotherapy drugs prophylactically can effectively reduce recurrence rates after mastectomy.

The ideal therapy plan in each case must be 'custom tailored,' if you will, to suit the clinical setting of the individual case scenario.

The side effects—both major and minor—are discussed for each of the chemotherapy agents in a later section of this book.

Management Team: The composition of the management team—as far as type of physicians is concerned—varies with the extent of disease at the time of diagnosis and with the type of treatment chosen for any given stage of the breast cancer. I feel that the ideal arrangement is to have all physician-members of the oncology team involved after a diagnosis is established and before a complete therapy plan is adopted.

Since some form of surgical biopsy is always required there will automatically be a surgeon involved early in any breast cancer case. Also, the surgeon should be the team leader until the recovery period is complete, and until any complications of the surgical procedure have been ameliorated.

Radiation therapy—which should only be given by a qualified radiation oncologist—may or may not be required in your breast cancer depending on the consensus opinion of the management team.

The same principles of the therapy management team hold true for chemotherapy whether given in the adjuvant setting or to treat obvious spread of the breast cancer. Most often chemotherapy is given by a medical oncologist but there are other types of qualified and experienced chemotherapists. The chosen chemotherapist remains involved for as long a period of time which is required to complete the course of chemotherapy or for as long as a risk of complications exists from the chemotherapy chosen.

Equally important in the plan is the follow-up period which may last for years or even for the remainder of the patient's life. Any and all types of physicians have been made aware, at sometime in their training ,of the proper means required to follow the course of breast cancer. Therefore, either the family physician, the surgeon, the radiation oncologist or the medical oncologist may be appropriately chosen to follow the patient's course. In this writer's opinion this period extends for the remainder of the patient's life.

The follow up program must include periodic and regular history and physical examinations, blood chemistry tests and occasionally x-rays and scans as indicated. A breast cancer patient must never be left to their own devices by their physician or be advised to "come back when you have any symptoms or other troubles." Such statements by a physician sometimes send the message that he has only a fleeting interest in the patient's welfare, or gives you the false sense of security which implies— "you're cured now." Even if the chance of recurrences is very low the physician must always act on the premise—hope for the best but expect the unexpected.

Chapter 25

Cancer of the Colon, Rectum and Anus

Anatomically speaking, the colon, rectum and the anus make up only a small portion of a single large organ system—the gastrointestinal tract. Nevertheless, cancers of these three sections comprise the most common cancers of that organ system. These cancers are, however, among the more easily prevented cancers and among those which lend themselves most readily to early detection.

Names and Synonyms: Some common lay-public and medical names for this cancer include colonic cancer; adenocarcinoma of the color or rectum; large bowel cancer or carcinoma; and colo-rectal cancer.

Incidence Rates: Cancers of these three anatomic sites will account for 14% of all cancers in males and 14% of cancers in females; and they will cause 11% of all cancer deaths in males in 1995 and 12% of all cancer deaths in females. Stated in terms of actual lives lost an estimated 58,300 Americans will die of cancers of these three sites in 1995. Two thirds of the cases will occur in the over 50 age group; men are afflicted equally as often as women; 50% of all these cancers will occur in the lower portions (rectum and anus) of the colon and are within easy reach of endoscopic detection or digital rectal examination.

Causes and Risk Factors: As in most cancers the precise cause(s) of colo-rectal cancer is not known but certain predisposing risk factors are recognized.

(a) Heredity : In this category are included only those cases with a definite family history of multiple colon polyps.

(b) Chronic Colonic Diseases: The risk of colon cancer is increased in cases of Chronic Ulcerative Colitis, which is a distinctive and specific type of colitis not to be confused with the more nonspecific and common conditions generally entitled "colitis." Ulcerative Colitis can only be diagnosed by colon x-rays or colonscopic examination with biopsy of the lining of the colon. Special emphasis is placed on this point because many intestinal disorders can be manifested by diarrhea, abdominal cramps, bloody stools and other common symptoms which have been dubbed "Colitis." The generic term 'Colitis' is a misnomer and unrelated to true "Ulcerative Colitis."

There are many other common colonic conditions which have *not* been shown to be associated with colon cancer such as diverticulosis, diverticulitis, chronic constipation, or hemorrhoids.

Polyps of the adenomatous type—which have a special appearance and are not related to the hereditary type of polyps—has sparked a long-lasting debate as to whether their presence is a pre-malignant condition. It would appear that the controversy is still not settled at this time. However, there is little debate over the question that these polyps should be removed when found. A very special and distinctive kind of polyp—called a villous adenoma—is clearly associated with an increased cancer risk.

(c) Diet: There is some very suggestive, but as yet inconclusive, evidence that diets high in fiber decrease the risk of colon and rectum cancer. The evidence is indirectly inferred from the fact that colon cancers are much more common in the western world than they are in rural Africa because of the high fiber content of the diet ingested by Africans.

Signs and Symptoms: The symptoms produced by colo-rectal cancers depends on the section of the colon involved in the disorder.

For example the right side of the colon is upstream, so to speak, and at this point stool material is still liquid and soft. As a result, cancers in this location seldom cause pain or changes in bowel habits.

The most frequent situations arise when the wise and thorough physician investigates an unexplained anemia due to blood loss, the presence of blood in the stools or black tarry stools and then he finds the colon cancer. The physician's general rule of thumb is to suspect colon cancer in any adult patient—especially postmenopausal females and males over 40—with unexplained anemia of having hidden colon cancer until proven otherwise.

On the other hand, in the left side of the colon—the more downstream portion—the fecal material is very much more solid and, therefore, more often produces signs of blockage which produces changes in bowel habits, pain, vomiting or it presents as an acute abdominal emergency.

It is the common, late and nonspecific nature of the above named symptoms and signs which makes the detection of colo-rectal cancers so difficult.

Screening for Colo-rectal Cancer: There are three basic procedures which are recommended for screening of the general population who have no symptoms of colon cancer. The three are: digital-rectal examination; chemical examination of the stool for blood; and proctoscopic or colonoscopic (endoscopic) examination of the colon. None of these procedures is fool proof or without drawbacks. But they are the best we have available at the moment.

The rectal (also called digital) examination by the gloved finger of the physician is advised on an annual basis for all patients over age 40. One-half of all the cancers of the rectum can be detected by this simple and inexpensive examination. The rectal exam should be an integral part of all routine annual physical examinations—at any adult age.

The chemical examination of the stool for unseen (occult) blood is advised for all patients over age 40 on an annual basis. The examination is also safe, simple and inexpensive. It is not without its own disadvantages, however. When done properly the patient must be on a meat-free, vitamin C-free, high fiber diet for at least 48 hours before the test otherwise false-positive results may occur. Two separate stool samples are required on each of three consecutive days. The paper slides with the stool sample cannot be stored for more than 4 days before they are tested and they must be kept dry before testing.

Unfortunately there is a high rate of false-positives with the occult blood test, at least in respect to detection of cancer, since the test only reveals the presence of blood in the stool. The test will be positive regardless of the cause of the blood in the stool sample. It is *not* specific for colon cancer. There are many other common conditions which can cause a positive test for occult blood which include: ulcers in the upper intestine (duodenal or gastric ulcers); hemorrhoids; anal fistulas or fissures; swallowed blood from nose bleeds or from bleeding gums. As indicated by the special requirements of diet before performing the test, false positives results occur frequently due to simple dietary factors. It is this large group of false-positive results which causes many physicians to remain skeptical about the stool test. The skepticism is especially significant since the consequence may be that many people are submitted to costly and risky tests such as endoscopy, and x-rays of the upper and lower intestines.

Nevertheless, it is this author's opinion that when accompanied by a complete history of digestive symptoms and a good digital examination of the rectum the test is still of value as a screening procedure.

Routine proctoscopic, sigmoidoscopic or colonoscopic examination is another matter entirely. It has been widely advocated by many physicians as an annual routine exam because two-thirds of all colo-rectal cancers are within the reach of the instrument. However, cost and safety are considered its major disadvantages. The general application of the procedure would require the examination of 4000 normal individuals before discovering one case of colo-rectal cancer. Some physicians feel that this is not cost effective enough to warrant its routine use. Your physician should discuss these points with you if you request the examination to allow you to take part in the decision. There is no doubt, however, the examination is indicated in all patients with a history of abnormal bowel function, a suspicious digital examination or in patients with an unexplained anemia. The endoscopy is also indicated on a routine basis for all patients with a past history of colo-rectal cancer, colon polyps, chronic ulcerative colitis, or a strong family history of colo-rectal cancer.

Blood Tests for Colo-Rectal Cancer: The blood test known as the CEA (carcino-embryonic antigen) has received considerable attention in the mass media as a 'screening test' for colo-rectal cancer. But the test has been considered too expensive, too nonspecific, and not sensitive enough for routine use. There are too many other cancers and noncancerous diseases which give a false-positive CEA test result and there are too many patients with cancer who have a normal result. Indeed, even heavy smokers without any detectable disease may have a positive CEA test. Therefore, the test is not considered to have any more screening value than a history and physical examination and other routine tests.

Regular routine x-ray examination of the lower bowel (barium enema) is also not considered useful except for specific findings such as a bloody stools, a positive test for occult blood, unexplained anemia, etc.

Diagnosis of Colo-Rectal Cancer: Biopsy is, of course, still an indispensable requirement for this diagnosis of cancer. But the methods by which such biopsy is obtained my vary for the individual case. The biopsy sample may be obtained through the examining proctoscope, sigmoidoscope or the colonoscope. Occasionally, abdominal exploratory surgery is required to obtain an adequate specimen for biopsy interpretation.

Staging Procedures: The following procedures are necessary for the adequate staging of colo-rectal cancer because precise staging dictates the optimal treatment plan and provides information for accurate prognostication of your colon cancer. These are:

1. Complete history and physical examination.
2. Barium enema (lower G.I. series).
3. Blood tests including complete blood count, liver function chemistries and CEA.
4. Chest x-rays.
5. Endoscopic examination; that is ,sigmoidoscopy or colonoscopy. Occasionally some other special procedures may be indicated and these might include:

1. Cystoscopic examination of the urinary bladder to determine presence of, and extent of involvement by the cancer of this close neighboring structure.
2. CT scans of the liver and other portions of the abdomen and pelvis.
3. Exploratory abdominal surgery as mentioned above.

Staging and Classification: The staging systems of colo-rectal cancer are recognized under various titles such as: the Duke's Classification; the AJC system or the TMN system. The differences between these systems are technical and depend on your physician's owns bias but they essentially all make the same statement which is—the extent that the disease exists beyond the local colon or rectal cancer.

Each staging system uses four basic findings to determine the degree of dissemination of disease. The first and second levels of staging depend on the depth of penetration of the cancer growth into the wall of the large intestine; the third level indicates profound depth into the colonic wall with involvement of some lymph nodes inside the abdominal cavity; and the fourth level indicates involvement of more distant structures, such as lungs, liver, bones, etc. The names of the systems, per se, have no other useful meaning to the patient. Whereas, your physician uses the information to determine the best treatment plan and the prognosis. The patient need not have these names or definitions but you are, of course, entitled to the information if you so desire.

The various tests and measures used in arriving at the stage of disease have been listed above under diagnostic procedures.

Prognosis: The overall *5-year-survival* for all stages of colo-rectal cancer is in the range of 45%. The 5 year *cure* rate is estimated to be about 25%. In 1995 in the United States it is estimated that approximately 156,000 new cases of colo-rectal cancer will occur and there will be 58,300 deaths in the same year. These figures have not appreciably changed in the last several years even with newer modalities of therapy but further research is being carried out with various combinations of treatments to improve these results.

As usual, cure rates, 5-year-survival rates and remission rates vary with the stage of disease and the above figures are overall averages.

It should be noted here that treatment results vary somewhat for cancers on the right side of the colon (the upstream end furthest from the rectum and closer to the appendix) as compared to those on the left side (the downstream end closest to the rectum) of the colon.

The *'true cures'* only occur in the earlier stages of the disease which means they are limited to the colon (large intestine) and the local lymph nodes within the abdomen. Surgical removal of all the visible cancer offers the only chance, at this writing, for true cure. Some research studies involving radiation therapy combined with chemotherapy are showing some promise for better treatment results in the more advanced stages. Most recently studies have shown a combination of chemotherapy and immunotherapy (Levamisole) in the early stages of colon cancer can reduce recurrence rates.

Sites of Spread and Recurrences (Metastases): Some of these metastatic sites have already been mentioned but they deserve further emphasis. These recurrences include: those locally within the remainder of the colon or the pelvis; the lymph nodes within the abdominal cavity; the liver; lungs; lymph nodes outside the abdomen; the bones and the brain.

Therapeutic Approaches to Colo-rectal Cancer: The four major options now open to the patient in managing colo-rectal cancer are the standard forms of surgery, radiation therapy, chemotherapy, immunotherapy or a variety of combinations of these.

As in many other cancers, surgery is the mainstay of treatment for almost all stages of disease. Even if the cancer is found to be widely disseminated at the initial time of examining the patient, surgery is often still necessary either to establish the diagnosis by biopsy, to relieve some kind of severely distressing symptoms or prevent some impending disaster and death.

When the patient presents with obstruction of the bowel, for example, or active, vigorous bleeding from the rectum, surgery is necessary to relieve these dangerous consequences of the cancer. Frequently it is obvious at the time of x-ray of the colon that only a small opening remains to allow the flow of intestinal contents and the surgery is necessary to prevent impending intestinal obstruction.

There are basically two kinds of surgical operations available to your physician. The first is simple removal of the cancer followed by rejoining of the ends of the colon to allow for normal passage of stool through the rectum. The other procedures used involve the need for a colostomy after removal of the cancerous growth. As a result of the colostomy a reservoir for the stool is used to collect the material after it drains through an opening (colostomy) made in the front wall of the abdomen. When colostomy is chosen its need is dictated by the technical limitations found at the time of surgery. In the cases requiring colostomy it is just not technically possible to rejoin the opened ends of the colon to allow normal passage of material through the rectum.

Radiation therapy is occasionally recommended as an additional treatment modality. But radiation therapy is seldom used alone as the only attack on the cancer. It may be administered prior to surgery or after surgery. In occasional cases it is used as the only means of treatment when the patient is so ill that surgery cannot be performed without endangering their life. The radiation therapy may be given in these instances to relieve—partially and temporarily—the distress of intestinal obstruction or active bleeding. Using this approach, it is sometimes possible to stabilize the patient's immediate distress and allow your physician time to improve their general condition so surgery can performed later with a lower and more acceptable risk.

In the case of severe pain or other distressing symptoms due to the spread of the cancer to more distant locations, say, to bone or lung, radiation therapy can be utilized to relieve the pain or other distress before undertaking the surgery.

Chemotherapy by itself, up to the present time, has not been found to be of great value in the treatment of colo-rectal cancers. There have been many research projects carried out to try to utilize these chemotherapy drugs to improve the survival rates with application of the drugs before and after surgery. Unfortunately very little benefit has been demonstrated from this approach. Some chemotherapy agents have been found useful for the relief of distressing symptoms not alleviated by surgery and radiation therapy. However, vigorous research is continuing in these areas to discover a combination of agents or in search of a totally new agent which might offer some hope.

Some of the chemotherapy agents presently utilized to treat colo-rectal cancer include: 5-fluorouracil (5-FU) which is the most common and most effective; methotrexate; vincristine, CCNU, BCNU, Methyl-CCNU, mitomycin-C. Some newer agents being utilized include; cisplatinum, Adriamycin®, fluoxuridine, streptozotocin, chlorozotocin. Various combinations of these agents given either in sequence or simultaneously are under study and do hold some promise for improvement of survival and remission rates.

There is one special method of treatment presently being used to treat the distant metastases of colo-rectal cancers when they have involved the liver called, regional perfusion with chemotherapy agents. In this method a plastic catheter is fed into a large artery carrying blood to the liver with its in dwelling cancer. The chemotherapy agents, such as 5-FU or fluoxuridine, are infused through the plastic catheter into the organ over an extended period of time. The method has been found useful in palliation of some of the discomforting symptoms of this metastatic stage of colo-rectal cancer. However, it is not clear if this approach has had any significant impact on length of survival or remission rates. It has certainly not produced any 'true cures,' as yet.

Immunotherapy has been utilized in colo-rectal cancer in the form of general, nonspecific stimulators of the immune system. Agents such as BCG, MER-BCG and levamisole have been tried and not found especially effective. Newer forms of immune therapy—interferon and interleukins—are presently under investigation. These are more accurately called Biological Response Modifiers.

Management Team: Since the vast majority of cases of Colo-rectal cancers require surgical therapy the general surgeon is the initial manager of the management team. In some cases the managerial role is shared by the surgeon and the radiotherapist, or by the surgeon and the medical oncologist.

When the cancer has spread to other areas in the body it is usually treated with chemotherapy and therefore the chemotherapist—either the medical or the surgical oncologist—leads the management team. He acts as the major problem solver and the first line of contact with the patient and family.

Follow-Up Examinations: In those cases which appear to have had a completely removable colo-rectal cancer it is mandatory that regular periodic examinations by a physician be carried out. Whether the follow up physician is your surgeon, family physician or medical oncologist depends on the point in time or the patient's personal choice. In either case, regular, standard periodic testing is advisable.

The comprehensive medical history and physical examination is still mandatory with particular attention paid to the areas mentioned above under the most common sites of recurrences or distant spread. These test usually include a repeat colonoscopy or proctoscopy; barium enema; CEA; chemistry profile to evaluate the function of other internal organs; complete blood count; chest x-ray; CAT scans of liver, bone scans, etc., as indicated by results of screening examinations.

There are some inconsistencies among physicians' opinions as to how often these examinations should be carried out. My personal preference is to vary the length of time between examinations based on the likelihood of relapse and the stage of the cancer at first diagnosis. So that, if a case had an early stage of disease with complete surgical removal of the cancer the patient is examined once a month for the first six months with plans for CEA blood test every 3 months, and a complete history, physical exam, and chest x-ray, etc. every year for the first 5 years after apparent cure.

The duration between examinations is progressively shortened as the stage of the colo-rectal cancer when from it was first discovered increases. In other words, the more advanced the disease the more likelihood of recurrences and therefore the more frequent the repeat examinations should be done.

Chapter 26

Cancer of the Prostate

Cancer of the prostate: cancers of this glandular organ are, of course, limited to males. It is one of the most common cancers in men over 50 years old. It is one of the few organs in humans which is very accessible for easy, frequent and inexpensive examination on a regular basis. It is sad to note, however, that the examination of this structure by digital-rectal examination is not carried out more frequently. It is recommended that the prostate examination is a mandatory requirement for all routine physical examinations. It should be done on a annual basis for all males over age 50.

Names and Synonyms: Cancer of the prostate; carcinoma of the prostate; adenocarcinoma of the prostate; cancer of the prostate gland are some of the more well known names for this cancer.

Incidence Rates: As I have previously stated cancer of the prostate is most common after age 50 and rare before that age. The median age of incidence is 70 years. In 1995 it is estimated it will be responsible for 12% of cancer deaths in males and will account for 23% of all cancers in men. In any one year there will be at least 36 new cases for every 100,000 population. It will cause, in 1995, 34,000 deaths and there will be 132,000 new cases discovered.

Causes and Risk Factors: At this writing there is no clear causative agent identified for cancer of the prostate although there may be some role played by male hormones. The relationship between male hormones (androgens), sexual activity or inactivity is not at all clear despite some of the 'old witches' and warlocks' tales' to the contrary.

Signs & Symptoms: Unfortunately the symptoms of cancer of the prostate may also be caused by many noncancerous conditions of the male genitourinary system. It is for this reason I feel that all bladder or urinary abnormalities must be investigated by a physician with cancer being the first consideration in men over age 50.

These common symptoms include: difficulty in passage of urine, including complete blockage of the passage of urine; partial obstruction of urine flow which produces a decreased force of the stream of urine or dribbling of the stream; passage of bloody urine; frequent and recurrent bladder or kidney infections.

Screening Tests: Unfortunately there is no ideal, inexpensive blood or urine test which can be utilized for early detection in large numbers of the population which is any more useful than the digital palpation of the prostate via the rectal examination. The prostate gland is examined for the presence of nodules or hardness. Over 50% of nodules in the prostate are cancerous which also means, of course, the other approximately 50% are not cancerous.

Not even simple urine analysis examination has been found useful for screening purposes. The urine analysis is, however, commonly utilized for diagnosing and screening for many other medical abnormalities but not cancer of the prostate.

Two more recent additions to the list of diagnostic procedures for cancer of the prostate are the ultrasonogram of the prostate and the prostate specific antigen (PSA) blood test. The precise role of these new modalities in screening and diagnosis is still under investigation.

Diagnosis: Biopsy tissue for diagnosis of prostate cancer can be obtained in a variety of ways. In the case of a palpated (felt) nodule within the prostate an adequate specimen can be obtained without major surgery in the form of a simple and safe needle biopsy via the rectal route.

In other cases of unsuspected prostate cancer the diseased tissue removed for relief of obstruction of the bladder by the prostate gland unexpectedly reveals the diagnosis. The procedure—called 'transurethral resection (TUR)—is performed through an optical instrument (the cystoscope) inserted into the bladder via the opening in the penis called the urethra. The obstructing tissue is removed by scraping or chipping away the excess pieces of the prostate gland. The removed fragments are then examined by the pathologist under the microscope to diagnosis the presence of cancer.

In still other circumstances a more extensive surgical procedure is required by removing the entire prostate gland via abdominal or pelvic surgery (Suprapubic prostatectomy). This type of operation is indicated in only 5-10% of patients with cancer of the prostate.

Under special circumstances—where the first sign of prostate cancer to be detected is in a focus of distant spread—a biopsy of the metastatic cancer tissue raises the suspicion of prostate cancer. These metastatic sites most commonly include spread to the bones, liver, lungs, lymph nodes or the urinary bladder.

Staging Systems: There are two staging systems presently in use for the classification of prostate cancer. Both systems are very complex and highly technical. Suffice it to say the disease staging progresses along the lines of more disease, size of individual tumors, involvement of lymph nodes and spread to more distant organs. In the system used by the American Urological system the letters A, B, C or D designate the stages of disease–with A being the least advanced and D the most advanced level of disease. This highly technical data is of little or no value to the patient but is essential for the physician.

The best therapeutic choice for each stage of prostate cancer is determined by the stage designation. Several types of tests are required to ascertain the extent, and therefore, the stage of disease. These include: examination; needle biopsy of suspicious nodules as described above; x-rays and scan of bones; blood acid and alkaline levels; excretory urogram to determine any involvement of the bladder and its outlets; complete blood count.

For certain special circumstances some special tests may be required, such as: x-ray examination of lymph nodes (lymphangiography), and subsequent needle biopsy of any suspicious lymph nodes found; needle biopsy of the bone and bone marrow; and, occasionally, exploratory surgery of the pelvis to locate involved lymph nodes.

Prognosis: The overall 5 year survival rate for prostate cancer has been slowly improving over the years from a low of 50% in 1963 to a high of 62% in 1986. However, these are again average figures or medians and the actual survival rate depends on the stage of each case of cancer. This is information your physician should be willing to discuss with the patients as it applies to their particular situation.

In general those patients in the group with less extensive cancer—stages A and B— survive longer than those with more extensive disease—stages C and D.

Stage A patients have a better than 90% five-year-survival rate. Stage B patients have approximately an 80% five-year-survival, Stage C patients have a 50% five year survival rate, and Stage D patients have less than a 10% five year survival rate.

Consistent and meaningful statistics are difficult to obtain for prostate cancer because of a lack of uniformity among physicians on how to measure response to treatment and disparity among the medical research community as to what constitutes standard therapy for various stages of this cancer. It is for these same reasons there is a lack of clear-cut uniform treatment recommendations given below in the therapy section.

Sites of Spread: The most commonly involved area of spread is found in the lymph nodes in the pelvis at the time of surgery. It is the finding of disease involving these lymph nodes which drastically changes the prognosis. Lymph node involvement in the pelvis automatically places a case into the Stage D category, the stage with the poorest prognosis and lowest five year survival.

More distant spread is most common in the bones, the bone marrow, lungs, liver and bladder. Bone metastases are, by far, the commonest form of distant spread.

Therapeutic Choices: Surgery is the mainstay in treatment of localized prostate cancer by 'Radical Prostate Surgery' being the most aggressive form of surgical treatment. However, this surgery is indicated only in those patients with confirmed localized disease, who are under age 70, and are otherwise very healthy without any other medical conditions which might shorten survival to under 10 years. Unfortunately, only 5 to 10% of patients qualify under these criteria. In some cases extensive removal of lymph nodes in the pelvis is recommended. It is still unclear if the addition of this maneuver improves the prognosis and survival rate. All patients experience sexual impotence after this surgery and 15% experience urinary incontinence (uncontrolled spontaneous evacuation of urine).

Radiation Therapy: Radiation therapy, in one form or another, can be utilized in those patients who do not qualify for the radical surgery discussed above. This is given in the form of external radiation applied to the prostate gland itself and to the local lymph nodes in the pelvis.

An alternative approach is to place radioactive chemicals (Iodine-125) in the area of the pelvic lymph nodes at the time of surgery, if such surgery is performed.

Radiation therapy is also useful in two other common clinical situations. The first is in the treatment of painful bone involvement. Seventy to 80 percent of patients experience dramatic pain relief within 24 to 48 hours after receiving radiation therapy.

The second area of usefulness is in the radiation of the male breast prior to prescribing female hormone therapy (estrogens) which results in the eventual pendulous enlargement of the male breasts. This is indeed a great source of embarrassment and emotional discomfort to the patient and every effort is made to minimize it.

Hormonal Manipulations: The most frequently applied form of this modality is given as estrogen (diethyl stilbestrol) tablets on a daily basis. As mentioned above impotence and enlargement of the breasts are common side effects. In addition, there is the potential for worsening of other medical conditions such as heart disease and high blood pressure. These adverse effects are easily averted by administration of diuretics (water pills) at the time of starting estrogen therapy.

Orchiectomy, or surgical removal of the testicles, is another form of hormonal manipulation utilized in patients who are not candidates for radical surgery or who cannot risk the side effects of estrogens.

This modality is often used as a means of palliation when all else has failed. Some physicians do, however, recommend that orchiectomy be performed at the same point in time that estrogens are prescribed. There is still some disagreement among physicians about this approach.

More recently newer approaches have been investigated with the resultant development of anti-androgen therapy with agents such as flutamide, cyproterone, and injections of luteinizing hormones. The value of these agents and their role in treating prostate cancer is still under study.

Chemotherapy: Strictly speaking this term refers to the use of chemotherapy agents which kill cancer cells and harm normal cells at the same time. There are very few chemotherapeutic agents which have been found useful for prostate cancer except, perhaps, for relief of discomfort. They have not been shown, thus far, to alter survival rate or duration of life, significantly.

A combination agent in which a hormone—estradiol and a true anticancer chemical, nitrogen mustard—are chemical united has been shown to have some limited value in palliation, also. The agent is called Emcyt® or estramustine.

Some of the newer chemotherapeutic agents under study for prostate cancer include, cisplatinum, bleomycin, doxorubicin, carboplatin and others. These agents are also being combined with more established and well known agents such as 5-FU, cyclophosphamide, methotrexate and others.

Some very recent work has revealed a possible beneficial therapeutic effect when chemotherapy drugs (vinblastine) are combined with a hormonal drug (estramustine) or with injections of biological response modifiers (alpha-interferon).

Significant advances in treatment have resulted in prolonged duration survival and increase in 5 year survival rates but none has proven to increase the 'true cure rate' of prostate cancer.

Chapter 27

Cancers of the Uterus

Cancers of the uterus are discussed in two parts based on their location in the uterus since they have different presentations and treatment. Some understanding of the structure of the uterus will clarify the discussion. If the reader thinks of the female uterus as being shaped like a common household light bulb its two divisions are easily recognized. The small end of the bulb that is screwed into the socket is called the cervix. The larger, globular end of the bulb is called the body of the uterus. We will first discuss the small end—the cervix.

Cancer of the Cervix: Cancer of the uterine cervix has two of the characteristics which make the physicians' task easier; (1) the uterine cervix is easily accessible to direct visual examination and diagnosis; (2) cancer of the cervix has a very high rate of curability, if detected early. The easy accessibility of the cervix is via the pelvic examination and the Pap (Papanicolaou) smear. Unfortunately too many women do not take advantage of this accessibility by having frequent pelvic examinations and the Pap smear. When cervical cancer is detected in this way— before symptoms appear (called cancer in situ)—there is greater than 90% cure rate by radiation therapy or surgery. The cure rate is so high that cancer of the cervix in situ (not invasive) is usually omitted from national death rates due to cancer. Sadly, the cure rate drops dramatically in those women who wait until they have symptoms of the disease before seeking the advice of a physician. In the advanced stages (called invasive cancer of the cervix) the cure rate by any treatment method is less than 10%.

Synonyms: Cervical Cancer, Carcinoma of the Cervix, Cancer of Female Organs (very general and nonspecific).

Incidence Rates: There are approximately 13,500 new case of Invasive cancer of the cervix in this country each year. Forty-five thousand of these patients ultimately die of their disease. It is the second most common cancer in women age 15 to 34, although it can be found in any age group. The incidence of the advanced or invasive stage has dropped dramatically from 23 cases per 100,000 population to just 12 per 100,000; the mortality has decreased from 15 to 6 cases per 100,000; and the incidence of the early cancer in situ has increased, all as a result of the use of regular pelvic examination and the Pap smear before symptoms appear.

Patients with cancer of the cervix tend to come from the lower socioeconomic levels of our society. Its mortality rate is higher in those women whose husbands are lower on the scale of socioeconomic strata for reasons that are not quite clear at this time.

Causes and Risk Factors: A single, clearly definable cause of cancer of the cervix has not been established but there are certain detectably significant risk factors. Some experts consider it a form of 'venereal disease' in that certain sexually transmitted infections seem to influence development of cervical cancer.

There are two viruses which cause sexually transmitted diseases which appear to increase the rate of cervical cancer. They are known as the herpes viruses and the papilloma virus. The Epstein-Barr virus—a member of the herpes family of viruses—along with other herpes viruses are known to produce certain types of cancers in animals. When women with herpes virus infection are examined over an extended period of time by Pap smears up to 25% of them develop in situ cancer of the cervix.

The papilloma viruses are the cause of clear cut human infections including genital warts, plantar warts, condyloma warts, and the common flat warts.

Other risk factors seem to relate to the sexual activity of the female. For example, cervical cancer is more common in women who have multiple sex partners during their teenage years, and is less common in women who have the cervix protected by a condom or diaphragm. This protective factor seems to implicate some role of the sperm or semen from the male partner in the causation of cervical cancer. However, the causative relationship has not been clearly established.

Signs and Symptoms: Most cases of the early, curable form of in situ cancer of the cervix are devoid of symptoms or signs. And their absence lends to the higher rate of cure but it also fails to alert the reader earlier of the presence of the cancer. Those cases without symptoms are readily detected by the routine, annual Pap smear.

When obvious symptoms do occur cervical cancer is too often far advanced. Sadly, most patients who have symptoms from cancer of the cervix when they first present themselves to the physician have invasive cancer of the cervix. The symptoms at this invasive stage include vaginal bleeding after intercourse or between menstrual periods; a watery, foul smelling vaginal discharge; painful or uncomfortable sexual intercourse; and in women after menopausal age any vaginal bleeding is highly suspect for cancer.

In very advanced cervical cancer—which occurs when the disease is beyond the confines of the pelvis (the borders of which are formed by the hip bones)—the symptoms include swelling (edema) of the legs, sciatica-type back pain, or inability to lie flat with legs straightened without causing severe pain. Most women with this advanced stage give a record of *never* having had a routine annual Pap smear or many report not having had the Pap test since their last child was born.

Screening Tests: As previously stated the ease and safety with which the vagina and cervix can be examined with the naked eye, palpated with the examining glove and sampled for cells makes it one of the more ideal areas for detecting early cancer and other diseases. However, this earlier detection is dependent upon the reader voluntarily coming to the physician to have the examination done. Nevertheless, I believe it is the job of the medical profession and its associates to disseminate these facts and to educate the public. Because the exam is such a direct method of surveillance via the pelvic examination and Pap smear it need not be bolstered with other miscellaneous blood tests, and the like. The Pap smear is actually another kind of biopsy in which cells are gently scraped from the cervix and placed of a slide to be stained and examined by the pathologist. Even a grossly normal appearing cervix may harbor the early changes of cancer in situ.

When your physician observes any suspicious changes on the uterine cervix a larger section of tissue can be obtained with a snipping-type instrument for further studies. Cells are also aspirated from the body of the uterus via a small suction device inserted into the opening in the cervix. This suctioning process can reveal evidence of any abnormal changes in the lining of the uterus (endometrium) which can then be examined for signs of cancer.

The vagina is also examined at the same time, both visually and manually, to detect the occasional case of cancer in this structure.

Many lives are being saved daily by this method of early detection and many more could be saved if the women readers would just present themselves on a annual basis for this simple examination. Statistically analyses indicate that only 10-15% of U.S. women get this recommend examination on a yearly basis.

Diagnosis: I think it is evident from the previous discussion that the diagnosis is usually established in most cases of cancer of the cervix without any further testing. And if the reader goes on to surgery for removal of the uterus (hysterectomy) along with its cervix these structures are examined by the pathologist to further substantiate the diagnosis and to look for evidence of local spread and deeper invasion. However, hysterectomy is not necessary for cure in all cases. The need for hysterectomy is discussed further under treatment options.

Stagings Systems and Tests: As in the staging of other types of cancer the designations for each stage are made in numerical and lettered fashion with several subdivisions. As usual, the earlier and less extensive levels of involvement receive lower Roman numerals—Stage I, II, etc.—and the subdivisions are indicated by attached small letters, such as Stage Ia, IIb, and so on.

The least extensive division in this cancer is designated Stage 0 which does not indicate 'no disease' but it simply indicates no disease is visible to the unaided eye and it is also not producing symptoms. Stage 0 signifies cancer of the cervix detected, and often unexpectedly, by Pap smear. Therefore, stage 0 is the same as Cancer in situ. The most advanced stage of cervical cancer is designated Stage IVb which indicates the spread of the cancer to distant organs far removed from the female reproductive system.

Other tests your physician recommends for complete staging may include: examination of the internal parts of the bladder (cystoscopy); kidney x-rays (Intravenous pyelography, IVP); blood tests to survey the functional integrity of the liver, kidney, bones, etc.; an x-ray of the chest; x-ray or scanning techniques to detect disease in any lymph nodes in the pelvis and abdomen (lymphangiography or CT scanning); further scanning of other organs if they are found to be abnormal by surveillance blood tests or by physical examination.

In addition, it is matter of routine to examine the internal organs and lymph nodes visually and manually if the patient undergoes surgery. Direct visual examination at surgery is routine because physicians are aware of the fallibility of any and all tests and x-rays. First hand direct visual examination helps to alleviate any concerns on your physician's part regarding the accuracy of the tests.

Prognosis: The survival and cure rate of cervical cancer are closely linked to the stage of disease and the type of therapy utilized. Overall, however, the 5 year survival rate for all stages of cancer of the cervix has increased from 55% in 1963 to approximately 65% without the including early cancer in situ since it is cured in greater than 95% of cases.

The following table lists the 5 year survival rates for each stage of cervical cancer:

Stage I	90%+
Stage II	75%
Stage III	40%
Stage IV	14%

The level of the staging and the cure rate usually parallel the time at which disease is discovered. Therefore, the readers who have regular annual Pap smear and pelvic examinations and those who present for examination as soon as symptoms appear have the earliest level of cancer and the greatest chance for cure.

Sites of Spread and Recurrence: Cancer of the cervix most often spreads and recurs within the area of the pelvis and its neighboring structures such as, urinary bladder, rectum and lymph nodes. It is unusual for cervical cancer to spread to distant organs but will sometimes involve liver, lungs, peritoneum (lining of the inner walls of the abdomen) and its lymph nodes, bone, and, rarely, lymph nodes above the clavicles (supraclavicular lymph nodes).

Prolonged survivals or even remissions in these later stages of cervical cancer are extremely difficult to obtain although other methods of treating these stages are being studied.

Therapeutic Modalities: As always the choice of the type of therapy or its combinations depends on the stage of the cancer, the age of and the health of the patient. In addition, because of the function of the uterus, the maintenance of reproductive ability can be important when cervical cancer occurs in women of child bearing age.

The earlier stages of disease—Stages 0 and I—can be cured with cryotherapy, Laser therapy, and conization surgery while preserving the child bearing potential in patients so inclined. These therapeutic choices in these early stages of cervical cancer are applicable and practical in 80% of cases. The remaining 20% of cases may choose hysterectomy because they have other gynecological problems present. But all patients in these two stages can be treated without hysterectomy.

In the subgroups Stages Ia and Ib—which have deeper invasion of the cancer—usually require some form of hysterectomy. In many of these cases radiation therapy is required in addition to surgery.

Stages IIb, IIIa, IIIb, IVa of cervical cancer require radiation administered via two radiation sources. One source is an external beam applied through the outer structures of the pelvis and abdomen. The second radiation source is an internal device which is temporarily inserted into the vaginal vault and later removed.

Stage IVb, the most advanced form of cervical cancer, is usually not amenable to radiation therapy or surgery. Many of these advanced stages of cervical cancer receive some chemotherapy for palliation. Unfortunately, no single chemotherapeutic agent or combinations of agents has been found very effective in this advanced stage of the disease but research in this area continues.

Management Team: There can be no doubt that the gynecologist should be the coordinator of the team for treating cancer of the cervix. Even during the brief period of the administration of radiation therapy the gynecologist is the most appropriate and best trained person to follow the response to treatment.

Of course, when surgery is part of the treatment plan the gynecological surgeon performs the operation with the assistance of others. Future examinations and regular periodic checkup's are best done by the gynecologist, where one is available. Where a gynecologist is not available a well trained and experienced family physician or the radiotherapist can perform the examinations.

In the rare instances of cervical cancer when chemotherapy is indicated for palliation the chemotherapist or medical oncologist should be in charge of the team. He provides the special techniques required to administer the chemotherapy and manages the side effects or complications.

Follow Up: Even in the early stages of cervical cancer in which a high cure rate can be expected, frequent and regularly scheduled repeat pelvic examinations must be performed. Occasional x-rays, and blood and urine tests are mandatory. The gynecologist originally involved in your case is the best professional person to perform the follow up exams but the family physician can also be involved.

Cancer of the Body of the Uterus: Cancer of the body of the uterus is more accurately called cancer of the internal lining of the uterus—or the endometrium. Endometrial cancer is the most frequently occurring form of gynecological cancer in mature American women.

Names and Synonyms: Cancer of the Uterus; Carcinoma of

the Uterus; Cancer of the Endometrium; Carcinoma of the Endometrium; Endometrial cancer; Endometrial Carcinoma. Sometimes the term "Cancer of the Female Organs " is erroneously applied to this condition as it is to cervical cancer. Since the 'female organs' are actually composed of many individual but interrelated structures the term is inaccurate and should be discarded because of the confusion it causes. If your physician uses this term ask him to specify the precise part of the organ system involved for the purpose of accuracy in reporting medical history.

Incidence Rates: Approximately 32,000 new cases of cancer of the endometrium occur each year in the U.S. Endometrial cancer will account for approximately 5,600 deaths in 1995. The incidence of this cancer has been steadily decreasing since the widespread use of estrogens has declined. Endometrial cancer occurs in about one of 1,000 women each year.

Causes and Risk Factors: As in the case of most cancers there is probably more than one cause of endometrial cancer. There are most likely a combination of causes rather than a single causative agent. But some clear and discernible risk factors have been elucidated. These risk factors include obesity, diabetes, high blood pressure (hypertension), infertility, irregular menstrual periods, menopause occurring after age 52, and the use of estrogens to treat menopause.

When menopause occurs after age 52 it is estimated that the risk of developing cancer of the endometrium increases three fold.

When multiple risk factors are combined the risk is even greater. For example when a woman has: weight gain beyond 15% of her ideal weight; late menopause and no pregnancies. When these factors are taken together the risk of cancer of the endometrium increases five fold.

When the use of estrogens to treat menopausal symptoms in women was very much in vogue—1960 to 1975—the incidence of endometrial cancer increased 91% in women aged 50 to 54. Since 1975 the incidence has been diminishing in parallel with the declining use of estrogens to treat menopause. However to put these statícts into proper perspective, only 1% of women taking estrogenic medication will develop endometrial cancer. Nevertheless, the female reader should be aware of these facts before deciding to use estrogens for postmenopausal symptoms.

For inapparent reasons endometrial cancer is found to be more common in Jewish women. However, endometrial cancer cannot be excluded as a cause for symptoms in any patient based simply on her race or ethnic background.

An increase in the estrogen naturally produced by the body is also considered part of the mechanism of developing endometrial cancer in woman who are at high risk. These factors which increase risk include: obesity; women with—cancer of the ovaries —which normally produce excess estrogen in all women; late menopause; and women who have not produced any children.

Signs and Symptoms: Vaginal bleeding which occurs in any woman after or during menopause should be considered to be due to endometrial cancer until proven otherwise. The production of a yellow or pink vaginal discharge should also be considered in the same light.

Although endometrial cancer has its highest incidence in postmenopausal women it must also be considered in younger women especially if they possess the other risk factors; i.e., obesity, hypertension, diabetes, Jewishness, etc. Statistical studies have shown that 25% of all cases of endometrial cancer are diagnosed in women before menopause (under age 52) and 5% of all cases occur under age 40. Other less common symptoms include pain in the pelvis during intercourse, with bowel movements, during urination or spontaneously. Low back pain is also a rare, nonspecific symptom of endometrial cancer.

Screening Tests: As discussed above under Cancer of the Cervix the annual pelvic exam and Pap smear are the best ways to screen large numbers of the female population. However, the complete history and physical examination are important for detecting the risk factors of hypertension, diabetes, infertility, etc. and must not be neglected.

There are some special maneuvers necessary, however, in screening for this cancer. In addition to scrapping cells from the cervix a sample of the cells shed by the internal lining of the uterus—the endometrium—must be obtained.

These cell samples may be obtained in a variety of ways in the screening process. Microscopic examination of the cells scrapped from the cervix or from the contents of the vagina or from the opening exiting from the uterus will uncover 50 to 75% of cases cancer of the endometrium. These methods are not infallible and more extensive sampling may be required in highly suspicious, high risk cases in which the simpler methods are not confirmatory. These are discussed further under the heading Diagnosis immediately below.

Diagnosis: As always, biopsy of the endometrial tissue provides the most precise method of establishing or ruling out endometrial cancer. There are two ways to obtain these biopsy samples of tissue.

The first method of biopsy can often be safely performed at an outpatient surgical suite. The endometrial biopsies are obtained by scrapping the lining of the uterus with small instruments called curettes (a spoon or scoop with a cutting edge). Local anesthesia is utilized to minimize the mild pain experienced during the procedure.

The most definitive method of biopsy is performed under general anesthesia so that more extensive sampling can be carried out. This procedure is called Fractional Dilatation and Curettage (D and C).

In certain rare instances—where the diagnosis of cancer has not been established but your physicians's suspicions are very high for malignancy—complete hysterectomy is often recommended for the sake of accuracy and for curative intent.

Staging Systems and Tests: Endometrial cancer has its stages named in a way similar to cancer of the cervix. That is, Stage 0 indicates in situ cancer with disease found only under the microscope. At the opposite end of the spectrum, Stage IVb is the most extensive disease which indicates that the endometrial cancer which has extended to distant organs outside the pelvis. All the stages in between 0 and IVb are determined by the degree of spread of disease within, or close to, the pelvis.

The tests recommended for complete staging include medical history and physical examination including a pelvic examination and Pap smear; and a fractional dilatation and curettage. The pelvic examination must be done meticulously to discover any local spread of disease to the vaginal structures.

Your physician may recommend routine examination of the bladder (cystoscopy); examination of the rectum and colon (barium enema contrast x-ray), and examination of the kidneys and its drainage system (the ureters) by x-ray examination (the pyelogram).

Optional tests include hysterography and hysteroscopy—to examine the interior of the uterus; lymphangiography to visualize the pelvic lymph nodes; and CT scanning of the uterus. However, the value of these tests as routine procedures is doubtful and debatable.

Surgical staging yields the most valuable and accurate information for determining; the stage, the best treatment options, and prognosis of your cancer. Surgery is the most accurate means of determining the depth of cancer growth into the muscular walls of the uterus; histological grade of the cancer; involvement of important structures like the cervix and endocervix; size of the uterus; involvement of the ovaries and fallopian tubes; the presence of cancer cells in the fluid in the abdomen (peritoneal fluid); involvement of the lymph nodes in and around the pelvis; and distant spread to liver and other intra-abdominal organs. All these findings can significantly alter the stage of the cancer and thus effect the cancer's prognosis.

Prognosis: The survival rate of endometrial cancer is dependent on the stage and the availability of modern therapeutic modalities in your local community. In the U.S. and other technically advanced nations the survival for Stage I endometrial cancer is as high as 90-95%. In some of the lesser developed countries it may be as low as 50-75%. Listed below are the 5 year survival rates for the other stages of endometrial cancer.

Stage II	50%
Stage III	27%
Stage IV	less than 10%

Sites of Spread: The recurrences of endometrial cancer usually occur locally within and around the pelvis to involve urinary bladder, rectum and anus, lymph nodes and other supportive structures within the pelvis. More distant spread might involve lymph nodes within the abdomen but outside the pelvis; and rarely more distant sites such as liver, kidneys, lungs, etc.

Treatment Modalities: Most cases of endometrial cancer are treated with surgery, radiation therapy or combinations of both. The therapy of choice for each stage is given below.

Stage Ia or Ib-total hysterectomy with removal of both ovaries.

Stage II - external beam and intracavitary radiation followed by total hysterectomy and removal of both ovaries.

Stage III and IV - these two stages are fortunately uncommon and the degree of surgery and radiation is individualized for each case. Chemotherapy is sometimes added in advanced cases. Radiation therapy alone is sometimes administered in advanced cases in which surgery is not indicated or is too dangerous to be carried out without a high mortality risk.

Chemotherapy in advanced cases of endometrial cancer has been disappointing with very little improvement of survival rate or prolongation of life. It has been useful in some cases for relief of symptoms and decreasing discomfort. Some of the chemotherapy agents presently utilized are: doxorubicin, cisplatinum, melphalan, 5-FU and combinations of these agents. These produce approximately a 25-35% response rate. Hormonal Therapy - Progestins and the anti-estrogen tamoxifen have been found to produce about 20% responses in endometrial cancer but for only short periods of time. These hormonal agents do have some value in palliation of distressful symptoms.

Follow Up Examinations: Repeat pelvic examinations every 6 months for the first two years seems prudent. Complete medical history, physical, pelvic exam, chest x-ray and blood tests are recommended at the same six month intervals.

Chapter 28

Cancer of the Ovary

Cancer of the ovary is a catchall term which actually consists of several cancer cell types and the terminology can be confusing. The statements given below apply to all the cell types which I have lumped together as a single group. It is estimated that these cancers will account for 4% of all female cancers in 1995 and for 5% of all cancer deaths in women in the same year.

Names and Synonyms: Cancer of the ovaries, ovarian cancer, carcinoma of the ovary, ovarian carcinoma, epithelial cancer of the ovary, adenocarcinoma of the ovary. There are also many cell types and substages of ovarian cancer each of which has its own designation.

Incidence Rates: It has been estimated that ovarian cancers will account for 4% of all female malignancies in 1995 and that it will cause 5% of the cancer deaths in women in the same year. These projections will total up to 21,000 new cases and almost 13,000 deaths.

Some types of ovarian cancers have a higher occurrence rate in industrialized countries such as the U.S.A. and Switzerland but are less common in Oriental and Latin American nations.

The overall cure rate for all types and stages of ovarian cancer is only 30% and the 5 year survival rate is only 40%.

Causes and Risk Factors: No definite causal relationships can be linked to the incidence of these ovarian cancers. But the ovary is indirectly exposed to the external environment through the fallopian tubes, uterus and vagina and is therefore subject to multiple infectious agents, chemicals and radiation.

Asbestos and talcum powder have been suspect when used as deodorant powders in the vaginal area.

Hormonal influences are also suspect as suggested by some clinical observations. Female readers who use oral contraceptive medications have a much lower risk of these ovarian cancers. Also, since ovarian cancer has its greatest occurrence rate right after menopause—when natural estrogen levels decline—this suggests a strong relation with hormonal substances. The observation that pregnancy seems to protect against these cancer of the ovary is noteworthy. Women readers who have had multiple pregnancies throughout their reproductive years have been found to have a lower incidence of ovarian cancers.

Signs and Symptoms: Unfortunately the location of the ovaries deep within the pelvis and their proximity to the highly mobile structures in the abdomen allows these cancers to grow to large size before symptoms appear. As a result over 70% of ovarian cancer patients present with advanced disease and usually report a 2 to 6 month history of vague abdominal fullness, bloating, early fullness after a partial meal, increasing abdominal girth, and sudden tightness of clothing.

Other late symptoms included shortness of breath due to (pleural) fluid in the chest and fluid (ascites) in the abdomen. In very advanced cases the abdomen may appear so large that the patient will present with a visibly enlarged abdominal tumor mass. Younger female patients will erroneously believe they are pregnant.

Physical examination of the abdomen and the pelvic examination will usually reveal the presence of an ovarian mass and this finding suggests ovarian cancer in a female in the right age group.

In women in the reproductive age group it is acceptable for your doctor to continue to examine you through two menstrual cycles before pursuing the possibility of cancer with other tests. Since some of the tests used to diagnosis ovarian cancer include x-rays which could damage an unborn fetus it is particularly important to be cautious.

Screening Tests: The pelvic examination and the routine Pap smear remain the most reliable and practical means of screening large populations of women for ovarian cancer. Sadly, there is not presently available any practical and reliable blood test or x-ray for detecting these cancers.

The recently developed ovarian cancer blood test called the CA-125 is best used to follow the course of diagnosed cases. Its use as a tool for screening high risk population groups is still to be determined. Transvaginal and external pelvic ultrasound examinations are also under study for use as screening tests.

Diagnosis: The definitive diagnosis of ovarian cancer is usually made by the pathologist after the surgical removal of a suspicious mass from the pelvis and abdomen. The main dilemma for your physician arises in trying to decide if surgery is indicated at all. The tests discussed below can help your physician make that decision.

Pap smear from the contents of the vagina and cervix will in some cases reveal the presence of cancerous cells suggestive of cancer of the ovary.

Culdocentesis is a method of removing a small amount of fluid from between the back wall of the uterus and the abdominal wall. If this fluid contains cancer cells and can be detected under the microscope it supports the need for exploratory surgery.

Any female found to have a large amount of fluid in the abdomen (ascites)—which can sometimes be demonstrated by x-ray or ultrasound—can have the fluid aspirated through a needle and the fluid can be examined for cancer cells. The same approach applies in the female patient who has excess fluid in the space between the lung and chest wall, called pleural fluid. Free fluid in this anatomic space can be easily detected by routine chest x-ray.

Laparoscopy is the insertion of an instrument into the abdominal cavity through which the physician can visually examine any suspicious areas of the female genital tract and biopsy them through the instrument to establish the diagnosis. This procedure can also help to determine if further surgery is necessary.

As always the basic requirement of obtaining cells or tissue by biopsy must be achieved in order to establish a diagnosis of cancer.

Staging Systems and Tests: Cancers of the ovary are staged by anatomic involvement as discussed under previous types of cancer and by histological (cell) type.

Histologic or cell type is an expression of the kind of cancer cells which are seen under the microscope. These cell types are divided into three major groups which are named according to the part of the ovarian tissue from which they arise; (1) the epithelial surface, (2) the sex cord-stromal cells, and (3) the germ cell layers. There are several cellular subtypes under each of these categories which results in more than 25 different types of ovarian cancer. These categories and subcategories are very complex and technical and are not necessary information for the readers to understand their cancer. The categories are, however, very important in helping the physician determine the best treatment plan and the prognosis for the ovarian cancer.

The anatomical staging system takes into consideration the extent of disease according to anatomic regions found to be involved with the cancer. In general, Stage I ovarian cancer is limited to the ovaries; Stage II disease extends to other gynecologic organs within the pelvis such as uterus and fallopian tubes; Stage III disease refers to involvement outside of the pelvis but still within the abdomen but below the diaphragm; Stage IV disease indicates spread to major organs such as liver, surfaces covering the lungs (pleural effusion), the bones, the lungs themselves, and lymph nodes outside the abdomen.

The following tests are required for complete staging of ovarian cancer. By and large the greatest amount of staging information is obtained when your physician performs surgical removal of the cancerous ovary(ies) and visually examines all the pelvic and abdominal organs She will then take a biopsy of certain organs and any other obviously diseased structures.

Many other tests are required, however, before performing major surgery. The comprehensive and detailed history and physical examination including the pelvic exam and Pap smear are a must. The chest x-ray, complete blood count (CBC), organ chemistries (Chemistry Profile), CEA, CA-125, and urine analysis are standard.

Other tests might be indicated in special clinical circumstances. Barium enema, small bowel series, upper G.I. series, proctoscopic examination may be needed to rule involvement of the gastrointestinal tract. Assessment of the urinary tract and kidneys (IVP) may be performed when indicated by symptoms or other abnormal tests.

Ultrasound of the abdomen and pelvis may be performed before surgery to assess other structures which your physician suspects may be involved.

Removal of pleural fluid by needle aspiration (thoracentesis), or removal of abdominal fluid (paracentesis) may be required before surgery if the fluid is detected by x-ray or ultrasound examination.

Laparoscopy and biopsy, as mentioned above, are helpful to determine if surgery is necessary.

Less often, lymphangiography is indicated to assess the status of abdominal and pelvic lymph nodes prior to surgery.

As stated above, complete staging at the time of surgery is the most accurate method of determining the extent of disease. However, some very special maneuvers must be done by your physician during the surgical procedure. These include; careful visual examination of the surface lining of the abdomen (the peritoneum), all the structures within the abdomen and pelvis—such as the diaphragms, liver, spleen, intestines, mesentery, and all the lymph nodes therein; as well as all pelvic structures—the other ovary, the uterus, the fallopian tubes, the urinary bladder, the rectum, etc. In addition, if any of these appear abnormal they must be biopsied to verify any cancerous involvement. If any free fluid is present in the abdomen it is removed and examined for cancer cells. If no free fluid is present the abdominal cavity is washed with a sterile salt solution (saline) and examined for cancer cells.

In many cases these maneuvers drastically change the stage of what appears to be limited disease when biopsy reports return after the completion of surgery. To emphasize the point about 56% of cases of ovarian cancer thought to be in Stages I and II are found to actual be in Stage III after pathological examination of organs which initially appeared to be normal organs at surgery.

Prognosis: The overall cure rate for ovarian cancer is about 30% for all stages and types of ovarian cancers. The overall 5 year survival rate is about 40%. Of course, the stage and the cell type ultimately determine the prognosis for individual cases, as listed below:

Stage I	40-82% 5 year survival rate
Stage II	17-53% 5 year survival rate
Stages III & IV	0-30% 5 year survival rate

Sites of Spread: All the possible sites of spread or metastases of ovarian cancer have already been mentioned in the discussion given above and need no further dissertation at this point.

Therapeutic Modalities: Because the group of ovarian cancers is so complex and subtyped and subgrouped it is not possible to give a detailed outline of all the treatment options for each type and stage. Each case must be managed according to its own characteristics and the choices of the treatment team. As usual, your physician must discuss and describe these treatment options with the reader before a final decision is made.

Surgery: Generally speaking, however, extensive surgery is not always necessary in ovarian cancer. But some surgery is nearly always indicated if for no other reason than to accomplish accurate staging; to clearly establish a diagnosis; and to reduce the bulk of the cancer which is present. Also, there is nearly always a combined treatment modality plan used which involves radiation and/or chemotherapy before or after surgery.

The primary goal of surgery, in addition to staging, is to remove all organs known or suspected of being involved by ovarian cancer when this is feasible. Such surgery usually includes removal of both ovaries, the uterus and the fallopian tubes (panhysterectomy), the omentum(the fatty apron hanging over the intestines), the lymph nodes around the pelvic area and certain select (peri-aortic) lymph nodes in the abdomen.

Below is a table of the generally recommended therapeutic program for each of the larger staging groups of ovarian cancer. However, there are individual special cases which may require 'custom tailored' therapy plans.

Stages I & II	Panhysterectomy followed by external beam and/or chemotherapy in select subgroups
Stage III	Panhysterectomy followed by external beam and/or single agent or triple agent chemotherapy
Stage IV	Panhysterectomy, external beam chemotherapy and specialized therapy based on type of distant spread (see below).

Special types of therapy, in addition to those given above, is often necessary for selected types of disseminated ovarian cancer. For example, when chest (pleural) fluid is present it is necessary to aspirate the fluid from the pleural space and then insert radioactive chemicals or chemotherapy chemicals into the space to prevent the re-accumulation of the fluid. The same type of local drug instillation therapy may be needed in the case of abdominal fluid (ascites).

It is becoming more common place in cancer research centers to check on the results of therapy to try to confirm apparent cure of ovarian cancer by so called "second look" surgery. In this second look surgery the abdomen is reexamined by the naked eye and select biopsies taken because of the inability of x-rays and other tests to reliably detect small amounts of residual or recurrent ovarian cancer.

Chemotherapy and radiation therapy are frequently given after surgery for known residual ovarian cancer. They are also commonly used in cases of suspected residual disease or in those advanced stages where the likelihood of recurrence is great—so called prophylactic or adjuvant therapy.

Many chemotherapy agents have been effectively used in treating ovarian cancer and have resulted in some rare cures. The more commonly chemotherapy used agents, given either alone or in combination, include: melphalan (Alkeran®), nitrogen mustard, chlorambucil (Leukeran®), cyclophosphamide (Cytoxan®), cis-platinum (Platinol®), carboplatin, etoposide, ifosfamide, doxorubicin (Adriamycin®), hexamethylmelamine, 5-fluorouracil, and other newer agents. Some of these agents are used in tablet form, some in injectable form, some as single agents, and some in combination. The chemotherapist should discuss these options with the reader as well as their side effects, their therapeutic/toxic ratio and the chances of responding before starting therapy.

Many new and experimental therapeutic modalities are presently under study and hold significant promise of effectiveness in treating ovarian cancer. Hormonal therapy is being investigated with agents such as tamoxifen (Nolvadex), progesterone (Megace) and combinations of these two in alternating sequences. Immunotherapy, biological response modifiers and monoclonal antibodies are also under investigation.

Among the newest endeavors to improve survival in far advanced and locally recurrent disease is the technique of adjuvant (see glossary) chemotherapy. In this technique chemotherapy agents such as cis-platinum or doxorubicin are inserted directly into the abdominal cavity so that the cancerous tissue comes in direct, close contact with the chemotherapy agent for an extended period of time. This procedure has produced palliation in some cases and holds much promise as an additional treatment modality. There is, as yet however, no unequivocal evidence that adjuvant chemotherapy has produced any cures or prolongation of survival.

Management Team: All of the usual medical and paramedical members of the team should be involved in the management of ovarian cancer. The leader of the team is undoubtedly the gynecologist, and preferably the oncologic gynecologist, where one is available. The team leadership may shift, temporarily, based on the type of therapy being administered at the time, i.e., the chemotherapist, the radiation, and so on.

Special consideration must be given to the cases of ovarian cancer in younger patients who are still in the reproductive years. Your physician must discuss with the reader the possibility of conserving the uterus, and one ovary and tube in order to retain the ability to reproduce children, if the reader so desires. Preserving the reproductive function of the patient may not always be possible or feasible because of the advanced stage of the ovarian cancer . When it is a consideration an obstetrician should also be a member of the management team.

Follow Up: As in most gynecological cancers regular periodic pelvic examinations and Pap smears are needed in follow up for the remainder of the ovarian cancer patient's life. In addition, the comprehensive history and physical examination, selected x-rays, scans, ultrasounds of the pelvis and abdomen, blood and urine tests are required on annual basis. Such follow up examinations can be accomplished solely by the gynecologist or with the assistance of a general internist or family physician, if the gynecologist and the patient are so inclined.

Chapter 29

Cancer of the Urinary Bladder

Cancer of the urinary bladder is the most common cancer of the urinary tract. In 1995 it is expected to occur anew in over 51,600 Americans of both sexes and cause almost 9500 deaths. Although the urinary bladder is an internal organ it is still one of the most easily assessed via the urine analysis, and one the most accessible via the cystoscope. For these reasons it is possible to detect more cases of bladder cancer in an earlier, curable stage.

Names and Synonyms: Carcinoma of the urinary bladder; Bladder cancer; Transitional Cell cancer of the bladder; papillary carcinoma of the bladder; adenocarcinoma of the bladder; squamous cell carcinoma of the bladder.

These different designations actually refer to the variety of cell types of bladder cancer in which Transitional cell type is the most common.

Incidence Rates: These bladder cancers are expected, in 1995, to account for 10% of all cancers in males and for 4% of all cancers in females. It will account for 5% of cancer deaths in men and 3% of deaths in women. Most alarming is the fact that the number of cases of bladder cancer and deaths caused by it appears to be on the increase with 37,000 cases diagnosed in 1982 and 51,600 cases which will be diagnosed in 1995. These changes may be partly related to the rising use of tobacco smoking especially in women.

Bladder cancers are most common in the 50-70 year age group although no age group is immune. It occurs more often in males as compared to females in a ratio of 2:1.

Causes and Risk Factors: As with other kinds of cancer a clear and direct causative agent has not been identified but the following agents are associated with a greater risk of developing bladder cancer.

The aniline dyes which are used in the rubber and cable industries appear to increase the risk in those workers so exposed. It apparently takes a long period of time to develop bladder cancer during exposure to these chemicals—6 to 20 years.

Tobacco tar, ß-naphthylamine, and 4-amino diphenyl are chemicals which are known to cause cancers in animals. Therefore, use of tobacco whether smoked, chewed or used in any other way appears to increase the risk of bladder cancer in humans. Large population studies have supported this contention linking cigarette smoking and bladder cancer.

Chronic infections of the bladder and chronic bladder stones may also increase the risk of developing bladder cancer.

Signs and Symptoms: The passage of grossly visible, bright red blood in the urine (hematuria) is the initial symptom in at least 75% of cases of bladder cancer which is the reason its appearance must always be investigated. The finding of microscopic blood—as opposed to gross blood—can also be detected by urine analysis in most cases of bladder cancer.

Unfortunately, the bleeding is intermittent in most cases of bladder cancer. Often, however, the patient delays seeking medical attention for a considerable length of time because of the intermittency.

Difficulty or painful urination with frequent irritability of the bladder occurs in about 1/3 of cases of bladder cancer.

Unfortunately, no ideal screening test exists, other than the routine urine analysis as done in most doctor's offices. The routine, periodic examination of the urine for cancer cells is recommended, however, in workers regularly exposed to the carcinogenic chemicals listed above.

Diagnosis: Direct visual examination of the urinary bladder with biopsy of suspicious areas of abnormal appearance establishes the diagnosis in the vast majority of cases of bladder cancer.

Staging Systems and Tests: The stages of bladder cancer are established through determination of the extent of disease and designated as follows:

Stage 0 Cancer is confined to the superficial, internal lining of the bladder (in situ)

Stage A Confined to the second deepest layer (submucosa) of the bladder lining

Stage B Invasion into the third (muscular) layer of the bladder lining

- **B1** superficial invasion of the lining
- **B2** deeper invasion of the lining

Stage C Extension into the outer most and deepest layer (serosa and fat layer) of the bladder

Stage D Spread beyond the bladder completely

- **D1** Spread to lymph nodes in the lower half of the abdomen
- **D2** Involvement of lymph nodes in the upper half of the abdomen and/or distant organs.

Other tests generally recommended for staging of bladder cancer are: comprehensive history and physical examination, urine analysis—especially for microscopic blood; pelvic CT scan to detect involved lymph nodes; blood tests of liver and kidney function, chest x-ray; cystoscopic examination and biopsy; IVP to assess integrity of the remainder of the urinary tract; bone x-rays and/or scans; and, when indicated, scans of the liver and other organs suspected of being involved with the bladder cancer.

Surgical staging to visually examine all the internal and pelvic structures mentioned above is the most crucial part of the staging process.

Prognosis: When treatments are combined to include removal of the bladder surgically (cystectomy) and radiation therapy are utilized the results are given below by stage of disease—as 5 year survival rates.

Stages 0, A, B1	12 to 80%
Stages B2, C	7 to 36%
Stage D	0 to 12%

The 5 year survival for all stages combined is in the range of 6 to 43%. If, and when, relapse of bladder cancer occurs in 90% of the cases it recurs within 50 months after initial treatment. And in 50% of the cases it recurs within 12 months of the initial diagnosis and treatment.

Sites of Spread: The most common form of recurrence is locally within the bladder itself if total cystectomy has not been performed. If no bladder tissue remains after total cystectomy the recurrence appears in neighboring structures within the pelvis and abdomen such as; the rectum, colon, lymph nodes and pelvic bones. Distant spreads is very uncommon.

Therapeutic Modalities: Generally speaking, the more aggressive and deeply penetrating the stage of the bladder cancer the more aggressive and extensive must be the therapy scheme. The following factors will influence the choice of treatment: the exact location of the cancer within the bladder; general health of the patient; associated diseases of the intestinal tract or urinary tract; the patient's ability to manage any of the artificial systems which are used to function in place of the removed bladder; previous recurrence rate of the patient's bladder cancer; and the training and experience of the surgeon.

Surgery: Several forms of surgical therapy are available for bladder cancer and are listed below beginning with the simplest method to the more aggressive schema.

1. Endoscopic surgery in this procedure the most superficial cancers are removed, under direct visualization through an instrument inserted into the bladder. The visible cancers are removed either by sharp excision or electrical cautery-type removal (fulguration).

2. Cystotomy--a surgical procedure done by opening the bladder to remove large, multiple, superficial cancers and for better control of

any active bleeding.

3. Segmental resection—is a procedure designed for the excision of the part of the bladder containing the large cancer but enough bladder structure is left in place to function as a normal urinary reservoir.

4. Total cystectomy—is the surgical removal of the entire bladder along with the cancer contained therein. This radical procedure is indicated when the cancer is deeply invasive, highly malignant, and has invaded most of the bladder including especially a section called the trigone. But the patient must have a good life expectancy with no distant spread of cancer and no other major life threatening illnesses to warrant this radical operation.

Of course, with removal of the entire bladder some other surgical procedure is required to form another artificial reservoir for the storage of urine. This can be accomplished in one of four ways: 1) the use of a segment of small bowel (ileum) or ileal loop to act as an external reservoir; 2) the use of a section of large bowel (colon) as reservoir; 3) the use of a section of rectum and 4) by simply allowing the urine to drain through the abdominal wall and into a plastic bag or other external receptacle. These surgical procedures are collectively called urinary diversion operations. They require a great deal of care for the new reservoir on the part of the patient.

Radiation Therapy: There is a great deal of research evidence that the survival rate is much better when radiation therapy is combined with surgery for bladder cancer. It may be administered before or after surgery depending on the stage of the bladder cancer.

The following table indicates the best choice of therapy based on the stage of the bladder cancer.

Stage 0, A, B1	Radiation therapy only after surgical therapy, and chemotherapy have failed to control the cancer
Stage B2 or C	Pre-operative Radiation therapy followed by surgical removal of the bladder
Stage D	Radiation Therapy used only as a measure to control pain or bleeding.

Chemotherapy has been very useful in cases of recurrent bladder cancer and in controlling distant spread. Unfortunately, no chemotherapy regimen has yet been found to increase the cure rate or to prolong the duration of survival. The chemotherapy agents most often used in bladder cancer include methotrexate, 5-FU, doxorubicin (Adriamycin®), cyclophosphamide, mitomycin C, cis-platinum, vincristine. Each can be used either alone or in combination.

These agents can be given systemically—by direct injection into the circulation, or topically by insertion into the bladder through a catheter.

A specific intravenous combination of methotrexate, vincristine, Adriamycin and cis-platinum (M-VAC) has been found to be especially effective.

In the topical method of treatment the chemical agent is inserted directly into the bladder through a catheter in order for the agent to directly bathe the cancer and kill the cancer cells. The topical method has been found very useful in local recurrences of bladder cancer. At least nine different agents have been studied for use in this way and have been found effective in treating superficial recurrences of bladder cancer.

Very recent studies have shown that immunotherapy agents or biological response modifiers can be applied topically into the bladder to control this cancer. These agents include the well known agent interferon, and the less well known but equally effective agent BCG vaccine which was initially used as a vaccine against Tuberculosis.

Naturally, there are investigational studies now in progress to determine if using all these agents sequentially or simultaneously will improve the cure rate or prolong the survival rate of bladder cancer.

Management Team: There can be no doubt that the 'quarterback' of this team throughout the course of the management is the Urologist. Of course, the urologist needs the assistance of the radiation oncologist and the medical oncologist when the different treatment modalities are being administered. Nevertheless, the urologist should remain in contact with and be available to the patient throughout the treatment period. The urologist is most suited to perform follow up examinations on the urinary bladder via cystoscopy to monitor the results of therapy and watch for local recurrences of the bladder cancer.

Follow Up: Periodic cystoscopic examinations are a must to watch for the early appearance of local and regional recurrences of bladder cancer. In addition, many urologists personally perform their own urine analysis and examine the urine specimen microscopically for the reappearance of microscopic blood. They also send a urine sample to the pathologist to be microscopically examined for cancer cells. The standard complete annual history, physical examination, routine blood tests and x-rays are also necessary.

Chapter 30

The Leukemias and the Lymphomas

Leukemias and lymphomas are a large, diverse group of cancers which are usually lumped together because they are considered to arise from the blood and blood forming organs and are called "Hematological Malignancies." This is a misnomer but it is useful for purposes of classification and discussion. However, in this section they are discussed in two separate groups for the sake of facility and ease of discussion.

As a group, leukemias and lymphomas constitute the most extensively studied and researched types of cancers. The large body of knowledge, the great variety of therapeutic choices, the complex mixture of the groupings and subgroupings, and the high rate of curability of these cancers has caused them to serve as the prototype for research teams investigating all other malignancies. The triumphs accomplished for this group of malignancies exemplifies the principle that the greater our understanding of a malady or group of maladies the greater will be our ability to affect cures. As a group they have acted as a springboard which has encouraged and inspired researchers and clinicians alike to pursue more enthusiastically the treatment and eventual cure of all other malignancies. The earliest and most frequent 'true cures' of any type of cancers have occurred in this group.

Occurrence Rates: In 1995 this collection of malignancies of the blood and blood forming organs will account for 9% of all cancers in males and 7% of all cancers in females. It will produce 9% of cancer deaths in men and 9% of the deaths from cancers in women. They will result in 60,900 cancer cases and 30,100 cancer deaths in 1995.

The Lymphomas: The lymphomas are a group of cancers which *originate* in the lymph nodes and lymph-like organs (such as the spleen). They are to be distinguish from other cancers which *spread* to the lymph nodes as opposed to this group which starts and has its primary origin of growth in the lymph nodes. The suffix -oma is, of course, a misnomer and a confusing one since all these cancers are malignant (see section on definition of terms).

Name and Synonyms: The Lymphomas were originally divided into three simple categories until an explosion of knowledge in research resulted in the recognition of literally dozens of groups and subgroups. The two major groups are currently called, A) the Hodgkin's Lymphomas and, B) the Non-Hodgkin's lymphomas. The nomenclature and subtypes of this group of malignancies can be very confusing and disorienting to the layman. An attempt is made to over-simplify and clarify its classification for the sake of discussion. Again, one need not have all this information to have the most basic questions answered regarding the treatment and cure of this kind of cancer.

(A) The Hodgkin's Lymphomas—also known as Hodgkin's disease is divided into 4 major cell types: the lymphocyte predominant; the nodular sclerosing; the mixed cellularity; and lymphocyte depleted group. The various stages and substages are discussed very shortly.

Incidence Rates: Hodgkin's lymphoma will account for 40% of all malignant lymphomas in 1995. There will be over 7400 new cases each year and it will account for approximately 1500 deaths each year. There will be 4200 cases in females and 3200 cases in males. The male affected with this malignancy will have a slightly poorer survival rate than the females. As one can see its one of the least common malignancies. Fifty per cent of the cases occur between the ages of 20 and 40. Less than 10% of cases have their onset after the age of 60 and another 10% or less before the age of 10.

Causes and Risk Factors: Because of some clinical features of the Hodgkin's lymphoma suggest an infectious illness—such as fever, chills and increased white blood count—a viral agents has been suspected as a cause for Hodgkin's Disease for many years. A close relationship with an agent known as the Epstein-Barr virus (a herpes-like virus) has been investigated intensely. However, although some patients with Hodgkin's disease do have increased antibody levels against the Epstein-Barr virus a direct causative association has not been proven. The report of some so called 'clusters' of Hodgkin's disease in closely associated groups of people have implied that social contact within these groups has led to increase risk of the disease but this has not been proven.

Since many Hodgkin's disease patients demonstrate a decreased immunity—as measured by blood tests for immunity and by their increased susceptibility to infection—some researchers have felt that the compromised immunity is the cause of the disease. An attractive theory but one not yet proved.

Signs and Symptoms and Screening Tests: In over 90% of cases of Hodgkin's the patient reports with the self-discovery of an enlarged, painless lymph node in the neck (80%) or in the armpit. The swollen lymph node may be accompanied by fever, chills, weight loss, night sweats, itching of the skin (pruritus), fatigue and a general rundown feeling (malaise). However, many other diseases, both minor and serious, may also have exactly these same presenting symptoms and same physical findings. In fact, most cases with this group of findings will not have lymphoma but some other minor infectious condition. Patients with simple viral throat infections have these same signs and symptoms. No ideal screening test has been discovered for mass surveillance of the population.

On physical examination several findings increase the physician's suspicion of lymphoma. These findings include the simultaneous presence of several other enlarged lymph nodes in the same anatomic vicinity, or in other distant lymph node areas such as the groin, axillae, elbow and abdomen. There may also be found enlargement of the liver and spleen which also increase suspicion.

Diagnosis: The diagnosis can only be established by surgical removal of an abnormal lymph node and its examination under the microscope. Some other tests help to increase or decrease the suspicion of Hodgkin's disease but do not replace the biopsy. The white blood count may be increased, there may be anemia, elevation of certain liver tests, the serum copper may be high, and the red blood cell sedimentation rate may by rapid. All of these only heighten the physician's suspicions but they prove nothing. Biopsy is still mandatory.

The only debatable question regarding the biopsy is the site from which the lymph node is excised. There are literally thousands of lymph nodes scattered throughout the body and any one or all of them may contain the disease. However, the choice of biopsy site is based on the most obviously diseased node and the largest one, and on the ease and safety of its removal. The safest nodes are those which can be removed without major surgery as might be required by abdominal surgery or chest surgery. Therefore, lymph nodes in the neck(cervical), just above the clavicles (supraclavicular), just above the elbow (epitrochlear), in the armpits (axillary) and in the groin (inguinal or femoral) are the easiest to remove. The choice, if all these areas have enlarged nodes, is based on those most likely to give a clear cut answer. They are, in the order of decreasing positive yield, the cervical, supraclavicular, axillary, epitrochlear, inguinal and femoral lymph nodes.

On occasion the lymph nodes which are more difficult to remove are the only choice because they are the only ones which are enlarged. These difficult nodes to reach include lymph nodes within the chest cavity (mediastinal, hilar, etc.), or within the abdominal cavity (mesenteric, omental, peri-aortic, etc.), or other intra-abdominal structures (liver, spleen, stomach, small intestine, etc.)

Staging Systems and Tests: Hodgkin's disease has served as the major prototype for staging of cancers. Hodgkin's disease research has demonstrated clearly the advantages and usefulness of a staging system in determining the best treatment and prognosis of any cancer. It was one of the first cancers extensively studied to divide groups of patients into subgroups to improve the accuracy of diagnosis, to customize the treatment plan and validate the results of treatment through meticulous restaging at the completion of a treatment course. The management plan of many other cancers have been modeled after that of Hodgkin's disease.

The clinical stages of Hodgkin's Lymphoma with their definitions are tabulated below.

Stage I	Single lymph node region involved.
Stage II	Two lymph nodes regions involved; both regions are above the diaphragm
Stage III	Two or more lymph node regions but they are above and below the diaphragm.
Stage IV	Extensive involvement of lymph nodes and other organs such as liver, bone, etc.
A & B	all stages are subdivided into A) *without* fever, weight loss, sweats or B) *with* fever, weight 1 loss, sweats.

For example, a patient with one involved lymph node in the neck and one in the abdomen, with fever, and weight loss is classified in Stage IIIB.

A second additional method of staging called histology or cell type—the description of the cellular structure of the Hodgkin's disease lymph node under the microscope—has added greater accuracy in treatment and prognosis. The four histological types of Hodgkin's Disease are: the lymphocyte predominant; the nodular sclerosing; the mixed cellularity; and the lymphocyte depleted.

The procedures recommended for accurate and complete staging of Hodgkin's disease are: the standard complete history and physical examination; complete blood count, liver and other internal organ chemistries, sedimentation rate; and bone marrow biopsy. An additional word about bone marrow biopsy seems appropriate here. The procedure is usually performed after confirmation of the diagnosis by lymph node biopsy and is mandatory before starting any treatment or before pursuing more extensive surgery, such as exploratory chest or abdominal surgery.

Certain x-ray examinations are also required for staging Hodgkin's disease. They are: chest x-ray with CT scan of the organs within the chest; lymphangiography to detect disease in any lymph nodes within the abdomen; CT scan of abdomen, liver spleen and pelvis. In special situations some unusual tests are required for staging such as; abdominal ultrasound, Gallium scanning, bone scans and bone x-rays.

Exploratory abdominal surgery (laparotomy) is a major staging operation and requires some detailed discussion. It is generally recommended that all Hodgkin's disease patients under age 40 who do not have any other serious diseases have their internal organs examined by the naked eye of the surgeon. At the same time the surgeon performs extensive biopsy of liver and lymph nodes, and the spleen is completely removed (splenectomy). The bone marrow biopsy is done before exploratory surgery to expressly avoid the laparotomy which is unnecessary if the bone marrow contains Hodgkin's Disease. Because if the bone marrow is positive for Hodgkin's Disease the case is automatically in stage IV and no useful purpose is served by the laparotomy.

The reason laparotomy is considered necessary for accurate staging is that the other methods for detecting intra-abdominal Hodgkin's disease have a large margin of error. This margin of error can adversely affect the choice of treatment and the accurate prognostication of the disease. There is now some disagreement among medical researchers of Hodgkin's disease regarding this dictum.

Of course, every effort is made to accurately stage the patient without abdominal or chest surgery whenever possible.

Prognosis: In the earlier stages of Hodgkin's disease (Stages I and II), and with the best histological cell type a 90% 'true cure' rate can be realistically expected with appropriate treatment. Even the more advanced stages of disease (stages II through stages IV A & B) can expect a high degree of long range survival.

The five year survival rate for all stages of Hodgkin's disease has demonstrated one of the most dramatic improvements in the last two decades. It has risen from 40% in 1963 to 75-85% in 1995. These astonishing accomplishments are a powerful testimonial for the improvement of life expectancy through classical scientific methods and the concerted efforts of traditional research. And there is every indication that further research and development of new therapies will continue to improve survival and increase cure rates in this and other forms of cancer.

Sites of Spread: It is the relatively predictable path of spread of Hodgkin's disease which has made the study of its natural course so amenable to the scientific method. Generally speaking, the path of spread is from one lymph node region to one of its 'upstream' or 'downstream' neighbors. As a result, a patient with a Hodgkin's disease lymph node in the left side of the neck is likely to later develop disease in the left supraclavicular (collar bone) nodes, left axillary nodes and nodes in the left side of the chest, and so on. Because of this predictable sequential spread, radiation therapy applied simultaneously to areas known to be involved and neighboring areas of likely involvement later has produce a high cure rate of Hodgkin's disease.

The other likely areas of spread of Hodgkin's disease coincide with those areas and organs which are examined during the staging process. These are the major lymph node regions—including the spleen—already discussed, and the other non-lymph node (extralymphatic) organs and structures, such as: liver, bone, bone marrow, stomach, small intestine, lungs, and rarely the testicles, the kidneys, the brain and its coverings (the meninges), the heart, the eyes, the skin, etc.

Therapeutic Modalities: The therapeutic principles and its triumphs over Hodgkin's disease have encouraged many researchers to continue to pursue the cure of other cancers with renewed hope and vigor. And this increased effort has resulted in much improvement in cure rates and survival times in many other types of cancer.

Surgical Therapy: Surgery is seldom used alone for the *therapy* of Hodgkin's disease today. In former times surgery was commonly used to remove as many diseased lymph nodes as possible. It eventually became apparent that this approach seldom produced any cures, or even any prolongation of survival. Currently surgery is used primarily for diagnostic and staging purposes. Surgery is frequently used to relieve life-threatening or very discomforting symptoms. Such surgery is often performed to relieve some kind of physical compression of an organ or blockage of the circulation by a enlarged Hodgkin's disease lymph node. It is also used in clinical staging such as the exploratory laparotomy as discussed above.

Radiation Therapy : Radiotherapy is the primary form of therapy for most cases of localized Hodgkin's disease i.e., stages I, II and some cases of IIIA disease. However, some special techniques are required to produce a cure. The first special technique modification is the use of modern radiation therapy equipment called, *megavoltage radiation.* The second modification is the application of the radiation to extended lymph node fields based on the predictability of the pathway of Hodgkin's disease mode of spread. Also, relatively high total radiation doses are given which were unthinkable in former days with older, less sophisticated equipment. Radiation therapy can by itself produce 90% cures in stage IA disease; 70% cures in stage IIA; and 40% cures in stage IIIA Hodgkin's disease.

Chemotherapy: One of the greatest advances and least heralded developments in chemotherapy was first applied successfully in Hodgkin's disease and has acted as a prototype for therapeutic approaches to other cancers. The administration of multiple drugs given simultaneously, and the use of relatively large doses of drugs given intermittently—with frequent long rest periods without therapy—has resulted in fewer serious side-effects, marked improvement in remission rates, and higher cure rates.

Usually a combination of chemotherapy agents with different toxicities are given by injection and by mouth twice a month for 6 to 12 months. The combinations utilized are often designated by an acronym to shorten the cumbersome communication of many long drug names and to reduce the staggering amount of paperwork required. The earliest and most common combination and its acronyms is: MOPP or nitrogen mustard, Oncovin® (Vincristine); Prednisone; procarbazine. The first two agents are given by intravenous injection twice a month and the last two agents are given by mouth for the first 14 days of each cycle. Each cycle is 28 days in length followed by no therapy—the rest period—for the last 14 days of each cycle. Each cycle is repeated for 6 to 12 times. This combination and many others like it have produced many excellent and sustained remissions, and possibly some 'true cures,' in far advanced stages of Hodgkin's disease such as stage IIIB, IVA and IVB.

Some other drugs and combinations used are: cyclophosphamide, CCNU, BCNU, vinblastine, doxorubicin, bleomycin, methotrexate, DTIC, and now the newer agents; cisplatin, etoposide, etc. Biological response modifiers such as Interferon and Interleukin 2 have shown some utility for relapsed or previously unresponsive Hodgkin's disease but are still under investigation.

The most common and troublesome side effects of these chemotherapy agents include: hair loss (alopecia); decrease in white blood counts, red blood counts and platelet counts; decreased immunity and increased risk of serious infections; nausea and vomiting; diarrhea; and fatigue. Most of these side effects are temporary and manageable with other medications. These chemotherapy drug combinations have resulted in up to 70% five-year survivals and as much as 58% of ten-year survivals. As many as three-fourths of the patients with complete remission go on to complete cures.

Management Team: The structure of the management team and its chairman vary with the stage of disease but a medical oncologist should always be involved since the application of adjuvant (prophylactic) therapy after radiation therapy is commonly required. Also, a specialist with a high degree of expertise and long experience with these types of cancers is the best physician to follow the patient with frequent subsequent physical examinations and yearly restaging procedures.

During radiation therapy the radiation oncologist is the best trained person for applying the radiation and observing the patient for complications and side effects of this therapy.

Follow Up: Frequent follow up office visits are required to detect any new disease or relapses in previously treated areas. The highest number of recurrences occur within the first two years after diagnosis and treatment. At least monthly visits are required in the first 6 to 12 months and no less than every two months in the second year. Most patients will require complete history and physical examinations annually in addition to repeat blood tests, x-rays and scans. But long term follow up for at least 5 years after therapy, and as much as 10 years after remission, is needed because late relapses can and do occur after the 5 year period. Frequent periodic examination is especially important since the early treatment of any recurrences can still result in a cure with appropriate treatments which are still being discovered. Some experts on the lymphomas feel that all Hodgkin's disease patients should maintain regular contact with their physician for the remainder of their lives.

(B) The Non-Hodgkin's Lymphomas: There is frequently a good deal of confusion in the terminology used in naming the lymphomas. The appellation of Non-Hodgkin's Lymphoma (NHL) is a prime example. However, if you remember that the precise name of the cancer is not important for the reader to be fully informed about their cancer there is much less apprehension about terminology.. But for the sake of clarity the following explanation is offered. The term 'Non-Hodgkin's Lymphoma' was coined so that physicians and scientist could distinguish it from Hodgkin's Lymphoma because the course, treatment and cure rate of these two lymphomas is so markedly different. To make matters worse some of the titles of the subgroup's of Non-Hodgkin's Lymphoma both of these entities are very similar. Thus medical science has created one of its many pigeon holes in which to categorize these cancers. In the early days of treatment of Non-Hodgkin's lymphomas there were practically no long remissions or cures but there were many cures in Hodgkin's Lymphoma, as discussed earlier. The determination of whether or not a biopsy specimen is diagnosed as Hodgkin's or Non-Hodgkin's Lymphoma can only be decided by examination under the microscope. The need and the rationale for this distinction will be made clear as our discussion proceeds.

These Non-Hodgkin's Lymphomas are also cancers which arise and originate in the lymph nodes—like Hodgkin's Lymphoma—and it usually spreads to neighboring lymph nodes. Non-Hodgkin's lymphoma is more common than Hodgkin's lymphoma and occurs in the older age groups.

Names and Synonyms: There are few, if any, common synonyms for this group of conditions except for the now outdated title, 'Lymphosarcoma.'

Incidence: In 1995 Non-Hodgkin's lymphoma is expected to occur in 41,000 individuals in the United States and cause 19,400 deaths.

The incidence of Non-Hodgkin's lymphoma is only slightly greater in males than females. The peak incidence period is later than Hodgkin's Lymphoma. Approximately 25% of cases occur in the 50-59 age group but the maximum risk period is in the 60-69 age group.

Causes and Risk Factors: There is no clear causative agent(s) of Non Hodgkin's lymphomas but a relation to the Epstein-Barr virus is also suspected.

Signs and Symptoms: The signs and symptoms of this group of Non-Hodgkin's Lymphomas (NHL) are similar to Hodgkin's Lymphoma with the following exceptions:

1. Early involvement in the nose and throat area, the skin, the intestinal tract and bone is common.
2. In children, early involvement of structures within the abdomen is much more likely.
3. NHL frequently (13% of cases) changes to a leukemia-type of disease.
4. Complicating infections are more often due to an immune deficiency state.

Unfortunately, no ideal mass screening method has been devised for Non-Hodgkin's lymphoma. The best advice I can give the reader is to have any lymph node enlargement examined by your physician as soon as practically possible.

Diagnosis: As in Hodgkin's Lymphoma the lymph node biopsy is the only reliable way of establishing the diagnosis of Non-Hodgkin's lymphoma.

Staging: The terminology of NHL is similar to that used in Hodgkin's Disease. However, many more patients with NHL (80%) have more advanced disease (stages III or IV) when first diagnosed.

To reiterate the staging divisions of NHL are as follows:

Stage I	Single lymph node region
Stage II	Two or more contiguous lymph node areas but on the same side of diaphragm
Stage III	Two or more node areas on different sides of diaphragm
Stage IV	Diffuse node involvement with other organs affected such as lungs, bone marrow, etc.
Substage A	Absence of fever, weight loss, sweats
Substage B	Presence of fever, weight loss, sweats

The tests recommended in staging NHL are similar to Hodgkin's Lymphoma with perhaps the exception of the staging exploratory laparotomy and spleen removal. Surgical staging is less often required in Non-Hodgkin's lymphoma because diffuse disease is usually apparent at the time of diagnosis and, therefore, exploratory surgery does not substantially influence the choice of therapy or prognosis. In addition, since many of these NHL patients are older they frequently have other majors health problems which make the risk of fatality from the surgery much greater.

Staging by cell type (histological) is extremely important in Non-Hodgkin's lymphoma as it is in Hodgkin's but the nomenclature has recently undergone radical and extensive changes. There are so many cell types and subtypes they are too technical to be of use to the reader in this book.

As recently as 1983 there were only 6-8 different types of NHL recognized. At the present there are at least 20 major types with several subtypes in each major group. The nomenclature is cumbersome, to say the least, but it is very useful. It is important for the reader to know that there are three major groups of NHL which are designated according to their risks of recurrence. These are simply called; low, intermediate and high risk groups.

I'm sure your physician will be willing to discuss these risk groups in detail in the reader's particular case but the technical details serve little purpose here. Suffice it to point out, however, that this information is extremely important for the oncologist to have in order to prescribe proper treatment and ascribe accurate prognosis to the NHL.

Prognosis: The author can recall when he started practice twenty-five years ago that patients with NHL had very little chance for even a short-lived partial remission, and absolutely no chance for a cure. At the present time, however, from 40 to 80% of NHL patients can be expected to achieve prolonged (5 to 10 years) disease-free remission. The actual cure rate of NHL is difficult to pinpoint because of the divergence in staging and cell typing around the world but it is probably in the vicinity of 30 to 40%.

Sites of Spread: The predictable route of recurrence of these NHL's is very similar to that of Hodgkin's Lymphomas. This fact of anticipated spread has also been put to good use in administering radiation therapy to produce good remission rates and cure rates in NHL. As I have pointed out above the sites of original appearance of NHL is very different than that of Hodgkin's Lymphoma but recurrences are quite similar and predictable.

Therapeutic Modalities: Surgery: The therapeutic use of surgery in these lymphomas is similar to Hodgkin's lymphoma. Surgery is seldom, if ever, used alone in therapy of NHL except to relieve obstruction or compression but is often used in obtaining biopsy material to establish diagnosis. Abdominal surgery is used often not for staging purposes but for diagnostic purposes. Since an abdominal presentation is so frequent in NHL the necessity for abdominal surgery is greater.

Radiation Therapy: Radiotherapy is very important in the management of these lymphomas but it is usually limited to the earlier stages of involvement, i.e., Stages I and II. However, since at least 80% of patients with NHL present with more advanced stages (i.e., Stages III and IV).

Chemotherapy: Great strides have been made in the development and advancement of chemotherapeutic agents in the treatment of NHL. Quite obviously it has been applied effectively since the remission rates and cure rates of NHL have improved so strikingly . In 1983 the remission rate and 5-year-survival rate of Non-Hodgkin's Lymphomas was approximately 30% but has risen to the previously stated maximum of 80% primarily due the improvement in chemotherapy.

Single drug chemotherapy agents may also be used in tablet form with effective response in the low risk groups. Some cases of low risk NHL are so dormant that no treatment need be given at all in the earlier stages. In those cases which do advance to later stages successful therapy is still possible.

Stages III and IV NHL are nearly always treated with combination chemotherapy in much the same fashion as in Hodgkin's Lymphoma. The list of chemotherapeutic agents now effective in NHL has become extensive indeed and continues to grow. When one considers the infinite number of ways in which these agents can be use in combination the varieties are innumerable. Some of the more commonly used chemotherapy combinations —with their acronyms—are given below:

COP Regimen	Cyclophosphamide (Cytoxan®)
	Oncovin® (Vincristine)
	Prednisone
C-MOPP	Cyclophosphamide or Mustargen
	Oncovin®
	Procarbazine (Matulane®)
	Prednisone
CHOP	Cyclophosphamide
	Doxorubicin (Adriamycin®)
	Oncovin®
	Prednisone
BACOP	Cyclophosphamide
	Adriamycin®
	Oncovin®
	Bleomycin
	Prednisone

In addition, many of these drugs can be used as single agents or in combinations of two. Other agents which can be used alone are; melphalan, chlorambucil, CCNU, cisplatinum, BCNU, etoposide, dacarbizine, methotrexate, Ara-C, Ifosfamide, 2-cDa, fludarabine and many others.

However, when used in first line therapy the combination regimens are much more likely to result in complete remission, prolonged survival or cure of NHL.

Management Team: The usual triumvirate of surgeon, radiation oncologist and medical oncologist is recommended with each individual physician acting as team leader during the period of his part of the therapy program. When treatment is completed the primary caregiver and follower of the course of NHLymphoma is the medical oncologist.

Follow-Up: During the period of treatment follow up medical examinations twice a month are advisable in order to monitor the rapid remission—or progression—of the disease and the side effects of therapy. Proper documentation by physical examination of changes in lymph node and other organ size is extremely important. After the completion of the NHL treatment plan a recommendation for regular visits to the medical oncologist is planned for at least the next two years. The follow up period corresponds to the duration of time during which relapses of NHL are most likely. During this period, and from then on, a yearly medical examination with repeat of appropriate blood tests, x-rays, scans and bone marrow biopsy are indicated.

The Leukemias: The multiple and varied definitions of leukemia can be very confusing to the reader when stated in scientific and technical terms. As a result I have oversimplified the definitions for the sake of ease and clarity in discussion.

The word leukemia was originally coined to designate a blood condition which was manifested by an excess of white blood cells in the circulation. Since some cases of leukemia have normal and even below normal white blood counts the term is no longer accurate but it is traditionally utilized in designating these diseases.

In general, Leukemia is the result of an uncontrolled, excessive growth of malignant white blood cells in the bone marrow and blood forming organs. The two major ways in which leukemia threatens the life of the patient is through the liability for overwhelming infection and massive hemorrhage. The leukemia does so by reducing the immunity of the subject, by suppressing the production of normal white blood cells and reducing the number of blood clotting cells called platelets. The mechanisms which lead to these liabilities are basically the same for all types of leukemia with some specific and unusual exceptions.

The Leukemias do not lend themselves to staging by anatomic involvement since they do no tend to form solid masses (tumors) as do the other cancers such as breast cancer, lung cancer, and so on. Leukemias are thus known as Non-solid cancers, and the others are known as Solid Cancers (Tumors).

The leukemias may be classified in several ways most of which are disorienting and highly technical. The chart which follows is my attempt to simplify and to clarify the terminology of the leukemias for practical purposes.

Acute Leukemias

Acute Lymphoblastic Leukemia (ALL)
Acute Myeloblastic (Granulocytic) Leukemia (AML)

Chronic Leukemias

Chronic Lymphocytic (Lymphatic) Leukemia (CLL)
Chronic Myelogenous (Granulocytic) Leukemia (CML)

The terms acute and chronic are more often chosen on the basis of the kind of blood cell that is growing wildly in the body rather than the rapidity of onset of the symptoms. But generally speaking the acute leukemias, if not treated, can lead to death more quickly than the chronic leukemias .

There are many other unusual types of leukemia which are too rare to discuss in detail here. These include; 'Hairy cell leukemia,' plasma cell leukemia, lymphoma-leukemia, monocytic leukemia, myelomonocytic leukemia, megakaryocytic leukemia, Sezary-cell leukemia, erythroleukemia and several others. These special cases should be discussed in detail by your physician with the reader where applicable.

Incidence: The leukemias are a relatively rare group of malignancies when compared to, say, breast cancer which has 180,000 new cases a year. The leukemias as a group will account for 28,200 cases a year and 18,200 deaths in 1995. When grouped together by cell type—granulocytic and lymphocytic—they occur with about equal frequency in males and female with no gender differences.

The age groups affected by the different leukemias, however, are striking and are of major clinical importance. Acute Lymphoblastic Leukemia is almost exclusively a disease of childhood; chronic lymphocytic leukemia is a disease of the aged; chronic myelogenous leukemia occurs most in middle life; and acute myeloblastic leukemia occurs with equal frequency in all age groups.

Causes and Risk Factors: Both environmental and genetic factors appear to be important in the causation of the leukemias. Nonetheless, a precisely identifiable cause can be found in only a small fraction of leukemia cases.

Environmental Factors: Exposure to large amounts of radiation, especially in pregnant mothers; high dose radiation exposure from nuclear explosions (Hiroshima, Japan); exposure to specific chemicals and drugs—benzene, arsenic, phenylbutazone, and rarely exposure to some chemotherapy drugs; early exposure to special viral illnesses in childhood; and any combination of these factors.

Genetic Factors: The presence of some genetically transmitted disorders are associated with an increased risk of leukemia. These genetic disorders include; Down's Syndrome, Fanconi's anemia, Klinefelter's Syndrome, and other rare genetic conditions. If an identical twin spontaneously develops leukemia the other member of the pair has a greater risk of contracting the same type of leukemia. There is also a slight increase in occurrence of leukemia in the siblings of a child with leukemia but there is no increased risk in their parents or aunts and uncles.

Others: Viral factors, immunological factors, and interacting factors.

However, it must be made clear that these factors are rarely identified as antecedent causes in the total number of cases of leukemia which are treated each year in the United States.

Signs and Symptoms: Because of the minor but distinct differences in the presentation of each leukemia the signs and symptoms are discussed separately for each of the four major types of leukemia.

1) Acute Myeloblastic Leukemia (AML)-Symptoms in this leukemia are usually slower in onset with early appearance signals for one to six months before the diagnosis of leukemia is made. These symptoms may include fatigue, shortness of breath with mild exertion, chest (heart) pain and palpitations of the heart, all of which are manifestations of the anemia (low red blood cell count) caused by the leukemia.

The diminished number of normal white blood cells in the circulation may produce a variety of infections, such as; skin abscesses, pneumonia, meningitis, blood stream infections (septicemia), and the like, with resultant fever, chills, weakness, lethargy and sweats.

Hemorrhagic manifestations due to the reduced platelets mentioned above may include nose bleeds, skin bruises, bleeding gums, coughing and vomiting of blood, bloody diarrhea and bloody urine. An enlarged spleen may produce the feeling of fullness in the left side of the abdomen and consequent weight loss.

2) Chronic Myelogenous Leukemia (CML or CGL)- The onset of this leukemia is often subtle. Many cases are discovered accidentally when performing routine blood counts for physical examinations prior to surgery, dental work, insurance examinations, etc. Most common are the symptoms of "feeling run down," easy fatigue, sweating, heat intolerance, easy bruising and abdominal discomfort due to enlargement of the spleen which occurs in almost all cases.

3) Acute Lymphoblastic Leukemia (ALL)- The symptoms of this leukemia are very similar to those of acute myeloblastic leukemia and are also produced by the diminished production of normal blood cells, i.e., anemia, low numbers of normal white blood cells and decreased platelets.

4) Chronic Lymphocytic Leukemia (CLL)- This type of leukemia causes signs and symptoms which are similar to those listed for chronic myelogenous leukemia and are also frequently discovered accidentally when routine blood counts are performed.

Diagnosis and Screening Tests: These testing and screening methods are essentially the same for all leukemias with simple screening often performed during annual physical examinations and other situations where routine blood counts are performed. It has not been common practice to screen large numbers of the population with blood counts except in high risk groups such as benzene workers, radiologist and radiology technicians, Down's Syndrome victims, atomic bomb victims, etc.

There is only one reliable method of establishing or eliminating the diagnosis of any kind of leukemia and that is examination of a specimen of the bone marrow obtained either by simple aspiration or needle biopsy of the bone marrow. There is no substitute for bone marrow examination no matter how characteristic a case of leukemia appears from routine blood counts or other signs and symptoms. Above all a patient should never receive treatment for leukemia without this test first being performed. The hazards of the test, in experienced hands, are too minor to exclude the bone marrow test.

As stated earlier the leukemias are not staged in the usual anatomic terms because they do not occur as solid, well demarcated masses.

Many other tests are required in assessing the status of a case of leukemia in order to detect unsuspected complications or to judge the function of other organs before beginning aggressive treatment programs. The ever-necessary complete history and physical examination is at the core of this process. Special blood tests for surveying the function of kidneys, liver, bones are performed. Radiologic studies of the chest and bones are sometimes required. In both forms of acute leukemia a lumbar puncture (spinal tap) must be done to obtain spinal fluid for examination which often contains evidence of occult leukemia involving the covering membrane of the brain—called the meningeal leukemia.

Prognosis: The prognosis for leukemia is discussed under the heading of each type of leukemia.

1) Acute Myeloblastic Leukemia (AML)- The median survival for untreated cases of AML is about 2 months. However, with contemporary chemotherapy of AML this survival can be increased to about 15 months in 50 to 70% of individuals. Survival is more likely in those cases of AML in patients under the age of 50 than for those over age 50. In recent times a significant 'cure rate' has been prophesied for AML. This prophesy remains to be demonstrated with long term studies.

2) Chronic Myelogenous Leukemia (CML)- The median survival of this type of leukemia is about 3.5 years whether treatment is administered or not. All the cases of CML which do not die of early complications will slowly deteriorate into a universally fatal, progressive phase called *acute blastic transformation.* Treatment of CML with appropriate chemotherapy does produce greater comfort, alleviates distressing symptoms, reduces the need for frequent blood transfusions and frequent hospitalizations, although, it does not prolong duration of survival. This dismal survival outlook for CML has been improved by some new approaches to treatment which are discussed in detail below.

3) Acute Lymphoblastic Leukemia (ALL)- The prognosis of this kind of leukemia is entirely different in childhood than it is in adults and, therefore, they are discussed individually according to age groups.

Childhood ALL - With proper therapy 80 to 90% of children with acute lymphoblastic leukemia achieve remissions lasting 3 or more years. About 75% of those cases of ALL which enter into remission have long lasting disease free periods and are probably eventually cured.

Adult ALL - In patients who are over the age of 15 years remission can be accomplished with chemotherapy in approximately 75% of cases. However, long disease-free survival is unlikely and the prospects of cure are very remote. Despite all our therapeutic efforts the median survival period in Adult ALL is less than 2 years. Here again, some new developments will be discussed later which may alter this poor prognosis.

4) Chronic Lymphocytic Leukemia (CLL)- In most cases of chronic lymphocytic leukemia the clinical activity of the leukemia is so very low—regardless of how high the white blood cell counts become—that treatment may never be required. Patients only require treatment under specific circumstances which will be discussed below. If the chemotherapy agents for CLL are given before they are really necessary they may have major complications themselves without improving survival for the patient or producing cure. Because of the diverse variability of criteria for treatment accurate figures for survival or cure rate are not available for CLL. But it has been estimated that less than 20% of cases of chronic lymphocytic leukemia become active enough to require treatment and the majority of these have a successful response to therapy.

Sites of Spread: Since these leukemias do not spread into other organs there are no real metastases or sites of spread. The disease progresses by driving down the levels of red blood cells, normal white blood cells and platelets.

Therapeutic Modalities: The choice of therapies for each of the leukemias depends on the type and the activity of the leukemia and they will be discussed individually by the type of leukemic cell.

1) Acute Myeloblastic Leukemia (AML)- In essence, chemotherapy is the only modality utilized to treat this leukemia with radiation therapy occasionally used as an adjunct. Surgery is not an integral part of the diagnosis or treatment of AML.

The first question to be addressed regarding treatment is whether to give any therapy at all, other than supportive care. This dilemma arises for two reasons. First, the disease occurs most often in the older population groups with other major medical problems, and secondly; the cure rates and remission rates for this leukemia are quite low with any kind of chemotherapy. The dilemma is compounded by the fact that the chemotherapy is so very toxic and often causes fatal complications itself in patients over 50 years, and is even worse in those over 60 years. These are emotionally charged choices in which the patient and family must take part in unless they completely delegate the authority for the decision to the physician. Who is to say how much time alive is worthwhile or what odds are not worth any effort?

In the age group under 50 years and childhood age groups the choices are somewhat easier but still difficult.

When the choice is made to give chemotherapy for AML it is given in two phases, an induction phase and a maintenance phase. Single agent chemotherapy is almost never used in this disease. Very powerful combination agents are given in a hospital inpatient setting. The patient is supported with blood transfusions, antibiotics and many other prophylactic measures. The most commonly used chemotherapy agents for the induction phase are doxorubicin, vincristine, prednisone, asparaginase, thioguanine, and others. For the maintenance phase methotrexate, mercaptopurine, prednisone and vincristine are also used.

Radiation therapy is an important part of both induction and maintenance therapy because involvement of the brain coverings (meningeal leukemia) is such a frequent problem both early and late in the course of AML. The radiation treatments are very effective in preventing and treating this complication.

The chances of major complications and even death are so very high with this anti-leukemia therapy that it must be spelled out clearly to the patient and family before embarking on therapy. Patients are told in no uncertain terms that they will become very ill with the therapy, they will require long hospitalization and they will have a greater risk of death from the therapy. Anything less is hedging. And any therapy of lesser potency is ineffective and wasteful.

Newer, more promising developments in therapy are discussed at the end of this section since they may be applicable to all forms of leukemia.

2) Chronic Myelogenous Leukemia (CML)- Chemotherapy, in a variety of methods, is the mainstay of treatment of this type of CML although surgery and radiation therapy are occasionally used in special circumstances. The therapy differs for the two stages of the disease; the chronic phase and the accelerated (-blastic transformation) phase.

In the chronic phase the sole intent of therapy is to produce patient comfort and reduce morbidity. No effective therapy has been found yet to prolong survival. The chemotherapy agents used, usually in tablet form, are busulfan (Myleran®), hydroxyurea (Hydrea®) and other similar classes of drugs. Now, however, alpha-interferon appears to be a promising agent in treating CML.

Radiation therapy is sometimes used to shrink the size of a large, painful spleen and also to improve the patient's blood counts. It does occasionally produce remission by itself but very infrequently. Other special techniques include extracting the excess white blood cells from the circulation (leukopheresis); extracorporeal irradiation (passing blood through a tube outside of the body and treating the blood with radiation); and removal of the spleen (splenectomy).

Accelerated Phase of Chronic Myelogenous Leukemia- Combination chemotherapy is applied in this phase much the same as it is in the Acute Leukemias. The results of treatment in this phase of CML are very poor, with few remissions and even fewer cures. Survival time is no more than a few weeks.

3) Acute Lymphoblastic Leukemia (ALL)- in the childhood cases of ALL the results of therapy of this disease are indeed gratifying. The therapy is applied in 3 steps: induction therapy; intensification therapy; maintenance therapy.

Induction therapy is started with the drugs vincristine, prednisone, and asparaginase or doxorubicin. In addition, the entire brain and spinal cord are treated with radiation therapy—since this is a sanctuary where leukemic cells are not effected by chemotherapy—to prevent or eliminate leukemic involvement in these structures.

Maintenance therapy is then given in the form of tablets of methotrexate as a once a week dose plus Purinethal® (6-mercaptopurine). This maintenance therapy combination is continued for an extended period of time, sometimes as long as two and one-half to three years.

Patients over the age of 15 years are treated more vigorously with a combination of agents such as; vincristine, prednisone, Cytosar®, doxorubicin; thioguanine, etc. rates are very discouraging, however.

4) Chronic Lymphocytic Leukemia - In most early cases, without other significant findings, treatment is often withheld for reasons previously stated. When treatment is indicated it is usually administered with oral agents such as; chlorambucil, cyclophosphamide, prednisone. When the disease does not respond to these agents or passes into a more aggressive phase combination injectable chemotherapy is administered with agents such as; vincristine, cyclophosphamide, bleomycin, prednisone; BCNU; Velban®, Adriamycin®, DTIC; and others.

In some cases when the major clinical finding is the presence of enlarged, troublesome lymph nodes it may be sufficient to simply shrink these lymph nodes with radiation therapy with good results. Occasionally, the only clinical difficulty is due to enlargement of the spleen. In this situation surgical removal of the spleen (splenectomy) may adequately alleviate the condition.

Other uncommonly utilized modalities for CLL include leukopheresis and low dose total body radiation therapy.

Special, New and Experimental Forms of Therapy for the Leukemias: Some of these forms of treatment are presently available for the treatment of the leukemias under special clinical circumstances. In some cases they are reserved for the aggressive phase of the disease; or when the disease has failed to respond to standard therapies; or when the likelihood of standard therapy producing remission is so small that one immediately enlists the experimental therapy. Some of these newer agents may even be available by the time this book is printed.

Interferons - this form of biological response modifier therapy is now possible through the recent advances made in genetic engineering and protein chemistry.

In the cases of Chronic Lymphocytic Leukemia which have failed to respond to standard therapy the Interferons—such as Recombinant alpha-Interferon-2-å—can produce gratifying responses in a modest number of cases in CML.

In Chronic myelogenous leukemia there is evidence accumulating that Interferon when applied early in the course of disease can prevent transition to the aggressive, accelerated phase of the disease. The early optimistic reports of treatment for CML remains to be verified.

In the situations of both of the Acute Leukemias adequate trials have not been conducted with the Interferons to make a judgement.

Bone Marrow Transplantation (BMT), one of the latest additions to the armamentarium of treatments of malignancy, is rapidly increasing in utilization, especially, but not exclusively in the leukemias. BMT is not yet considered first line, standard therapy, but it is utilized for cases of otherwise hopeless status in each disease. It is most commonly applied to: childhood acute leukemias which have relapsed and have no other chance of remission; adult acute leukemias with poor prognosis regardless of treatments available; and the adult chronic myelogenous leukemias in younger patients.

Age is the most troublesome contraindication to BMT since patients over the age of 50 years have little chance of recovery and higher risk of death from the transplant. The same statement is true of those patients with other serious maladies such as heart disease, chronic lung disease, liver disease, kidneys disease and any other major medical afflictions which would be worsened by the trauma of the bone marrow transplant's taxing of the body's healing powers.

Management Team and Follow-Up: In the vast majority of instances the management team and follow up examination is handled by the medical oncologist or hematologist. Other specialists may be called in for special procedures. Of course, the usual diverse support team is involved when the leukemia progresses to the aggressive phase.

Chapter 31

Multiple Myeloma

Although not a true leukemia multiple myeloma is discussed here because it does originate in the bone marrow cell known as the plasma cell.

Multiple myeloma (more correctly known as Plasma Cell Myeloma) is greater in frequency than Hodgkin's Disease and at least equal in frequency to each of the more common leukemias. It arises as a malignant, uncontrolled, neoplastic proliferation of the plasma cells of the bone marrow which most commonly produces severe bone pain, bone fractures and anemia.

Names and Synonyms: Multiple myeloma, plasma cell myeloma, broken bone disease, immunoproliferative disorder, bone cancer, bone marrow cancer.

Incidence Rates: In 1995 multiple myeloma will effect 12,500 Americans and cause 9,200 deaths. It will occur with equal frequency in males and females. It is the most common malignancy of the bone marrow in nonwhites and the third most common in whites. Over 90% of the cases of multiple myeloma occur after the age of 40, and rare cases are seen in teenagers.

Causes and Risk Factors: No precise cause is known for multiple myeloma but prolonged immune stimulation with a final inappropriate response has been suspected. Virus particles have been seen in both human and animal plasma cell neoplasms but are not clearly considered to be causative.

Signs and Symptoms: Back pain is the most common presenting complaint of patients with multiple myeloma. When X-rays are taken of the painful bone areas they may reveal either fractures, osteoporosis (thinning of the bones), or a punched-out, Swiss cheese appearance of the bones.

The profound anemia of multiple myeloma produces a variety of complaints including easy fatigue, weakness, shortness of breath, swollen ankles, etc.

Repeated and frequent major infections such as pneumonia, meningitis, and the like, are a result of the deficiency of production of immunity supporting proteins caused by multiple myeloma.

Abnormal bleeding tendencies including nose bleeds, skin bruising, bleeding in urine and stools may result from abnormal clotting due to excess abnormal protein (myeloma proteins) and low platelet counts.

Kidney failure is seen in some cases of multiple myeloma due to direct involvement of the kidneys (Myeloma Kidneys), or indirect damage to kidneys due to infection of the kidneys, high blood calcium and deposition of an abnormal substance called amyloid in the kidneys.

Screening Tests: Although a true specific screening test is not available for multiple myeloma the commonly used chemical blood analysis (Chemistry Profile) can detect excessively high serum protein content in the blood which strongly suggests multiple myeloma to your physician.

Diagnosis: Clear cut, unequivocal diagnosis of multiple myeloma can be difficult to establish since many other conditions can cause the above described constellation of findings. In most cases, however, a combination of anemia, high serum and abnormal proteins, and an excess of plasma cells on bone marrow examination can secure the diagnosis in 99% of cases. One thing is certain, nevertheless, the diagnosis of multiple myeloma cannot be established or ruled out without a bone marrow examination.

Other necessary tests in multiple myeloma include a complete blood count, serum and urine protein electrophoresis, bone x-rays, and other specific tests as needed to rule out any other diseases which may be confused with multiple myeloma.

Staging: True anatomic staging is not used in multiple myeloma but a form of staging to determine the likelihood of response to treatment and remission is used in some medical centers. The staging system incorporates; the degree of anemia, the degree of kidney impairment, the amount of abnormal protein in the serum, and the presence of high serum, calcium to determine the likelihood of response to treatment. There is some disagreement among experts as to the utility of this system.

Prognosis: Although the five year remission rate has increased from 12% in 1963 to 30% in 1983 precise statistics are difficult to obtain.

Response rates to chemotherapy have been reported to be as high as 75% and the median duration of survival has been as high as 80 months. However, complete remission with disease free survival is defined in terms of 2 year spans. More than 80% of myeloma patients can expect good quality survival of 2 to 3 years. True 'cures ' seldom, if ever, occur.

Sites of Spread: Aside from the bones and kidneys true spread or metastases from myeloma rarely occur to other organs. However, many myeloma patients are in grave danger of death from some of the other manifestations of this disease if they are not corrected expeditiously.

Serious and life-threatening infections, bleeding syndromes, kidney failure, and coma from high calcium in the blood are immediate major complications of Myeloma requiring emergency treatment interventions.

Therapeutic Modalities: General and vigorous supportive care to treat the immediate complications of myeloma discussed above are top priority and they may even supersede the specific therapy of the multiple myeloma. Once the myeloma patient's condition is stabilized chemotherapy is the primary staple of therapy in this disease since the bone marrow is a diffuse organ and the pockets of myeloma are also diffuse. Therefore, the application of chemotherapy agents which can diffuse into the many reaches of the bone marrow through the general circulating blood can effectively control the wildly proliferating culprit. . . the plasma cell.

Many chemotherapy drug agents have been found effective in treating multiple myeloma, these include: melphalan (Alkeran®); cyclophosphamide (Cytoxan®); prednisone; BCNU; doxorubicin; bleomycin; vincristine; dexamethasone, and others. The combination of these agents, in a variety of mixtures, has also been used in cases of multiple myeloma resistant to standard single agents. None of the combinations has yet been found to supplant the standard single agents given as tablets.

Radiation Therapy: Although radiation therapy is an indispensable part of the therapeutic armamentarium used against multiple myeloma it is in no sense ever curative. Radiotherapy is extremely useful for rapid and effect relief of severe bone pain due to multiple myeloma bone lesions and other localized forms of the disease but has no systemic effect against the widely disseminated malignant plasma cell.

Surgery: Surgery has no applications by itself in the treatment of multiple myeloma except in the occasional case of spinal cord compression.

Special Therapies: Plasmapheresis—the mechanical removal of excess blood proteins—is necessary in a special situation in multiple myeloma called the 'Hyperviscosity Syndrome.' The serious consequences of this syndrome— coma, massive bleeding, and death—are directly related to the circulating amounts of abnormal protein in the blood stream. The concentrations of this abnormal protein can be quickly reduced by this mechanical method of removal to allude death until any effective chemotherapy agent can have time to produce a remission.

Biological Response Modifiers: Up to the present time the interferons have only been superficially studied in cases of multiple myeloma which have relapsed or have failed to respond to standard therapy. Preliminary reports, however, indicate some considerable promise for the future of these substances in the therapy of multiple myeloma.

Management Team: The chemotherapist, either a medical oncologist or hematologist, is absolutely necessary to lead the management team in multiple myeloma. One of these specialists should also act as the coordinator of the rest of the team which often needs the services of the radiotherapist, the transfusionist and others. In the beginning weeks of the treatment multiple myeloma often daily and at most weekly measurements of the activity of the disease are required during acute threats to the life of the patient. Except in the most benign of cases of multiple myeloma is longer than monthly doctor visits acceptable.

Chapter 32

Skin Cancers

Skin cancers comprise the most common and yet the most curable cancers affecting the human race. The skin cancers grow slowly, seldom spread to neighboring lymph nodes, and more rarely do they spread to other distant organs, they are easily examined and readily detected, they are easily treated, and they rarely produce fatalities. All the information which is given below pertains to all types of skin cancers except the rare but very serious Malignant Melanoma which is, therefore, discussed separately in this book.

Names and Synonyms: Skin cancer is seldom known by other titles except for the two main cellular types of squamous cell carcinoma or basal cell carcinoma.

Incidence Rates: Skin cancers are estimated to develop in 600,000 Americans annually. It is estimated that 40-50% of all people who live to the age of 65 will develop at least one skin cancer during their lifetime. It is the most common 'second malignancy,' in that, a person with any other malignancy has a 50-60% chance of developing another type of cancer and it is usually a skin cancer.

The annual death rate from skin cancer is around 2,100 and most of these are preventable if the patient seeks early medical attention for suspicious skin changes.

Certain ethnic groups with a low pigment content of the skin have a higher risk of skin cancer such as the Irish and the Scots. However, no race is immune to skin cancer not even the highly pigmented black or brown races.

Causes and Risk Factors: The major causative factor in skin cancer is excessive sun exposure and sun damage. The ultraviolet radiation responsible for sun tan and sunburn seems the main culprit in the causation of skin cancer. The risk is especially high for the exposed, unprotected portions of the body such as hands and face.

Occasionally certain chemical agents have been known to increase the risk of skin cancers. For example, in chimney sweeps the higher occurrence rate of cancer of the skin of the scrotum seems related to the exposure to coal tar from this occupation. Other suspected chemicals in the cause of skin cancers include: arsenic in agricultural sprays; coal tars in petroleum occupations; the fumes and frequent burns in those who work with molten metals.

Radiation exposure has been a long recognized risk factor for skin cancer since the early days of x-ray diagnosis, especially in radiologist. Today this risk of skin cancer is limited to patients who receive excessively high doses of radiation for other malignancies.

There are also rare genetic defects which are associated with other skin conditions—such as xeroderma pigmentosa and basal nevus syndrome— which have a greater risk of developing skin cancer.

The destruction of the ozone layer of the atmosphere will allow more ultraviolet rays to reach the populous and therefore hypothetically can increase the risk of skin cancer.

Signs and Symptoms: The skin cancers are the most difficulty cancers on which to advise the public since virtually everyone alive has had some skin blemish or skin growth which they have been aware of from time to time.

The American Cancer Society uses the generalization of 'any sore that will not heal.' This is an acceptable statement but I believe it is not inclusive enough or clear enough. A more useful guide warns the public to be wary of any skin growth which doubles its size in a month or less; or begins to bleed; or changes color substantially. Granted these are vague and imprecise to the reader but they are the best guidelines medical science has at the moment. I can only direct the readers to seek the advice of a physician if they have any doubts about a skin blemish. They should have very little reason to delay since the curability of skin cancers is so very high.

There are some specific skin diseases which are felt to either be pre-malignant or have a high propensity to become cancerous which deserve mention here. Of course, physicians are aware of these skin lesions but I believe the reader should be aware of them as well. As a result, the public should realize the importance of frequent follow up visits to their physician and repeat examinations of suspicious lesions.

These pre-cancerous skin lesions include: Actinic and senile keratosis; seborrheic keratosis; arsenical keratosis; Bowen's disease; radiation dermatitis; xeroderma pigmentosum; scar carcinomas; basal cell nevus and keratoacanthoma. The technical description of these lesions is not germane here but at least their names are now recognizable.

Screening Tests: As such there are no useful testing measures other than a high index of suspicion by the physician and a high level of awareness by the public through education.

Diagnosis: As always, diagnosis skin cancer requires some kind of biopsy. Either a complete removal of the lesion (excision), if it is small enough, or removal of small portion of a larger lesion (incisional) is an appropriate method of biopsy. An assumption of benignity or malignancy should never be made on the basis of gross appearance of the skin blemish alone since the surgery is simple, safe and conclusive.

Staging and Testing: Anatomic staging of skin cancer utilizes the standard TNM system. The T indicates the characters of the primary Tumor or cancer; N refers to any lymph nodes which are involved; and M stands for any distant Metastases, which seldom occur in skin cancer.

The chart below defines these stages:

T1 Tumor less than 2 cm. (3/4 inches) in diameter

T2 Tumor is between 2 and 5 cm in diameter.

T3 Tumor is larger than 5 cm in diameter.

T4 Extension of tumor into local bone or muscle

N1 Nodes involved on the same side of the body as the primary lesion

N2 Nodes on the opposite side or both sides

N3 Nodes that are adherent or fixed to underlying tissues

Staging tests and x-rays, other than physical examination and measurement of the skin tumor, are seldom required in these skin cancers.

Histological Staging: Histological staging of skin cancer refers to the description of the cellular structure of the skin cancer since it does have major prognostic significance. The chart below lists the (histological) cell types of skin cancer:

Cell Type: Basal Cell Carcinoma

1. Superficial, multicentric type
2. Morphea type
3. Fibroepithelial

Cell Type: Squamous Cell Carcinoma

1. Adenoid squamous cell carcinoma
2. Spindle cell type

Other Less Common Cell Types:

Metatypical Carcinoma
Sweat Gland Tumors and related lesions
Sebaceous Gland Tumors
Tumors of Hair Follicle
Paget's Disease of Skin
Undifferentiated Carcinoma

Prognosis: After adequately performed surgical treatment and accurate staging are carried out a 90-95% cure rate can be anticipated when all cell types and stages of skin cancer are considered together. Basal cell carcinomas which are less than 1 cm. in size approach 100% in cure rates. Squamous cell carcinomas cure rates vary from 75-90% depending on the stage and size of the skin cancer.

Sites of Spread: Even though metastases are rare , they do occasionally occur. The lymph nodes and lungs are the most common sites of spread. Local recurrences are more common than distant spread. The recurrence rates are a direct function of completeness, or incompleteness, of initial surgical excision of the skin cancer.

Therapeutic Modalities: Surgery is the treatment of choice for skin cancer even if local invasion is present. In some cases radiation therapy may be added. In areas of the body such as the face and hands plastic surgery techniques may be indicated. The most important aspect of surgery is that wide excisional margins must be accomplished which go beyond skin tumor edges and well into normal skin tissue.

Radiation Therapy: In some skin cancer cases radiation therapy can be used in place of surgery to improve cosmetic result. Also, in cases where complete excision of the skin tumor is technically not possible total cure can be accomplished with the addition of radiation therapy. (page 291)

Other types of therapy: Chemosurgery, electrosurgery, chemotherapy and immunotherapy have all been successfully applied to treat skin cancer.

Management Team: The dermatologist, or plastic surgeon when required, is the primary team member in skin cancer management with the addition of the radiation therapist when necessary. A follow up period of 2-4 years is usually recommended.

Chapter 33

Malignant Melanoma

Malignant melanoma is discussed separately here because of its high mortality rate and aggressive nature. However, malignant melanoma is most often curable if diagnosed and treated early and adequately.

Although the average person has 20 moles on their body, each year only 4 out of 100,000 of those people develop a malignant melanoma. However, the incidence of this cancer is rapidly rising and about 30-40% of those persons who develop malignant melanoma will die of the disease. Nevertheless, with early diagnosis and wide excisional treatment a 100% cure rate is possible. The key to cure of malignant melanoma is in early diagnosis, and wide surgical excision.

Incidence Rates: It is expected that in 1995 thirty-two thousand new cases of malignant melanoma will be diagnosed and about 6,700 people will die of the disease. Males and females are effected to approximately the same degree. Fair-skinned and red-haired individuals have a greater risk of developing malignant melanoma. In the United States the incidence continues to rise with the occurrence rate doubling every 15 years since 1925.

Causes or Risk Factors: Excessive sunlight exposure is a definite risk factor. There is a clearly demonstrated increased occurrence of malignant melanoma on skin surfaces exposed to excessive amounts of sunlight. The incidence of malignant melanoma in whites increases as one's country of residence approaches the equator. Australia, therefore, has the greatest rate of malignant melanoma in the world.

The great majority of malignant melanomas arise from a benign skin lesion called a nevus. Therefore, these skin lesions must be reexamined frequently and carefully by a physician for changes in appearance. Malignant melanomas occur in all races but they are rare in blacks and when do occur they are limited to the non-pigmented regions of the skin such as the soles of the feet or palms of the hands. Malignant melanomas are most common in middle age and almost never occur before puberty.

Signs and Symptoms: The most frequent findings in malignant melanoma are: a darkening; a change in color; or increase in size of a mole or colored skin patch which has otherwise not changed since birth, or at least for many years. Sometimes the skin lesion bleeds, never seems to heal, or forms a persistent ulcer.

In males, the most common locations of malignant melanoma are the skin of the trunk, head, neck and arms. In females the skin of the legs, arms, trunk and neck are the most common locations.

Screening and Early Detection: Effective screening and early detection for malignant melanoma can only be accomplished effectively by education of the public and physicians in order that they may recognize suspicious skin lesions as early as possible. Some countries (Australia for example) have circulated a color photo-atlas of skin lesions to the public and physicians with a resultant improvement of 81% in five year survival rate.

Unfortunately no other simple effective screening tests are yet available for malignant melanoma.

Diagnosis: Wide excisional biopsy of the malignant melanoma with large margins of normal skin tissue is strongly recommended. The microscopic examination of the specimen establishes the diagnosis; it also determines the stage which will be discussed below.

Staging: The staging system of malignant melanoma is one of the few staging systems in which the mortality and risk of recurrences can be accurately estimated from microscopic examination of the cancer. Obviously this can only be done after surgical excision of the skin tumor. The penetration of the cancer into the skin layers is actually measured under the microscope and can consistently predict outcome. The table below lists these stages according to *thickness* of the cancer and the *penetration* into the skin:

Level I	indicates less than 0.75mm thickness
Level II	indicates greater than 0.75 mm
Level III	indicates 0.75 mm to 1.5 mm.
Level IV	indicates 1.5 mm to 3.00 mm
Level V	indicates greater than 3.00 mm

Further complete staging of malignant melanoma requires comprehensive history and physical examination with special attention to; lymph nodes in the neck and axilla, lesions in the lungs, liver, brain, and bones. Appropriate x-rays, scans, blood and urine test are done in any patient with symptoms suggestive of distant metastases to these organs with special attention paid to bone, liver and brain.

Prognosis: Prognostication is most closely related to the thickness, and level of penetration of the original skin tumor. As stated previously, cure rates would be higher if earlier diagnosis and more complete excision of the skin cancer were carried out. Delay in diagnosis and treatment, therefore, is the greatest encumbrance to cure with a 100% cure rate not an unrealistic goal.

The 5-year survival rates, as related to level, are given below:

Level	Disease-Free 5-Year Survival
II	94%
III	71%
IV	43%
V	27%

and survival rates as related to thickness of tumor:

Thickness	Disease-Free 5-Year Survival
0-0.75 mm	100%
0.76-1.49 mm	66%
1.50-2.25 mm	69%
2.26-3.00 mm	37%
greater than 3.00 mm	23%

Sites of Spread: Locally recurrent skin nodules, involved local lymph nodes, other local skin lesions and new lesions just beneath the original skin tumors are quite common. Distant metastases from malignant melanoma may appear in any and all organs but the more common sites are the liver, lungs, brain and bones. Significant remission rates are practically nonexistent when distant metastatic disease occurs.

Therapeutic Modalities: Complete, wide surgical excision of the non-metastatic malignant melanoma is most important. The excision must have at least a 2 mm margin of normal tissue removed along with the original skin cancer.

In certain cases of malignant melanoma and in certain medical centers prophylactic removal of local and regional lymph nodes is recommended. The issue of prophylactic removal of lymph nodes is still controversial and it remains to be determined if this additional surgery improves survival or cure rates.

Radiation Therapy: Most malignant melanomas are considered resistant to radiation therapy but research on this point is continuing. Some melanomas which have spread to other organs can respond enough to radiation therapy to achieve some degree of palliation and relief of symptoms such as those in; brain, bone, soft tissues and lymph nodes.

Chemotherapy: Many types and combinations of chemotherapy agents have shown some moderate activity in malignant melanoma but none have consistently produced prolonged survival. Some of the chemotherapy agents used include; cisplatin, carboplatin, DTIC, BCNU, methyl-CCNU, thio-TEPA, melphalan, dibromodulcitol, mitomycin-C, methotrexate. Response rates to any chemotherapy drugs seldom exceed 10 to 20% and the responses are of short duration.

Immunotherapy has been found to have some utility in malignant melanoma with 12 to 18 month remission possible in some cases.

Hormonal therapy: It has been observed that an anti-estrogen, such as Tamoxifen as used in breast cancer, does produce some .

Special Modalities: More recently the biological response modifiers, specifically alpha–Interferon and interleukin-2 (IL-2), have been found to produce 20 to 30% remission rates in recurrent and metastatic malignant melanoma.

Management Team: The dermatologist, pathologist and plastic surgeon all have important roles to play in the management of malignant melanoma.

Their roles fluctuate but ultimately the dermatologist is the coordinator of the effort until locally recurrent or distant metastases occur.

Recommendations for follow up visits consist of regular monthly examinations in the first year after treatment and complete history and physical examination with appropriate laboratory and x-ray examinations. The need for special testing and x-rays may require the help of an internist, medical oncologist or family physician.

Chapter 34

Cancer of the Major Digestive Glands: A) Pancreas B) Liver and C) Gallbladder

Cancers of these abdominal organs are among the most difficult to treat, with the poorest outcome and the lowest survival rates. The 5-year-survival rate has been less than 3% for decades and shows little sign of improving. These cancers are usually first discovered at a very advanced stage and are insidious in onset. All of the symptoms they produce are very common, nonspecific and vague. The only good thing one can say about these cancers is that they are relatively rare.

Of the 1,130,000 new cancer cases expected in 1995 cancers of the digestive glands will account for only 43,700 cases. Obviously, this is still too many cases but still a small percentage of the whole.

(A) Cancer of the Pancreas: The pancreas is one of the free-floating structures in the abdomen which is connected through a duct system to the intestinal tract to aid the digestion of food. It also produces insulin which it excretes through the blood circulation which is considered as a separate, non-digestive function.

Names and Synonyms: Cancer of the Pancreas, pancreatic cancer, carcinoma of the pancreas, pancreatic carcinoma, adenocarcinoma of the pancreas, cancer of the exocrine pancreas.

Incidence: In 1995 cancer of the pancreas will account for 28,300 cancer cases and 25,000 cancer deaths. The incidence is steadily rising having tripled in the past 40 years. Pancreatic cancer is the fourth most common cancer in men and the fifth most common in women. It accounts for 2-3% of all forms of cancer but for about 10% of all fatal cancers in the abdomen.

Males are stricken 3-4 more often than females. Pancreatic cancer occurs most often between the ages of 35 and 70 with the peak incidence around age 60. Incidence rates are more common in blacks than whites.

Causes and Risk Factors: Although no clear cause has been discovered, cigarette smoking has been implicated in pancreatic cancer. Certain chemicals and occupational toxin exposures have been suspected as a risk factor for pancreatic cancer among chemists, and coke, and metal workers.

Coffee (with caffeine) drinking was suspect in pancreatic cancer but has not yet been found to have a clear consistent association.

Signs and Symptoms: Pancreatic cancer usually begins with the insidious onset of weakness, anorexia, weight loss, nausea, indigestion and 'gas pains.' Pain occurs in 70-80% of cases of pancreatic cancer and is located high in the center of the abdomen just below the end of the breast bone (sternum) or in the lower back (lumbar spine). Blockage of the flow of the bile from the liver by the pancreatic cancer produces jaundice of the skin and eyes, and severe itching of the skin. The clinical setting of unrelenting jaundice and weight loss in an elderly individual immediately raises the suspicion of pancreatic cancer in your physician's mind.

A satisfactory screening test has not yet been developed for this cancer.

Diagnosis: Sadly, over 90% of cases of pancreatic cancer have already spread (metastasized) beyond the confines of the pancreas itself once the diagnosis is suspected. Ordinarily some indirect tests which support the diagnosis of pancreatic cancer are done before subjecting the patient to surgery and biopsy. Included among these many tests are: upper intestinal barium x-ray; ultrasound of the abdomen; CT scans of the abdomen; pancreatography; and fine needle biopsy of the pancreatic mass through the abdominal wall. Eighty-seven percent of cases can be diagnosed by a combination of the above methods without the need for major surgery. Several other tests may support the suspicion of pancreatic cancer. These tests include angiography, tumor markers (CEA and) in the blood but they are frequently not helpful.

Finally, exploratory abdominal surgery and biopsy may be required to unequivocally establish the diagnosis of pancreatic cancer.

Staging: The universal TNM system is currently used in staging pancreatic cancer. A staging system utilizing Roman numerals has not yet been establish in pancreatic cancer since it does not facilitate the prognosis or the choice of treatment at this time.

The TNM system is given below:

T1 Indicates cancer less than 2 cm., limited to pancreas
T2 Indicates 6 cm cancer, limited to pancreas
T3 Indicates Cancer over 6 cm.
T4 Indicates Cancer outside pancreas but extending only into 'local' structures
N0 Indicates no involvement of lymph nodes
N1 Indicates involvement of one group of local nodes
N2 Indicates more than 2 node groups involved
N3&4 Indicates more extensive involvement of many lymph nodes within the abdomen
M metastases to more distant organs

Other testing studies needed for staging pancreatic cancer include the comprehensive history and physical examination, blood and urine tests, chest x-ray, liver scan. The major information for staging is obtained by exploratory surgery with direct examination of the pancreas, lymph nodes and other abdominal organs, and liver biopsy.

Prognosis: Thus far the results of all forms of treatment of pancreatic cancer have been disappointingly poor. Over 90% of patients with pancreatic cancer are dead within one year of establishing the diagnosis. Newer treatment programs under study do not even speak of survival durations of greater than one year. Therefore, remission times for pancreatic cancer are spoken of in terms of months rather than years and 'true cures' are practically unheard of.

Treatment Modalities: Surgery is the only definitive treatment available for pancreatic cancer and even then most of the cancers of the pancreas cannot be completely removed for technical reasons. Therefore, simple maneuvers are performed to attempt to relieve symptoms and reduce complications. Rarely is any case of pancreatic cancer cured with surgery.

Radiation Therapy: Using a variety of techniques there has been some modest successes in treating pancreatic cancer with radiation therapy. An attempt has been made to improve the response rate by administering radiation therapy simultaneously with, or subsequent to, surgery and chemotherapy.

Chemotherapy: Only a few chemotherapy agents have been found useful in the treatment of pancreatic cancer. There has been some modest improvement of survival when these drug agents are combined with radiation therapy, and when the drugs are used in combinations. The most commonly used chemotherapeutic agents are: 5-FU, doxorubicin, mitomycin-C, streptozotocin administered singly or in combination. More recently, newer agents such as cisplatinum are being studied but reports are too preliminary to be meaningful.

In some cases the chemotherapy agents for pancreatic cancer have been given directly into the circulation system of the pancreatic cancer (intra-arterially) with some slightly better results.

Response rates to these different maneuvers have varied from 15% to 65% but median duration of survival for pancreatic cancer is seldom greater than 10-12 months.

A great deal of research work remains to be done in pancreatic cancer to try to improve the discouraging prognosis.

Management Team: The general surgeon or the oncologic surgeon is the main signal caller in pancreatic cancer. The medical oncologist and radiation oncologist provide assistance in their specialties when indicated. Pain relief and comfort are the primary goals of the team in pancreatic cancer. Therefore, decisions regarding treatment choices must be weighed against the short term gains which can be accomplished without adding to the patient's suffering. Since survival periods for pancreatic cancer are so brief frequent visits to the doctor are required to maintain close contact with the physician in charge.

B) Cancer of the Liver: In order to clarify confusion which exists when discussing liver cancer it should be emphasized that the term 'cancer of the liver' refers to cancers which *originate* in the liver. The confusion arises from the common situation in which the liver cancer has spread from another organ—i.e., the colon, breast, rectum, lung, etc.—to the liver. This is usually called 'metastatic cancer of the liver' and is not the same as a cancer which starts in the liver—so called *primary liver cancer*. Of the two situations 'metastatic cancer of the liver' which has spread from other sites is the most common malignancy of the liver.

The remainder of this section deals only with *primary liver cancer*. Primary liver cancer is a very rare form of cancer which accounts for only about 2% of all cancers in the United States each year.

Names and Synonyms: Cancer of the liver, primary liver cancer, carcinoma of the liver, primary hepatoma, hepatocellular carcinoma, are some of the other appellations used for this cancer.

Incidence Rates: As stated above, primary liver cancer will account for only 2% of all cancers. Liver cancer is so infrequent, its fatality rate and occurrence rate (often given in actual numbers of cases instead of percentages) and is combined with cancers of the gallbladder and bile ducts. Together, as a group of three, in 1995, they are expected to account for 15,400 cancers and cause 12,300 cancer deaths.

True primary liver cancer , alone, is much more common in Oriental peoples and the Bantus of South Africa. It is 6-10 times more common in males than females. The average age of occurrence of primary liver cancer in the United States is 60-70 years.

Causes and Risk Factors: About 70% of patients with Primary Liver Cancer have preexisting cirrhosis of the liver. There has also been noted a close association of cancer of the liver with tropical infestations and parasitism of the liver especially schistosomiasis; with a rare iron deposition disease called Hemochromatosis; with viral hepatitis B; and with a peanut mold call aflatoxin. Cirrhosis of the liver, however, is the most common predisposing factor for Primary Liver Cancer. There are two kinds of cirrhosis which are most frequently in Primary Liver Cancer, they are, alcoholic cirrhosis and viral hepatitis B leading to cirrhosis.

Signs and Symptoms: Initial presenting complaints in liver cancer are often mild and nonspecific, they include; weakness, loss of appetite, abdominal fullness and bloating, dull aching pain in right upper abdomen.

Signs found on physical examination in Primary Liver Cancer include enlargement and tenderness of the liver with hard masses felt within the liver. Sometimes several small cancer nodules can be felt within the liver. Ascites—fluid accumulation within the abdomen—is often detectable. Yellow jaundice, if it occurs at all, is very mild.

Unfortunately all of the above signs and symptoms can occur with any cancer that has spread to the liver (metastatic liver cancer) from elsewhere and can only be distinguished from the primary form of liver cancer by biopsy and microscopic examination.

Screening Tests: No ideal screening test for surveying large numbers of the population for liver cancer is available. In suspected cases a special blood test—the serum alpha-fetoprotein—can be used to bolster your physician's suspicion of primary liver cancer. Liver scans can be performed if there is any doubt about the presence of cancer.

Some routine laboratory studies which may raise the suspicion of liver cancer include serum bilirubin (a reflection of yellow jaundice), abnormal liver function tests such as alkaline and several others.

Diagnosis: As always, biopsy is the only acceptable method of confirming the diagnosis of primary liver cancer. The biopsy can be accomplished either through exploratory surgery and direct visualization of the liver; or needle biopsy guided by CT scan, peritoneoscopy or blindly by feel.

Staging: No specific anatomic staging systems has been found useful in primary liver cancer. However, accurate assessment of any local spread, the multiplicity of tumors within the liver and distant spread are important to determine at the time of surgery in case the liver cancer has the rare chance of cure by surgical removal.

Prognosis: The overall 5-Year survival rate for primary liver cancer is less than 1% for all stages. If the liver cancer is not solitary and totally removable most patients will be dead within 6 months. Usually the liver cancer is present as multiple growths within the liver by the time of discovery and thus, cannot be totally removed surgically (completely resectable). In the rare case of resectable, non-disseminated liver cancers a 33% 5-year-survival rate has been reported.

Therapeutic Modalities: Surgical removal of the entire tumor is the only hope for cure in primary liver cancer but, unfortunately, most cases do not meet the criteria for surgery. These criteria are: a solitary or very localized tumor within the liver; no lymph node involvement; and no distant spread. Of course, the patient's general health must be adequate to make the extensive surgical operation safe.

The surgical operation recommended is called lobectomy i.e., removal of the entire lobe of the liver containing the cancer. The mortality from the operation itself is at least 20%. However, it is technically possible to remove up to 80-90% of the liver but operative mortality is unacceptably high.

Total liver removal with transplantation of a donor liver is being performed but is still under investigation and does hold some promise.

Radiation therapy is considered to be of little use in primary liver cancer since the liver cancer cells are not sensitive to x-ray energy.

Chemotherapy: Several chemotherapy agents have been found to be partially effective in treating primary liver cancer. Some are more effective when administered via infusion directly into the tumor area and others are under investigation for intravenous injection. However, the effect on overall survival in liver cancer has been minimal but other chemotherapeutic agents continue to be investigated. Some agents used are: 5-FU, fluoxuridine (FUDR), doxorubicin, streptozotocin and cisplatinum.

Of more recent vintage is the study of the interferons which seem to hold some promise in the treatment of primary liver cancer.

Special therapies now under investigation include immune therapy combined with different forms of radiation therapy, and do seem promising.

Management Team: In the cases of primary liver cancer not amenable to surgery the team coordinator is the medical oncologist who can only offer some palliation with chemotherapy.

(C) Cancer of the Gallbladder and Bile Ducts: Cancer of these two closely related anatomic structures are very rare. They will therefore be discussed together.

Incidence Rates: Together, gallbladder and bile duct cancer will account for about 6000 deaths in 1995. Gallbladder cancer will cause about 5000 of these fatalities and bile duct cancer will cause the remainder.

Causes and Risk Factors: No clearly defined cause for cancer of the gallbladder and bile ducts has been identified. However, approximately 5 to 20% of patients with cancer of the gallbladder and bile ducts are found to have gallstones or inflammation of the gallbladder (cholecystitis). About 1% of patients operated on for gallstones or infection of the gallbladder (cholecystitis) will be found to have an unexpected cancer of this type.

Signs and Symptoms: In gallbladder cancer weight loss, loss of appetite and vague abdominal pain are frequent symptoms. Nausea and vomiting are also common and jaundice eventually occurs in 60% of cases but appears late in the course of the disease.

In bile duct cancer jaundice is a very early sign and there is little pain in the early stages. Severe itching of the skin secondary to the jaundice is common and quite distressing to the patient.

In both kinds of cancer the gallbladder enlarges enough to be felt by the physician in 30-50% of cases.

No satisfactory screening tests for cancer of the gallbladder and bile ducts is available.

Diagnosis: In both cancer of the gallbladder and bile ducts diagnosis is usually established at surgery, unexpectedly.

In gallbladder cancer the liver function tests are often discovered to be abnormal prior to surgery. Gallbladder x-rays may simply show gallstones or a poorly functioning gallbladder neither of which are harbingers of cancer.

In bile duct cancer when blockage of the bile duct system is suspected the blockage can be demonstrated by injecting dye into the bile duct system. This can be done through a needle inserted into the liver and into a bile duct (transhepatic cholangiography), or by feeding a catheter through the small bowel and into the bile system (ERCP). These special x-ray tests might raise the suspicion of cancer but do not yet establish the diagnosis.

Staging: No detailed anatomic staging systems has been found useful in either gallbladder or bile duct cancer. However, extensive local invasion or distant spread of the cancer portends a poor prognosis and far advanced disease.

Prognosis: The outlook for gallbladder cancer is dismal with most patients succumbing within one year of diagnosis and less than 3% surviving for 5 years.

In bile duct cancer those few patients who do have surgically resectable disease have a 33% five year survival rate. However, most patients have distant spread by the time of diagnosis of the bile duct cancer and are dead within one year.

Therapeutic Modalities: Surgical removal of all the tumor offers the only hope for cure in these cancers. Unfortunately, complete removal is rarely possible. For most cases some form of palliation is accomplished through surgical relief of obstruction to the flow of bile with subsequent alleviation of pain and the severe jaundice and skin itching.

Radiation therapy can offer some palliation of symptoms with as many as 92% of patients receiving some benefit, albeit temporary.

Chemotherapy: Chemotherapeutic agents can also offer some benefit in those patients who relapse after surgery or radiation, or who fail to respond to these forms of treatment at all. Among the chemotherapy agents used are: 5-FU, BCNU, methyl-CCNU, streptozotocin, and others. Local infusion of chemotherapy drugs and biological response modifiers are under study in this group of cancers.

Management Team: The surgeon is most often the first line of attack with the radiation therapist and chemotherapist lending support.

Chapter 35

Cancers of the Head and Neck

The imprecise and blurred boundary lines of human anatomy, as applied in medical science, are exemplified by the title of this section. It is obvious to everyone that the 'head and neck' are not separate and distinct organs but are composed of many structures with different and unrelated functions. The eyes, for example, do not need the tongue in order to see and perceive images. Conversely the tongue does not require the integrity of the eyes in order to function in perceiving taste. Yet these structures each occupy a special place within the boundaries of the head and neck. The designation of 'Head and Neck Cancers' is purely an artificial one created by medical science to facilitate the study of the diseases in this anatomic area.

By arbitrary agreement cancers of the head and neck excludes cancers of the eye, the skin covering the head and neck, the thyroid gland, the bones of the neck and the skull, the brain and the internal organs of the ear.

Head and Neck Cancer essentially does include cancer of all the structures which are functionally part of the upper respiratory passages and the upper digestive tract.

The parts of the respiratory passages included in Head and Neck Cancer are such structures as the nasal cavities, the sinuses, the voice box (larynx), the throat (pharynx), the tonsils, etc.

The parts of the upper digestive system are represented by the mouth and its parts such as the tongue, the salivary glands, the gums, the lips, etc. There is obviously a good deal of overlap in these artificial boundaries.

Since all the anatomic parts of the head and neck, along with all the stages, subdivisions, cell types and substages of their cancers can become quite unwieldy the following discussion generally applies to all of the head and neck cancers as a single group.

The reader can safely assume that all the cancers considered to fit under the category of 'head and neck' cancers are discussed in this section. Any other cancers which appear to have been excluded conforms with the traditional manner of discussion. However, all of these other cancers are discussed in other sections of this book.

Cancers of the head and neck are relatively uncommon malignancies but they have very special significance because of the effect they have on the cosmetic integrity of the individual and because of the disruption of the important functions of eating and breathing which they can produce.

Incidence Rates: Head and neck cancers will account for about 3% of all malignancies or about 31,000 new cases in 1995, and a total of 8,000 deaths. Cancers of the voice box (larynx) are the most common type of the head and neck cancer group followed by the mouth, throat and salivary glands.

Causes and Risk Factors: No precise cause is known for head and neck cancers but there are several clearly defined risk factors.

Smoking tobacco and alcohol abuse, especially when used in combination, are extremely high risk factors. Poor oral hygiene seems to increase the risk of these cancers as well.

Occupants of southern China have a high risk of cancer of the nasal passages (nasopharynx) which seems to be environmental rather than genetic or ethnic in origin.

There is a high association between the presence of the Epstein-Barr virus and cancers of the nasopharynx.

There is a high incidence of nasopharynx cancer in furniture workers which may be associated with the inhalation of high concentrations of wood-dust.

Cancers of the lining of the oral cavity are very common in India and are associated with the chewing of the betel nut, a habit which is peculiar to this ethnic group.

Chronic iron deficiency, caused by inadequacy of dietary iron and worm infestations, seems to be associated with a higher incidence of cancers of the throat.

Prior to the antibiotic era the third stage syphilis was often associated with an increase in the incidence of cancer of the tongue.

Signs and Symptoms: The most common symptom of head and neck cancers is that of an ulcer growing on the inner lining (mucosa) of the mouth and throat. Raised, cauliflower-like masses in the mouth are also a common finding.

The location of the head and neck cancer growth influences the symptoms and signs the patient experiences. In the oral cavity the tumor may appear as an ulcer which fails to heal for a long period of time but has very little associated pain. In the throat there may be difficulty or pain on swallowing and pain referred to the ear during the act of swallowing. Sometimes an enlarged painful mass is visible on the external portions of the neck and throat.

Hoarseness of the voice, painful swallowing, obstruction to breathing and ear pain are frequently seen in the cancers of the larynx or voice box.

Chronic nose bleeds, obstructed nostrils, facial pain, hearing loss, double vision and a painless neck mass are common in the nasopharynx cancers. However, these symptoms are not caused by head and neck cancer.

The nose and sinus cancers may also produce nose bleeding, nasal discharge, nasal obstruction, facial pain, facial swelling and double vision.

Visible, painless swelling of the face or neck may be caused by cancers of the salivary glands such as the parotid gland—located in front of the ear where mumps occurs; or the submandibular glands—located just below the jaw on either side of the neck.

On occasion, the first clue of the presence of head and neck cancer is the enlargement of lymph nodes in the neck due to local spread of the invisible cancer from any of the above mentioned sites.

Screening Tests: No ideal screening test is available for head and neck cancers such as blood tests, x-rays or scans. The best method of early detection and general screening is a thorough mouth and throat examination during a complete physical examination. If suspicious changes or masses are found by your physician a more complete examination by an ear, nose and throat specialist (Otolaryngologist) is indicated.

Diagnosis: Biopsy of suspicious lesions is indicated but not until a more thorough examination is carried out by an expert in this type of examination such as an Otolaryngologist or an oral surgeon.

The surgeon must perform a careful inspection of all the internal structures of the nose and throat by direct visualization and indirectly via a mirror or fiber-optics. Then complete palpation of all the non-visible structures must be done with the gloved fingers. Only then can logical biopsy procedures be carried out. Even if the first biopsy is negative or inconclusive your physician may advise repeat biopsy for extremely questionable lesions.

Staging Systems: Because of the very complex nature of the head and neck cancers the complete anatomic staging system will not be discussed in detail. The standard TMN system is most often used and is the most practical system.

Stated in an oversimplified way the system is applied as follows: the primary (cancer) tumor (T) is designated T0 to T4 based on its measurement in centimeters. For example a cancer of the oral cavity measuring less than 2 cm. is designated T1; and a cancer measuring over 4cm. is designated T4.

If the cancer has spread to lymph nodes (N) the extent of their involvement is designated from N0 to N3, and so on.

If the cancer has extended to any area or organ below the collar bones (Clavicles) it is given the designation M for metastases.

The tests needed for staging head and neck cancers begins with the physical examination, extends through the surgical removal of apparent and suspected areas of cancer and concludes with the microscopic determination of the depth and extent of involvement.

Prior to the surgery of head and neck cancers some routine tests must be performed such as chest x-ray, blood count, and blood chemistry. Special x-ray examination requirements are dictated by the individual needs of each case and may include: x-rays of the skull, sinuses, and facial bones; CT scans of the nasopharynx, larynx; bone scans; and liver.

Of special importance is the detection of other unrelated serious diseases since their presence has such a large impact on the survival of patients with head and neck cancers. The mortality and morbidity rate is much higher for any patient with evidence of emphysema, coronary artery heart disease, cirrhosis of the liver, tuberculosis, lung cancer and syphilis. The mortality rate with these intercurrent diseases is reported to be 10-30% higher than in patients without these complicating illnesses.

Prognosis: It is sad to note that the 5-year survival rate for head and neck cancers, in general, has not improved much since 1960.

Important prognostic factors in head and neck cancers include anatomic site of the primary cancer lesion, and the size (T-stage) of that lesion; involvement of lymph nodes in the neck with cancer; and the presence of coexistent diseases mentioned above. Some representative examples of overall 5-year survival statistics are given below.

Cancer of the tongue	43% five-year survival
Cancer of the lip	85% five-year survival
Cancer of Tonsil	45% five-year survival
Cancer Floor of mouth	50% five-year survival
Cancer of Nasopharynx	43% five-year survival
Cancer of Larynx	60% five-year survival
Cancer of Sinuses	25% five-year survival
Cancer of Salivary Glands	45% five-year survival

Sites of Spread: Most often cancers of the head and neck recur within local neighboring structures as well as in the lymph nodes of the head and neck area but above the clavicles (collar bones). Distant spread beyond these boundaries has become more common in recent years because of longer overall life span of the population because of better treatment of cardiac and lung diseases. Thus, cases with metastases to the lungs, liver or lymph nodes below the clavicles are more frequently seen.

Therapeutic Modalities: Before discussing some of the treatment choices in head and neck cancers it should be pointed out that there are some special goals which are unique to treatment of the head and neck cancers. These special considerations are: eradication of the cancer; but with maintenance of the normal functions of swallowing, chewing and breathing; and the most important achievement, a socially acceptable cosmetic result.

The achievement of a good cosmetic result is a difficult one since, by necessity, the complications of the surgical treatment of the head and neck cancers can be quite disfiguring. Because of this cosmetic disfigurement your physician must take the time and trouble to explain, and even diagram, the possible alterations of appearance the patient will have to live with. Only the patient can decide if the preservation of his life is worth the cosmetic and social price to be paid.

Treatment decisions by your physician must take into consideration patient factors such as; age and general health; coexistent medical diseases; habits and life style; occupation; patient special needs and desires.

Surgery and radiation therapy are the primary treatment options in the head and neck cancers. Chemotherapy may add an additional dimension by upgrading the stage of disease and make it more amenable to the first two options. The use of chemotherapy to improve surgical cure is still under clinical investigation.

Small head and neck cancers of the T1-T2 category with no lymph node spread can be treated with one modality—surgery or radiation. The same size cancers with involved lymph nodes usually require a combination of surgery and radiation therapy.

In the larger head and neck cancers of the T3-T4 class with lymph node involvement surgical removal of the primary cancer and the lymph nodes is usually coupled with radiation.

Triple modality therapy utilizing surgery, radiation, and chemotherapy, in a variety of sequences and combinations, has shown some promise for increasing survival rates and cure rates of head and neck cancers. A great deal of research on this approach is still in progress and the final decision is not yet in.

Several chemotherapy agents have been found effective for head and neck cancers, both alone and in combination. The agents include; methotrexate, cis-platinum, carboplatin, bleomycin, 5-FU, and others.

Some effective combinations have reported to produce from 50-95% response rates but the duration of response has been short—6 months or less. The most active combinations are:

cis-platinum+bleomycin+vincristine;
cis-platinum+bleomycin+methotrexate+vinblastine;
bleomycin+vincristine+methotrexate;
bleomycin+vincristine+methotrexate+doxorubicin+5-FU.

The best responses have been with those combinations containing the agent cis-platinum.

Immunotherapy with BCG vaccine and other immunomodulator agents initially did show some responses but the procedure has been essentially abandoned in head and neck cancers. The newer biological response modifiers, namely the interferons and interleukin-2, are presently under intense investigation for treating head and neck cancers.

Management Team: The head and neck surgeon who has had specific training in oncologic surgery of this region is the ideal leader of the management team for head and neck cancer. There is no adequate substitute for this specially trained surgeon. Of course, along the way he may call on the medical oncologist and the radiation oncologist for assistance. Ideally, each case should be assessed by the entire team before offering treatment options to the patient. Unfortunately, the team concept has not taken a firm hold in the U.S. except for the large university cancer centers.

As always, careful and frequent follow up by the otolaryngologist (Ear, nose & throat specialist) is mandatory including regular, periodic examinations of the previously diseased areas of the head and neck. Most head and neck cancer recurrences appear within the first two years after treatment and seldom appear after the fourth year. But in this author's opinion annual complete physical examination and follow up are needed for the remainder of the patient's lifetime.

Chapter 36

Cancer of the Endocrine Glands: Thyroid, Adrenal and Pituitary Glands

It seems wise at this point to clarify before discussing these cancers what the endocrine glands actually are. These endocrine glands constitute a group of separate organs which influence various functions of the body by secreting chemicals (hormones) into the general circulation to maintain the integrity of the entire body. By mutual, arbitrary agreement the group does not include the sex hormones, insulin and several other minute but crucial hormones.

The group of endocrine glands does include the three organs listed above in the subheading.

Names and Synonyms: This relatively rare group of cancers has not yet suffered the burden of common names and synonyms.

Incidence Rates: As a group the cancers of the endocrine glands are by comparison quite uncommon. In 1995 they will account for only about 13,900 new cancers and for about 1,650 deaths. Thyroid cancer is the commonest of the group accounting for 12,500 cases and 1,000 deaths. As a result thyroid cancer will receive the most attention in the following discussion.

(A) Thyroid Cancer:

Causes and Risk Factors: Radiation exposure, both accidental and therapeutic, has been clearly associated with a higher incidence of thyroid cancer. After the Hiroshima atomic bomb explosion a major increase in the incidence of thyroid cancer in adults has been observed. In former times when radiation therapy was used to treat tonsil and adenoid diseases in infants it was not appreciated that the risk of thyroid cancer would increased in later years. A latency period of 5 to 30 years is needed between exposure to the radiation and occurrence of the thyroid cancer. Every effort should be made by physicians and hospitals to contact the adults who received such radiation therapy in childhood to advise them that careful and frequent thyroid examinations is necessary. On the other hand, no clear relationship between diagnostic x-rays and thyroid cancer has been found.

Other less clear risk factors which increase the risk of thyroid cancer include: the relationship between long standing goiter and cancer; benign adenomas of the thyroid; and the role of genetics and inheritance.

Signs and Symptoms: Hoarseness of the voice, difficulty in swallowing, pain or pressure sensation in the thyroid gland area of the neck, difficulty with breathing, increasing thyroid size, single or multiple lumps (nodules) in the thyroid, accidental discovery by physician on routine examination—all of these, alone or in combination, have been noted as initial findings in thyroid cancer.

Screening: Screening is now limited to routine physical examination of the thyroid gland and close surveillance of persons known to have been exposed to therapeutic and accidental radiation. No useful screening blood test or x-ray examination has been developed for thyroid cancer.

Diagnosis: Biopsy of any suspicious change in the thyroid gland is an obvious approach but deciding which patients need biopsy and when to perform the biopsy can be difficult. This dilemma is caused by the fact that there are so many people who have thyroid nodules which are not growing and are not causing symptoms. However, there are some generally accepted guidelines which the physician follows in solving this dilemma.

All solitary nodules or multiple nodules in the thyroid which are changing in size; any thyroid nodules is infants, or young adult males should be suspected and watched carefully.

Sometimes thyroid x-ray scans or CT scans are helpfully in deciding to biopsy a changing thyroid nodule. The use of thyroid blood tests to measure the glands functional status are seldom useful in thyroid cancer.

Biopsy is obtained by fine needle sampling through the skin; surgical excisions of the suspected nodule(s); or complete surgical removal of a lobe of the thyroid gland or the entire gland.

Staging: The standard TMN system is most often used in staging thyroid cancer.

The best prognosis is for Stage IA thyroid cancer which indicates there is a single thyroid cancer nodule, without involvement of any lymph nodes, or without distant spread to other organs. The worst outcome is seen in Stage IV thyroid cancer with distant spread to other major organs.

As part of the staging process the major organs are surveyed for distant metastases, and the local lymph nodes in the head and neck area are examined carefully. Chest x-ray, bone x-rays and bone scans, complete blood count, chemical profile and scanning of the thyroid gland with radioactive iodine are useful tests in thyroid cancer.

Prognosis: Long term survival studies indicate that about 20% of cases of thyroid cancer will eventually die of the malignancy. Nevertheless, there will be a 90% ten year survival rate, and a 60% twenty year survival rate in thyroid cancer.

Sites of Spread: The most common site of recurrence of thyroid cancer is in the lymph nodes in the neck, and in any thyroid tissue left after surgery. Other distant sites frequently found to have metastases from thyroid cancer include the lungs, bones, and liver.

Therapeutic Modalities: The choice of primary therapeutic attack of thyroid cancer varies with the cell-type of thyroid cancer, the number and size of cancer nodules found and the functional activity of the cancer nodules.

Either surgical removal of the diseased lobe of the thyroid is performed, or the entire thyroid gland is removed if the cancer is limited in extent and without distant metastases.

Radiation therapy can be applied to treat thyroid cancer in two fashions. The first is the standard x-ray external beam radiation source. The second method is via the administration of radioactive iodine orally by capsule which is then absorbed by the thyroid cancer. As a result the cancerous thyroid nodule is then slowly destroyed by the radiation energy.

Chemotherapy drugs have found only limited use in thyroid cancers. Doxorubicin is the most promising chemotherapy agent utilized. Combination therapies with surgery, radiation and chemotherapy are being explored.

Management Team: The special additional physician to this team is the Endocrinologist whose expertise lies in the area of diseases of the endocrine glands. The thyroid surgeon is an indispensable member of the team in order to establish the pathological diagnosis. The roles of the radiation oncologist and medical oncologist are obvious.

Follow Up: Regular physician examinations of any remaining thyroid tissue, lymph nodes and endangered distant organs is advised for the life of the thyroid cancer patient because recurrences as long as 20 or 30 years later are common.

(B)-Cancer of the Adrenal Gland: Since adrenal gland cancer is a very rare cancer it will be treated here in short summary form. It accounts for less than 0.2% of cancer deaths and it occurs in only 2 persons for each 1 million population.

Most often cancer of the adrenal gland is already disseminated to other organs by the time of its discovery. No distinct causes or even risk factors for adrenal gland cancer have become apparent. The most predominant symptom is abdominal pain due to the tumor mass which lies just above the kidney(s). Other more complex signs and symptoms result from the excess hormone production by the tumor or from symptoms which are due to a deficiency of that hormone.

Both the diagnosis and treatment of adrenal gland cancer are usually accomplished via surgical removal of the cancer mass. Radiation therapy has limited usefulness in adrenal cancer and can only be used to achieve palliation and does not result in remission or cure. Chemotherapy has even less application in adrenal gland cancer with short lived palliation and relief of symptoms.

The prognosis of adrenal cancer is at best very poor. The average duration of survival in the best hands is seldom beyond 3 months.

(C)-Cancer of the Pituitary Gland: In actual fact most growths within the pituitary gland are benign tumors (adenomas) based on their appearance under the microscope but they can produce severe symptoms and death by their strategic location within the brain. The pituitary tumors are located in the brain close to a point where the two optic nerves from the eyes intersect on their way to carrying the visual images to the brain. The other symptoms are produced by hormonal aberrations caused by the pituitary tumors, more accurately called adenomas.

Pituitary tumors account for only 10% of tumors in the brain substance. It is therefore also a rare kind of tumor. Thus, they are also discussed in summary fashion.

The proximity of the pituitary adenomas to the optic nerve often cause alterations of vision. These alterations include a loss of the same portion of a field of vision in each eye. This symptom of visual field loss is the most common vision change.

Aberrations of pituitary hormonal function cause symptoms which include: Acromegaly (a form of gigantism); Cushing's syndrome (caused by an excess of cortisone production), and many others.

Confirmation of the presence of the tumor mass within the pituitary gland is first required before undertaking the delicate surgery needed for cure. The tumor mass is usually well defined by x-rays, MRI scans and CT scans of the pituitary gland area of the brain.

Most types of pituitary tumors are treated with surgery or radiation therapy, and sometimes a combination of both. The results of these appropriate treatment plans is not precisely known but it has a high rate of success. Statistics suggest successes in the area of 70-90% long term survivals and are reasonable estimates.

Chemotherapy in the form of chemical agents to kill cancer cells (cytotoxic drugs) have very little if any value in pituitary gland cancers. But other non-chemotherapy drugs with properties for controlling the hormonal imbalances of these tumors have played a large part in improving the quality of life and long term survival.

Chapter 37

Cancers of the Brain and Spinal Cord

The brain and spinal cord jointly compose a system called the 'central nervous system' in order to distinguish it from the nerves which are located in the arms, and legs–called the peripheral nervous system . And all central nervous system cancers have the unique property of never spreading outside the anatomic confines of the central nervous system. These cancers may locally invade and penetrate deeper in their own neighborhood but do not disseminate outside it via the blood stream or lymphatic system as most other cancers do.

The discussion in this section contains only information about cancers which arise in the central nervous system. Many varieties of cancers commonly spread to the brain and spinal cord from their primary sites elsewhere in the body—i.e., breast cancer, lung cancer, prostate cancer, and so on. Approximately 20- 40% of brain cancers are due to dissemination of cancers from other sites. The remainder of the central nervous system cancers, about 60-80%, are 'primary' cancers of the central nervous system .

Names and Synonyms: The names and synonyms given for primary cancers of the central nervous system are actually a compilation of the various cell types of cancers in the central nervous system. Glioma, astrocytoma and meningioma are the more commonly known types of cancers.

Incidence Rates: In 1995 cancers of the central nervous system will account for 16,900 cases of cancer and cause 11,800 deaths.

Eighty percent of these will be brain cancers and 20% will be spinal cord cancers.

In children brain cancer is second only to leukemia as a cause of cancer deaths in children. It kills 1,600 children and young adults each year.

In adults the majority of all these central nervous system cancers are accounted for by three types: gliomas, meningiomas, and neurilemmomas.

Causes and Risk Factors: Genctics: In childhood, brain cancers are considered to be developmental in origin and are associated with several chromosomal disorders and genetic defects.

Chemical and viral Agents: There is little evidence for chemical and viral causes of brain cancers in humans but some agents can be made to induce central nervous system tumors in animals. The relation this laboratory finding has to central nervous system cancers in man is not clear at this time.

Signs and Symptoms: The symptoms of these central nervous system cancers are produced by increasing pressure caused by the cancer within the skull; or by directly compressing, invading or irritating regions of the brain. As a result, a large variety of nonspecific complaints are possible in the central nervous system including headaches, nausea and vomiting, convulsive seizures, changes in vision, paralysis of extremities, loss of sensation in extremities, difficulty in speaking, swallowing or hearing. Unfortunately these symptoms have so many varied causes it is difficult to now how to alert the reader as to the seriousness of the symptoms. Persistent and long lasting complaints of this type need the evaluation of a physician by appropriate testing.

Screening Tests: The complete history and physical examination remains the basic, major screening procedure to detect the possibility of brain and spinal cord cancers. When suspicious findings are evoked referral to a neurologist is indicated. The neurologist then performs a thorough examination of the entire nervous system by simple office procedures. If the likelihood of cancer is very high specific x-rays and scans of the central nervous system are indicated.

Diagnosis: Since the confirmation of the diagnosis requires major brain or spinal cord surgery there must be strong evidence from other tests that a cancer is indeed present. This strong evidence includes abnormal visual field examination, funduscopic examination, skull x-rays, electroencephalograms (EEG), lumbar puncture (spinal tap) for spinal fluid analysis, cerebral angiography, CT brain scans, MRI scans etc. But the major and most accurate methods have now become the computerized tomography (CT) scans of the brain and the more recent Magnetic Resonance Imaging (MRI). Both of these latter two imaging methods are highly sensitive and discriminating but they do not replace the need for biopsy confirmation.

Staging: Since these central nervous system cancers do not spread to either lymph nodes or distant organs the TNM systems has no application in central nervous system cancers. Instead, they are staged according to the size of the cancer; its confinement to one side, or its extension to the other side of the brain, and other factors. Stages I, IA and IB of central nervous systems tumors have the best prognosis and Stage IV has the worse prognosis.

Prognosis: Approximately 40% of people with brain cancers can be returned to a useful life style. Another 30% of patients can be given good palliation but with some physical disability or limitation of life style. The outcome varies with cell type of cancer, stage of cancer, response to treatment, etc. Below is listed some of the survival statistics for the various types of central nervous system cancers:

	Survival Percentage	
	5 yr.	**10 yr.**
Astrocytoma		
Stage I	50-100%	40-100%
Stage II	15-45	8-15
Stage III	10-30	0-10
Stage IV	0-10	0-1
Medulloblastoma	40-50	20-30
Ependymoma	40-55	35-45
Oligodendroglioma	50-80	20-30

Meningiomas	70-80	50-60
Craniopharyngioma	80-90	65-80

Therapeutic Modalities: The choice of therapy for central nervous system cancers depends on the cancer cell-type, the cancer stage and general health factors of the patient associated with their age.

Surgery is almost always required for establishing the diagnosis of central nervous system cancers unless even minor surgery for biopsy carries with it a very high risk of fatality.

The following chart lists the most optimal therapy for each type and stage of the central nervous system cancers:

Astrocytomas-Stages II, III & IV	= Radiation Therapy
Astrocytomas-Stage I	= Surgery+Radiation Therapy
Medulloblastoma	= Radiation Therapy
Meningiomas	= Surgery+Radiation Therapy
Ependymomas	= Radiation Therapy

Of course, in cases where complete surgical removal of the tumor is not possible radiation therapy is often added as an adjunct or a palliative measure. On the other hand, if high intracranial or spinal pressures is causing symptoms surgical relief of that pressure maybe indicated.

Chemotherapy: Chemotherapy (cytotoxic) agents have not produced any cures in central nervous system cancers by themselves but they have been useful in palliation. The application of chemotherapy drugs as additional therapy after surgery and/or radiation to improve survival and cure rates is under investigational research. The combination of these different modalities appears to have moderately improved survival rates, but not cure rates.

The effectiveness of many of these chemotherapeutic agents is limited by the fact that many do not penetrate into the brain or spinal cord in sufficient quantities to be able to destroy the cancer cells, although some authorities dispute this point. Some of the compounds which can achieve adequate central nervous system levels in quantity include procarbazine, VM-26, BCNU, CCNU, methyl-CCNU, vincristine, methotrexate, cisplatinum and VP-16. Also, several combinations of these drugs and newer single chemotherapeutic agents are being studied.

Intra-arterial infusion of these chemotherapy agents directly into the brain substance is also being investigated.

Immunotherapy, biological response modifiers, and their combination with standard chemotherapy and radiation therapy have also stirred recent interest.

Management Team: The neurosurgeon is the prime mover in the initial operative and postoperative period, if the cancer is cured or arrested by surgery alone. If radiation therapy and/or chemotherapy are indicated as additive or adjunctive therapy then the appropriate specialists will provide assistance.

Follow Up: At least monthly follow up visits to your physician are required, even in cured cases, for the first 12-24 months. Annual complete examinations should be done, thereafter, by the neurologist or neurosurgeon.

If chemotherapy and radiation therapy are administered, very close follow up by the chemotherapist or medical oncologist is mandatory.

Chapter 38

Cancers of the Bones

Most cancers of the bone are those that have spread (metastatic) from some other primary organ site, i.e., breast, lung, kidney, etc. The metastatic bone cancers constitute 60-65% of all bone cancers. The metastatic bone cancers most often occur in the bones of the spine and pelvis. Their spread to bones outside the trunk are much less likely. It is an accepted axiom that metastatic cancer of bone occurring beyond the elbow or below the knee is extremely rare. Whereas primary tumors of bone are more likely in these peripheral locations.

The remaining 30-35% of bone cancers actually arise within the bone substance and therefore are primary bone cancers. These primary bone cancers comprise the major subject of discussion of this section.

Names and Synonyms: Bone sarcoma, chondrosarcoma, osteosarcoma, osteogenic sarcoma, Ewing's tumor, malignant giant cell tumor, histiocytoma, fibrosarcoma, chordoma. Rather than the preceding being a list of true synonyms these are actually some the various cell types of the different bone cancers.

Incidence Rates: The primary bone cancers are relatively rare cancers occurring in only 3 persons per 100,000 of the general population, at least in adolescence; they account for 3.2% of cancers in childhood; in the age group 30-35 the incidence falls to 0.2 per 100,000 people. In the over 60 age group the incidence again rises to 3 per 100,000.

In 1995 there will only be 2,100 new cases of primary bone cancer diagnosed and 1,050 deaths will occur from these cancers. They are slightly more common in males than females. (The most common type of bone cancer is Multiple Myeloma which I have classified under Hematologic cancers and have discussed under that heading. Multiple myeloma will account for 35-43% of all primary bone cancers.)

Osteosarcoma (osteogenic sarcoma) is the most common primary bone malignancy comprising 28% of the entire group. The incidence of the other types of primary bone cancer are: chondrosarcoma 13%; fibrosarcoma 4%; the remainder is composed of many uncommon types listed above.

Causes or Risk Factors: Because of the relatively high incidence of primary bone cancers in children its is assumed these arise in areas of rapid growth. Other implicated, but unproven, causative factors include prolonged growth or over stimulated bone metabolism; mal-development syndromes; radiation exposure; and bone infections.

Signs and Symptoms: Bone pain is the most prominent symptom in the typical case of primary bone cancer. The pain is especially more severe at night than it is during the daylight hours. This nonspecific and common type of pain is the only symptom in most cases of bone cancer which makes early detection so difficult.

Screening: Plain x-rays of the limbs and a high index of suspicion by your physician are the only means of screening for bone cancer. The possibility of a primary bone cancer is usually triggered by your physician's suspicion of the appearance of the changes seen on x-rays of the bones. The characteristic x-ray appearance is that of a destructive bone lesion.

Diagnosis: The plain x-ray usually reveals the destructive lesion with a leading edge demarcating the true edge of the cancer; a so called 'moth eaten' appearance to the tumor mass; a permeating cancer extending in a longitudinal pattern along the length of the bone. MRI or CT scanning of the bone cancer mass is often helpful in distinguishing a benign from a malignant lesion.

Biopsy is, of course, the inevitable means of establishing a diagnosis of bone cancer. Sometimes the biopsy can be accomplished by needle aspiration of the bone lesion without major surgery but this procedure has a 25% rate of false-negative results.

Other tests are those which a reflection of bone metabolism, such as acid and alkaline, which are of only limited value. These tests of bone metabolism are more useful for detecting a metastatic bone cancer as opposed to a primary bone cancer.

Staging: A TNM system has not been developed for primary bone cancers because of its limited utility in this type of cancer. A staging system based on the size and local extension of the primary bone cancer has been devised and found helpful. Stage I bone cancers are those which are the smallest and have remained local and superficial.

Stage IV bone cancers—the most advanced—are the largest, the most extensive locally, and are those with distant spread to other organs, and as a result have the worse prognosis.

Prognosis: The prognosis of primary bone cancers depends on their cancer cell type, stage of disease and certain host factors. The following table lists some average 5-year survival treatment results by primary bone cancer type:

Bone Cancer Type	5-Year Survival
Osteosarcoma	5-20%
Chondrosarcoma	25-50%
Fibrosarcoma	20-25%
Ewing's Sarcoma	0-12%
Giant Cell Tumor	0-25%

Sites of Spread: The pattern of spread of primary bone cancer, in the early stages, is ordinarily directly along the longitudinal axis of the bone originally involved. Later, spread may involve other bones, lymph nodes and occasionally distant organs such as lungs and liver.

Therapeutic Modalities: Surgical removal of all visible bone tumor with at least a 10 cm. margin into normal bone is the primary form of treatment for bone cancer. Sometimes the extent and size of the original bone tumor occasional requires amputation of the limb, although, limb sparing surgery has its proponents if the cancer size and extent allows. In some cases limited excision of the cancer is possible with implantation of a bone graph or a prosthetic device.

Radiation Therapy: Unfortunately, most types of primary bone cancer, such as osteosarcoma, chondrosarcoma and fibrosarcoma are resistant to radiation therapy and is, therefore, of little use. Radiation therapy has been of some limited value in Ewing's sarcoma and other bone cancers.

Chemotherapy has played an increasingly more important role in the treatment of the primary bone cancers. Initially, the response to single chemotherapy agents was poor at best. The results with combinations of agents have shown more promise especially in osteogenic sarcoma.

In *Ewing's sarcoma,* characteristically a cancer with a very poor prognosis, combination chemotherapy in an adjuvant or preventative program has shown much promise. The 5-year survival rate with local treatment only—surgery and radiation—is less than 15%. When combination or single agent chemotherapy is added to surgery and radiation therapy a response rate of 40-60% is seen. Adjuvant (prophylactic) chemotherapy, when added to local therapy for Ewing's sarcoma, has shown marked reductions in local recurrences and dissemination of the primary bone cancer.

After removal of the Ewing's sarcoma a program of radiation to the primary site, along with radiation of both lungs, and chemotherapy with a combination of dactinomycin, vincristine, doxorubicin, and cyclophosphamide has resulted in a 58% response rate with median survival of over 3 years. Some research centers have reported a 5-year survival rate of over 75% with this and similar programs. Therefore, progress is being made in Ewing's sarcoma.

Immunotherapy of an older vintage-form such as BCG vaccine and others have been disappointing in improving response rates. However, in the newer forms of biological response modifiers such as Interferon, Transfer Factor and Tumor Necrosis Factor there is renewed hope and great promise for bone cancers.

Management Team: Total management team cooperation, especially before any definitive surgery, is most important in the care of the primary bone cancers. This statement is especially true now that adjuvant programs of chemotherapy and radiation therapy have shown such great promise for higher response rates and longer survivals. The orthopedic surgeon usually forms the first line of attack on these bone cancers with the radiation oncologist and the medical oncologist close at his side.

Follow Up: Very close follow up by a physician for the first 2-3 years after diagnosis and treatment is mandatory and lifetime follow up examinations are necessary. If recurrences or metastases appear there is still a good chance for remission, if the metastases are detected early enough.

Chapter 39

Soft Tissue Sarcomas

The soft tissue sarcoma group is actually composed of a mix of cancer types which are related in, essentially, two ways. First, they have the same cellular appearance under the microscope. Second, they clinically behave the same in the habits of growth and modes of spread. Actually, the soft tissue sarcomas are a conglomeration of similar cancers which appear to arise in the soft tissues not previously discussed elsewhere in this book. These soft tissues include muscle, fat tissue, joint spaces (synovia), nerve tissue (not including brain and spinal cord) blood vessels (called angiosarcomas) and fibrous connective tissue (fibrosarcomas).

Synonyms and Other Names: Liposarcoma, rhabdomyosarcoma, synoviasarcoma, neurofibrosarcoma, fibrosarcoma, angiosarcoma, leiomyosacroma, mesenchymoma, histiocytoma.

Incidence Rates: As a group the soft tissue sarcomas are quite rare cancers. They account for 1% of all cancers in men and 0.6% of cancers in women. The incidence rate is approximately 2 cases per 100,000 population. In the U.S. There are about 5,600 new cases a year and about 3,000 deaths. They are more common in children than adults and are ranked fifth as a cause of death in the age group below 15 years. The Fibrosarcomas are the most common type of soft tissue sarcomas composing 25% of the total group.

Causes and Risk Factors: No significant evidence points to a single causative agent in soft tissue sarcomas has been uncovered. Rarely, the soft tissue sarcomas will arise in old scars. However, high doses of radiation to treat other cancers can increase the risk of soft tissue sarcomas.

Signs and Symptoms: The symptoms produced by soft tissue sarcomas are usually insidious and quite nonspecific which makes their early detection very difficult. Occasionally, a hard and rapidly growing mass on one of the extremities or on the trunk is noted by the patients themselves. Too often, however, the tumor masses are hidden deep within the soft tissue of the muscles of the thigh, forearm or leg; deep in the abdomen; or in the joints.

Screening Tests: Generally speaking, there are no useful or reliable screening tests available for soft tissue sarcomas. Simple x-rays of suspicious areas are performed based on your physician's judgement and on her findings on physical examination.

Diagnosis: In appropriate cases of soft tissue sarcomas specialized studies such as CT scans, MRI scans, arteriograms can be helpful. However, open biopsy or excision of the tumor mass is usually diagnostic.

Staging Systems: The versatile and ubiquitous TNM system is used in most parts of the world for staging soft tissue sarcomas.

T-for tumor, is graded according the size of the original cancer mass in centimeters. N is for lymph nodes and M for distant metastases.

The various stages are designated based on the anatomic TNM group and a grading of the aggressive nature of the cancer by microscopic analysis.

The various stages of soft tissue sarcoma are: Stages I, IA, IB; II, IIA, IIB; III, IIIA, IIIB, IIIC, IV, IVA, IVB; progressing from the least extensive down to the most extensive disease.

Prognosis: As in most cancers the survival rates for soft tissue sarcomas vary with the stage of the cancer and type of treatment used. Surgery is the mainstay of treatment in these cancers and, unfortunately, the most radical surgery, namely amputation, is associated with the lowest recurrence rates. Recurrence rates based on the type of surgery used is given below:

Surgical Procedure	Local Recurrence Rates
Incisional Biopsy	100% local recurrences
Excisional Biopsy	80-100% local recurrences
Wide Excision	50% local recurrences
Radical Resection	10-20% local recurrences
Amputation	5% local recurrences

In general, recurrence rates of soft tissue sarcomas are relatively high ranging from 33% to 77%. Five year survival is approximately 60% after primary excision of the soft tissue sarcomas and drops to 30% if repeat excision of a local recurrence is required. However, with the addition of radiation therapy and chemotherapy these statistics are improving.

Approximate 5-year survivals of soft tissue sarcomas, by stage, are as follows:

STAGE	**5-year survival**
Stage I	75%
Stage II	55%
Stage III	30%
Stage IV	7%

Sites of Spread or Recurrence: The most common relapse of soft tissue sarcomas is in the form of local recurrence (unless amputation is performed) at the original primary tumor site. The distant recurrence sites are the lymph nodes, lungs, and liver.

Therapeutic Modalities: Surgical removal of all the tumor is the primary mode of attack on the soft tissue sarcomas. Amputation of the limb is most often recommended if an extremity is involved. However, there is some evidence that since the advent of combination therapy with radiation therapy and chemotherapy after wide excision that limb sparing surgery may be possible without a great reduction in survival rates. However, all the research data are not yet in on this question.

Radiation therapy has unequivocally improved disease control by reducing local recurrences and improving 5-year survival rates. However, the cure rate of soft tissue sarcomas has not yet been substantially altered by its addition to surgery.

Chemotherapy is useful both for recurrences and in the adjuvant setting for soft tissue sarcomas. Since the introduction of the drug doxorubicin into combination chemotherapy the response of the soft tissue sarcomas has increased considerably. Other useful chemotherapeutic agents include DTIC, cyclophosphamide, vincristine, cisplatin, ifosfamide.

Management Team: Initially, the surgeon is the primary team leader both in establishing diagnosis and in providing definitive therapy for soft tissue sarcomas. The specialty of the surgeon depends on the location of the primary soft tissue sarcoma. If the soft tissue sarcoma is located in the limbs then the orthopedic surgeon will prevail as team leader; if it is in the thorax the thoracic surgeon; if it is in the abdomen the abdominal surgeon, and so on.

Since combined modality approaches are the most frequently used treatment strategies for soft tissue sarcoma the support of the radiation oncologist and the medical oncologist are required at some point.

Follow Up: As always regular, meticulous follow up visits with annual complete restaging examinations are mandatory.

Chapter 40

Cancers of the Eye

When the common benign tumors of the eye are excluded malignant cancers of the eye are among the rarest forms of cancer. And when the various cancers of the lids are excluded—which are actually skin cancers—the number becomes even smaller. The discussion in this portion of this book will be limited to 'true cancers' of the eye itself (called intraocular cancer) but does not include cancers of the eye lids.

There are, essentially, only two 'primary cancers' of the eye; they are retinoblastoma and melanoma. They will be discussed separately.

Incidence Rates: In 1995 true cancers of the eye are expected to account for 1,700 cases and cause 275 deaths. The incidence is the same in both sexes. The kinds of eye cancers that occur in adults behave very differently from those which occur in children. Cancer masses in the orbit of the eye in adults are usually disseminated (metastatic) from a primary cancer found somewhere else.

Causes and Risk Factors: Aside from the cancers which occur on the skin of the eyelids and its relation to sun exposure there are no clear causative or risk factors known for the other cancers of the eye. The most common types of intraocular cancers are metastatic cancers.

(A) Retinoblastoma: Approximately 6% of retinoblastomas

have a tendency to be familial in nature. A person who survives a sporadic retinoblastoma of both eyes has a 50% chance of bearing a child with the same eye cancer. It is one of the truly inherited cancers.

Retinoblastoma is an eye cancer limited to childhood. It occurs in 1 in 23,000 live births. It is more common in whites than in blacks, with 86% in former and 14% in the latter. However, the mortality of retinoblastoma is twice as high in blacks as in whites. In most cases it is discovered by the age of 2 years and is rarely seen after age 6 years. There is a 5% association of retinoblastoma with other congenital defects such as mental retardation.

Signs and Symptoms: Retinoblastomas are typically detected on physical examination of the eye and are obvious by the whitened appearance of the pupil. Routine examination of the eyes at birth detects many cases of retinoblastoma.

Screening Methods: A high index of suspicion on the part of your physician is the best screening device especially in children whose parents or siblings have a history of retinoblastoma.

Diagnosis: Retinoblastoma is one of the few cancers in which biopsy is *not* required and is even considered hazardous and is more likely to cause spread of the cancer. But the accuracy of diagnosis with other tests is so very high the avoidance of biopsy is acceptable. Your physician can be virtually 100% certain of the diagnosis of retinoblastoma before treatment by surgical removal of the eye with the following tests: careful examination with specialized eye equipment (slit lamp microscopy) which is usually performed under general anesthesia to eliminate technical problems; CT scans of both eyes; and, occasionally, ultrasonic examination of both eyes.

Staging: Staging of retinoblastoma has an entirely different system of grading or staging other than the usual TNM system. The retinoblastomas are categorized as Group I through Group V based on the size and depth of the cancer within the eye. Group I retinoblastomas have the best prognosis and Group V the least favorable prognosis.

Other tests are used in staging to determine local extent of the cancer, its extension into the central nervous system, and its occasional distant spread into other organs. These staging tests should include: CT scan of the orbit including the optic nerve, bone and base of the brain; x-rays of the skull and bony orbits; lumbar puncture (spinal tap); when indicated scans of the entire brain, bone and liver; complete blood counts; and chemistry profile.

Prognosis: The prognosis is of course dependent on the Grouping, presence of disseminated disease, and appropriate treatment. The mortality for retinoblastoma is still an unacceptable 20%. The rates of cure based on Grouping is given below:

Grouping	Cure Rates
Group I	80-85%
Group II	65-70%
Group III	60-65%
Group IV	25-30%
Group V	15-20%

Those cases of retinoblastoma with distant spread to the brain or other organs have a very poor prognosis.

Sites of Spread: These have already been alluded to above.

Therapeutic Modalities: Surgical removal of the entire affected eye along with 10-15mm of the optic nerve is the treatment of choice. In the cases where both eyes involved with retinoblastomas only the eye with the largest cancer is removed in order to attempt to preserve some sight. Further attempts to control the retinoblastoma in the other eye are carried out with radiation therapy and chemotherapy.

Radiation therapy may also be used after surgery if residual cancer was found in the optic nerve examined by the pathologist on microscopic examination.

Some cancer research centers are now attempting to treat very small retinoblastomas with radiation alone in an attempt to preserve the sight in the involved eye. However, this approach is still under research investigation.

Chemotherapy: When chemotherapeutic agents are used in combination with surgery and radiation to treat retinoblastomas the use of adjuvant, multiple chemotherapy drugs appears to improve survival and cure rate substantially.

Management Team: The special physician additions to this management team are the ophthalmologist and the pediatrician. Frequent and careful repeat examinations of the orbit of the removed eye, the remaining eye, the nervous system and general physical status are mandatory.

(B) Intraocular Malignant Melanoma: Malignant melanoma of the eye is the most common primary intraocular malignancy. It is strictly a cancer of adults with the average age about 50 years. It occurs in only 0.05% of the eye patient population and is extremely rare in blacks. There are no sex or genetic predilections. It also has no association with other malignant melanomas which occur in the skin or elsewhere.

Signs and Symptoms: Unfortunately changes in vision may not occur until late in the course of intraocular malignant melanoma. Routine ophthalmological examination with the instruments used to examine the back of the eye (the retina) usually uncovers the unsuspected tumor mass. Ordinary eye chart examination will not detect this cancer. When vision changes are noted it is usually reported by the patient and is characterized as a 'loss of side vision.' Secondary consequences of melanoma of the eye may be glaucoma, retinal detachment, cataracts, and inflammatory changes.

The best screening procedure for malignant melanoma is a thorough ophthalomoscopic examination of both retinae.

Diagnosis: Again biopsy of a suspicious mass is *not* indicated in malignant melanoma of the eye. But diagnosis is virtually 100% accurate with other testing coupled with thorough ophthalomoscopic examination. When the results of CT scans of the eye and orbit, and ultrasonic examinations are combined the diagnosis of malignant melanoma is usually clear and unequivocal.

Staging Systems: No useful anatomic staging systems is applied in intraocular melanoma. When distant spread of malignant melanoma does occur almost any organ can be involved but the liver is the most common site. Blood tests of liver function, x-rays of lungs and ,occasionally, scans of liver are indicated.

Prognosis: Precise statistics on 5-year survival rates and cure rates for malignant melanoma are difficult to obtain in this rare cancer. But the prognosis is related to the size of the original tumor; anatomic extension into other portions of the eye; distant spread, if any; cancer located in the iris and other anterior parts of the eye; the time lapse between surgical removal and appearance of the first symptoms; and the age of the patient. Some very rough figures for survival rates are listed below but are, however, a general compilation of all types and grades of malignant melanoma, and for all treatments :

5-year survival	55%
10-year survival	38%

Sites of Spread: These have already been discussed.

Therapeutic Modalities: Surgical removal of the entire eye is the treatment of choice except when the melanoma is located in the iris only where it can be treated with excision of the tumor only. There has been some controversy among medical experts whether or not the surgery helps to spread the cancer—which is generally not considered a risk in other cancers—but many authorities disagree with this claim in malignant melanoma of the eye.

Radiation Therapy: Melanomas are generally resistant to radiation therapy but radiotherapy may sometimes be considered in the cases of patients with only the one remaining eye which contains the tumor.

Proton Beam: Proton beam energy is a special type of radiation therapy which can produce 90% control of malignant melanoma of the uveal tract.

Cobalt-60 discs, another special form of radiation, are useful and can deliver 4 to 5 times more radiation to the cancer than other forms of radiation therapy.

Radioactive radon seeds have produced some temporary arrest of malignant tumor growth when implanted in the sclera of the eye.

Other forms of Radiotherapy:

Iodine-125 plaques have also had limited utility.

Helium ions as a radiation source is being studied and holds some promise. The same can be said for Photocoagulation and Cryotherapy.

Management Team: The prime movers in intraocular malignant melanoma are the eye surgeon (ophthalmologist) and the radiation oncologist. Careful, frequent follow up visits with thorough eye examinations and general physical examinations are important.

Chapter 41

Cancers of the Kidney

This chapter will only discuss adult kidney cancer. Childhood kidney cancer, which has some very unique features, is taken up in another section, i.e., "Cancers of Childhood."

Names and Synonyms: Carcinoma of the kidney, Clear Cell kidney cancer, Renal Cell Cancer, Hypernephroma, Adenocarcinoma of the kidney.

Incidence: In 1995 there will occur an estimated 26,500 new cases of kidney cancer and it will cause 10,700 deaths. Kidney cancer comprises 2% of all cancers, has a 2 to 1 male predominance and the average age effected is 55-60 years. Eighty per cent of the cases occur as a single type called 'Hypernephroma' and thus most of the following statements refer to this type of kidney cancer.

Causes and Risk Factors: No definite cause of kidney cancer is known but there is a high correlation with its occurrence and cigarette smoking.

Signs and Symptoms: The most common presenting complaints and findings of kidney cancer are: bloody urine (hematuria); abdominal or flank pain; enlarged mass felt in the abdomen; high circulation red blood cell count (polycythemia); and fever. Since kidney cancer can exist for a prolonged period before symptoms occur approximately one-third of cases already have distant spread to other organs when first discovered.

Screening: Mass screening of the population for kidney cancer is not practical or productive. In suspected cases with characteristics symptoms and signs, the excretory urogram (IVP or Intravenous Pyelogram) with the improved modifications of MRI and CT scan, and nephrotomogram are the best screening tests for kidney cancer.

Diagnosis: Obtaining cancer cells via a biopsy of the kidney is required and is usually obtained by needle biopsy or major surgery. However, some of the following tests can be helpful in supporting the diagnosis of kidney cancer before surgery. Urine analysis for the presence of red blood, IVP, of the kidney, needle aspiration of kidney cysts or masses, scans, arteriorgraphy, and microscopic examination of urine for cancer cells.

Staging System and Tests: Staging methods used for kidney cancer are the TNM system and an A,B,C,D system. Both systems are based on the size of the cancer, its local extension, and distant spread of the cancer. Stage A is the least advanced and has the best prognosis. Most of the determination of the stage of the cancer is accomplished at surgery since local extension is so important and so common.

Other testing procedures for staging for kidney cancer include history and physical examination, complete blood count, blood chemistry analysis, chest x-ray, x-rays, CT scans, MRI and scans of the bones and the liver.

Prognosis: With appropriate therapy the following results can be expected in treatment of kidney cancer. In the early stages A and B there is a 5-year survival of 30-50%, and a 10-year survival of 15-30%; stage C has a 5-year survival 10%, and a 10-year survival of 5%; stage D has a very poor prognosis of probably less than 1% one year survival.

Sites of Spread: Local invasion by the kidney cancer into the soft tissue around the kidney and into lymph nodes, large blood vessels within the abdomen—such as renal vein and vena cava—are all very important prognostic factors. Spread to distant by kidney cancer organs includes the liver, bones, lungs and brain.

Therapeutic Modalities: Surgical removal of the entire kidney (nephrectomy) containing the tumor is the best treatment in early

Stage A cases of kidney cancer. Radiation therapy to the kidney bed after nephrectomy is added in Stages B and C. Stage D is treated with palliative intent only since long survival is not very likely.

Chemotherapy has found very little place in treating the kidney cancers at this time. There have been occasional responses with hormonal therapy in the form of an agent called Megace, and similar compounds.

Along the lines of newer developments the interferons, interleukin -2 (IL-2), and other biological response modifiers appear to offer some hope for the future. Complete remissions in metastatic kidney cancer can be accomplished with these agents in 10 to 20% of patients.

Management Team: The management team for kidney cancer is usually headed by the urologist with the additional assistance of the radiation oncologist and medical oncologist.

Follow Up: Careful follow up visits with repeat urological examinations and general medical surveillance are important in kidney cancer.

Chapter 42

Cancer of the Testicles

Although testicular cancer is one of the least common kinds of cancer it deserves special mention for several reasons. It is among the most curable types of cancer; it is easily detected by self-examination of the testicles; it is one of the most easily monitored cancers through simple blood tests; and it is one of the most sensitive to chemotherapy.

Names and Synonyms: Testicular cancer, cancer of the testis, carcinoma of the testicle, seminoma of the testicle, germ cell cancer of the testicle, non-seminomatous cancer of the testicle.

Incidence: Testicular cancer accounts for only 1% of all cancers. It is restricted, of course, to males. In 1995 it estimated that there will be 6,300 new cases but there will only be about 350 deaths caused by this cancer. The average age of onset of testicular cancer is 32 years. There is an increased incidence of testicular cancer in conjunction with the congenital abnormality called "Undescended (Cryptorchid) Testicle."

Causes and Risk Factors: No clear-cut cause for testicular cancer is known and the above mentioned cryptorchid testicle is the only known risk factor.

Signs and Symptoms: There are usually no symptoms such as pain or any other distress in the majority of cases of testicular cancer except for a vague tenderness in the testicle. In 96% of the cases a lump or mass is accidentally felt by the subject himself or by the physician on routine examination. Early detection is, therefore, possible through regular periodic self-examinations of the testicles.

Screening: No practical method of mass screening is available except for education of the general population emphasizing self-examination of the testicles which can significantly improve the early detection rate and therefore the cure rate.

Diagnosis: Biopsy is the ultimate answer to any diagnostic questions about a testicular mass. Your physician can be relatively certain of the diagnosis through special testing before proceeding with surgery. The following tests do help bolster your physician's clinical impression. These tests include: Thorough physical examination of both testicles and the abdomen; specific blood tests for human chorionic gonadotrophin (ß-HCG) and alpha-fetoprotein; ultrasound of the testicles; MRI and CT scans of abdomen; lymphangiograms of abdominal lymph nodes; chest x-ray; excretory urogram (IVP). The surgeon must have a very high degree of certainty of the diagnosis by this point since the entire testicle must be removed for biopsy.

Staging: Most of the tests required for staging of testicular cancer have been listed under the heading 'Diagnosis' above. Either the standard TNM system or an A,B,C,D system is utilized.

Stage	Definition
Stage A	Cancer confined to one testicle; none in lymph nodes
Stage B1	Lymph nodes involved minimally (less than 6 nodes)
Stage B2	more than 6 nodes involved
Stage B3	massive node involvement
Stage C	distant spread to nodes above diaphragm or to other organs.

Prognosis: With the advent of newer therapies and new applications of older approaches the prognosis for testicular cancers is steadily improving. The advancements are so rapid that the figures given below may already be outdated but they give the reader a general idea of prognosis.

Stage	5-year survival
Stage A	95%
Stage B1,2,3	80-90%
Stage C	70%

Sites of Spread: The most common site of spread of testicular cancer is the lymph nodes within the pelvis or abdomen. The more distant organs which may be involved are the lungs, and mediastinum (soft tissue substance in the center of chest).

Therapeutic Modalities: Surgical removal of the cancer mass and the entire testicle is the first priority. In many cases removal of local lymph nodes is carried out at the same time to determine the presence of cancer spread in these areas since it is helpful in determining accurate staging.

Radiation therapy is used in many cases of testicular cancer after surgery especially in the more common cell type known as 'Seminoma.' Very often prophylactic radiation therapy is administered to high relapse areas such as the mediastinum and abdomen. In the other common cell type—Non-seminoma— chemotherapy has largely replaced radiation therapy as the treatment of choice.

Chemotherapy, given both prophylactically and in known disseminated disease, has had a major impact on the cure rate of testicular cancers. Upwards of 90% of patients with testicular cancer, even those with distant spread to other organs, can anticipate significantly prolonged life expectancy without evidence of cancer. The more common agents used in testicular cancer are: cis-platinum, carboplatin, bleomycin, vinblastine, actinomycin-D, cyclophosphamide. These chemotherapy drugs are usually used in combination rather than as single agents.

Although precise statistics are difficult to obtain for testicular cancer there has most certainly been a major improvement in 'true cure' rates in testicular cancers because of these new combinations of therapy.

Management Team: The urologist and the medical oncologist are the primary team managers in the testicular cancers. Of course, the help of the radiation oncologist ,and sometimes that of the general surgeon , although they are rarely necessary. Long term follow up visits are mandatory with careful, regular monitoring for recurrence of disease by means of physical examination, the simple blood tests for ß-HCG and for alpha-fetoprotein.

Chapter 43

Gestational Trophoblastic Cancer

Although these rare cancers of the afterbirth (placenta) account for only a small number of cancers each year they deserve special mention because they occur during pregnancy and are highly 'curable' with chemotherapy.

This malignant growth actually occurs in the substance of the placenta during pregnancy and occurs in three forms. The first, and most common, is called "Hydatidiform" mole (80%); the second, locally invasive Hydatid moles (15%); and the third, the more aggressive choriocarcinoma (5%).

Names and Synonyms: These have all been mentioned in the above discussion.

Incidence Rates: In the U. S. the trophoblastic cancers occur in 1 out of every 2000 deliveries or 1 in 1,200 pregnancies. There is a racial and socioeconomic variation of this cancer with a higher incidence in the Orient, and in Mexican-Americans living in Southern California. It is more common after multiple pregnancies and in women over age 40. Although it can occur at any time during pregnancy it is most often found after a spontaneous miscarriage in the second trimester (the middle-third time period) of pregnancy.

Signs and Symptoms: The most common presentation of gestational trophoblastic cancer is as a spontaneous miscarriage in the second trimester of the pregnancy. Your physician notes on examination of the pregnant mother the absence of fetal heart tones and a uterus which is larger than expected for this mid-stage of pregnancy. The gestational trophoblastic cancer is sometimes suspected because of prolonged vaginal bleeding after the miscarriage, or because of the vaginal passage of grape-like tumor material.

Screening: Massive screening of all pregnancies for gestational trophoblastic cancers is not practical at this time.

Diagnosis: The diagnosis can only be established by examination of the spontaneously passed placenta but your physician's suspicions can be bolstered by the physical examination, and some special blood and urine tests.

The level of a hormone (ß-HCG) in the urine or blood is exceptionally high when gestational trophoblastic cancers are present and suspected cases can be screened with these tests. Pelvic ultrasound and amniography are also helpful visualizing tests.

Staging: An anatomic TNM staging system has not been applied in gestational trophoblastic cancers. However, certain examinations are mandatory to determine extent of disease. The cancers are then placed into 'Groups' to classify them and to estimate the risk of recurrence or spread. They are as follows:

Group I	Non-disseminated and limited to uterus
Group II	Low risk-duration less than 4 months and low titers of ß-HCG; spread limited and excluding liver or brain
Group III	High risk-distant spread but not to liver or brain Duration greater than 4 months High titers of ß-HCG in urine
Group IV	Very High risk-distant spread to brain or liver

Prognosis: Remissions for trophoblastic cancers are as high as 92% for all stages of disease from Group I to IV. Group I patients can expect to have a 100% disease-free, long term remission. Complete remission with treatment by combination chemotherapy occurs in 70% of the Group IV patients.

Sites of Spread: The sites of spread have already been alluded to in the above discussion.

Therapeutic Modalities: Surgery is carried out by the technique of suctioning out all of the unevacuated material from the uterus and is mandatory. In older patients, where reproductive function need not be preserved, total hysterectomy may be an acceptable alternative surgical procedure.

Radiation therapy: Radiation therapy plays only a small role in treatment of the trophoblastic cancers except when there is already spread of the cancer to the brain. Whole brain radiation therapy in these cases is very useful.

Chemotherapy: The successful application of chemotherapy in trophoblastic cancers remains a land mark event in the history of cancer chemotherapy. Complete eradication of all evidence of cancer—in both locally invasive cancers and those with distant spread—is very possible with single agent or combination agent chemotherapy with the exception of perhaps in cases of spread to the brain. This was the first such accomplishment in any solid cancer in the history of human cancer treatment. The chemotherapy agents which are used, singly or in combination, include: methotrexate, actinomycin-D, chlorambucil, hydroxyurea, cyclophosphamide, vincristine, doxorubicin and others.

Most significantly, and unusual in cancer, is the ability to determine complete eradication of disease based on a simple and reliable test, i.e., the analysis of the ß-HCG in the urine or blood. The test is so sensitive and so accurate that it can assure your physician that if it remains negative for several successive months all the gestational trophoblastic cancer has been eliminated. If the ß-HCG is still positive there is still definitely cancer remaining and further chemotherapy is needed.

Management Team: The primary guardian against recurrent gestational trophoblastic cancer and the physician responsible for the initial treatment is the Obstetrician-Gynecologist. Of course, the medical oncologist plays an important co-leadership role in administering the chemotherapy.

Follow Up: Regular periodic follow up visits to your Obstetrician-

—Gynecologist with pelvic examinations, and repeat blood and urine ß-HCG titers is mandatory.

Chapter 44

Cancers of Childhood

In spite of the fact that childhood cancers are quite rare they offer a unique opportunity to study cancer. They have been the seed bed of many of the current great advancements made in the understanding and treatment of cancer. There are only about 7800 new cases of cancer, including all types, diagnosed in children each year. However, it is the second leading cause of death in children ages 1 to 14 years. Over half of these are solid cancers and they are highly malignant. The trend, because of modern therapy advancements over the last few decades, has been one of increasing cures and decreasing mortality. The previous death rate of 83 per million childhood population has fallen to 33 per million in the last several years.

The major changes in mortality of childhood cancer has resulted from the use of combination of therapeutic modalities which had its beginnings with childhood cancer. This principle of combination therapy has improved greatly our ability to cure cancer. And, the ideal manner of researching cancer—multicenter cooperative studies—was first applied in childhood cancers. The following is a list of the ten major developments which have resulted from the study of childhood cancers:

1. Extirpative surgery
2. Postoperative radiation therapy
3. Effectiveness of single agent chemotherapy
4. Effectiveness of combinations of chemotherapy agents

5. Combination of modalities, i.e., surgery, radiation, chemotherapy
6. Desirability of multidisciplinary teams of physicians
7. Devising and refining staging systems
8. Identifying and refining prognostic indicators
9. Application of different treatment modalities based on stage and prognosis.
10. Widespread application of these new techniques to other cancers

The following section will discuss only the so called 'Solid Cancers' of childhood to differentiate them from the non-solid (Hematological) cancers which have been discussed elsewhere in this book. Some of the solid cancers of childhood have also been touched on in other sections of this book and are excluded here because they behave the same as the adult variety.

A special dimension is needed in the management of childhood cancer because of the fragile and sensitive constitution—both physical and psychological—of children. When the reader considers that even when children do survive their cancer their lives are permanently altered—such as their ability to have children of their own—one realizes the unique impact cancer will have on these delicate beings.

Late effects of Therapy: Since children with cancer may have a potentially longer normal life expectancy than adults many late effects of the anticancer therapies have become apparent 30 or 40 years after cure. These late effects need special consideration and must be discussed with the parents and the children when they are old enough to understand.

Some of the more common late problems anticancer therapies are:

1. Radiation therapy can cause retardation of bone and cartilage growth with resultant diminished physical stature, intellectual impairments, impaired bone marrow function, permanent damage to kidneys, liver and lungs.

2. Chemotherapy can produce impaired bone marrow function, functional damage to kidneys, heart, intestinal tract, brain, lungs, and reproductive organs. Damage to reproductive organs may lead to ste-

rility in males and infertility in females.

3. Combined modality therapies may result in enhancement of all the above listed late onset possibilities. They also increase the risk of second malignancies appearing later.

The risk of late second malignancies, especially leukemia, is a major concern, even though the risk is small. The risk of developing a second malignancy is usually far less than the risk of death from the first malignancy. Nevertheless, this point must be addressed. Parents and patients seldom have any other choice than to choose the potentially curative therapy but they must be made aware of the risks involved.

Psycho-social aspects are even more important not only for the child but for the parents and the rest of the family. Divorce rates tend to increase in families which have a child with cancer. Parents suffer special forms of guilt complexes by blaming themselves or the other spouse for; inadequate care, bad genetic inheritance, environmental pollution they should have recognized, fear of having more children with cancer, etc. Thus, the child and the remainder of the family have some special needs which must be recognized and addressed by the management team.

Only two of the four major childhood cancers are addressed in the following discussion—i.e.,1) Wilm's Tumor and 2) Neuroblastoma— since the other types have been discussed elsewhere in this work. The remaining two of the four are, Non-Hodgkin's Lymphoma and Soft tissue sarcomas, which are discussed in their respective chapters.

(1) Wilm's Tumor (Nephroblastoma): The treatment and cure of this form of cancer of the kidney is the classic model for the development of the many milestones of cancer therapy listed above. As a result of these developments one can track the 5-Year survival of Wilm's tumor from a low of 8% in 1920 to over 95% in 1980.

Incidence: The occurrence rate of Wilm's Kidney tumor is a low 7.6 cases per million population. It occurs slightly more frequently in blacks than in whites. The sex incidences are equal. The peak age incidence is 1-3 years and 90% of cases occur in children under age 7 years. Wilm's Kidney tumor is usually present in only one kidney with involvement of both kidneys found in only 5% of cases.

Causes and Risk Factors: There is no clear cut single cause of Wilm's tumor. Genetic makeup and inheritance factors are suspected of playing a strong part in the causation of Wilm's tumor. All the cases in which both kidneys are involved, and in 30% of those which are one sided cancers, Wilm's tumor is found to be inherited. This inheritance concept is supported by the finding of Wilm's Tumor in association with other genetically inherited abnormalities such as: Aniridia; hemi-hypertrophy; and other congenital abnormalities of the genitourinary systems.

Signs and Symptoms: The most frequent presenting finding of Wilm's Tumor is the detection of a large mass felt in the abdomen by your doctor on physical examination. In some cases the mass is so large it can be seen protruding against the abdominal wall. Abdominal pain occurs in only 37% of cases, fever in 23%, bloody urine in only 21% of cases in Wilm's tumor.

Screening Tests: The best available method of screening for this type of cancer is the physical examination of the abdomen and the routine urine analysis.

Diagnosis: The initial impression of a tumor mass and the localization of the mass which is felt can be confirmed with plain abdominal x-rays, excretory urogram (IVP), ultrasound and CT or MRI scans of the abdomen. Before surgical removal of the mass is planned a routine history and physical examination, complete blood count, blood chemistry profile, urine analysis, and chest x-ray are mandatory. Scans of the liver, lungs and bones may be needed in cases of suspected distant spread to these structures. Biopsy of the mass of the kidney tumor is performed by complete surgical removal of the mass. Needle biopsy of the kidney tumor mass or other forms of incomplete excisional removal are not advised.

Staging: Final and complete staging of Wilm's tumor is accomplished at surgery to confirm and define the local invasion of the cancer into surrounding structures. Distant metastases are usually discovered in pre-surgical staging tests.

The various stages of Wilm's tumor are outlined and defined below:

Stage I	Cancer limited to kidney with no local invasion. Tumor mass was not ruptured at surgery and is *completely* removed.
Stage II	Cancer extends beyond kidney but can still be completely removed. The extension of the tumor is limited to *local* structures.
Stage III	After surgery there is some residual cancer that could not be removed.
Stage IV	Distant spread to lung, liver, bone and brain.
Stage V	Cancer involves both kidneys.

Prognosis: As previously stated Wilm's tumor has an excellent prognosis presuming accurate staging is performed and meticulous treatment is exercised. The chart below outlines the 5-Year survival rates of Wilm's tumor by stage:

Stage	**Two Year Survival Rate**
Stage I	97% two year survival
Stage II	86% two year survival
Stage III	70% two year survival
Stage IV	80% two year survival
Stage V	53% two year survival

Age of the child at the time of diagnosis appears to be a major factor in prognosis in addition to stage in Wilm's Tumor. Age of the child below 2 years improves prognosis except in Stage I disease where it appears to have no bearing. Of course, administering proper recommended therapy is of major importance in prognosis.

Therapeutic Modalities: Surgery : Complete surgical removal of all the local Wilm's Kidney tumor mass is mandatory when technically possible. All of the surrounding tissue and the other kidney must be examined for completion of staging. All efforts must be made to avoid rupturing the tumor and to prevent spilling the contents into the abdomen. Silver clips are placed around the margins of the area which contained Wilm's Kidney tumor so that radiation treatment can be precisely applied to that area after surgery.

Radiation: Radiotherapy's primary goal is to prevent local recurrences of the Wilm's tumor. Whether radiation therapy is used or not is based on stage of the Wilm's tumor and age of the child. For example, in stage I Wilm's tumor in a child below the age of 2 years radiation is not necessary. However, radiation is indicated in children in this same stage I in patients over the age of 2 years. In stage II Wilm's tumor radiation therapy is used but is limited to the bed of the Wilm's tumor within the area of the silver clips mentioned above. Stage III patients should receive radiation therapy to the entire abdominal cavity as well as the tumor bed. Stages IV and V Wilm's tumor are usually treated with chemotherapy only after surgical removal of the tumor. Stages II through IV also receive chemotherapy after their radiation therapy and surgery.

Chemotherapy: As stated above, chemotherapy is used in Stages II through IV Wilm's tumor and results in a high rate of response. The two primary, and most effective, chemotherapy agents used are actinomycin-D and vincristine. Several other agents have been found to be active in treating Wilm's tumor and they include: doxorubicin, cyclophosphamide, methotrexate, and several others.

The most important factor in treatment of Wilm's tumor is accurate staging and application of combined modality therapy according to stage of the tumor and age of the child.

Side Effects of Therapy: The family and the patient must be made to realize that the cure of Wilm's tumor may have special consequences especially in the sensitive, rapidly growing, and developing organ structures of children. These consequences usually are a result of both the chemotherapy and radiation therapy. These consequences can include: impairment of physical growth resulting in scoliosis of the spine, small physical stature and skeletal deformities; damage to nerve and brain tissue with physical and intellectual impairment; destruction of ovaries and testicles with resultant loss of reproductive ability; lung damage with impairment of respiratory capacity and function; and even, rarely, second malignancies.

Indeed, the vast majority of the children treated for Wilm's tumor do not develop these late consequences but the parents and the child, when he or she is old enough to understand, must be made aware of these possibilities.

Management Team: The ideal management team of Wilm's tumor consists of a pediatrician, medical oncologist, radiation oncologist, or pediatric surgeon, and family physician. The psychologist's or psychiatrist's role in this team is indispensable in the management of the psycho-social problems which every family will have to face. The optimal approach to the management is discussion of the case by the entire team before any definitive treatment plan is put into effect.

Close, meticulous and multi-discipline follow up to the physician and careful physical examination is obligatory.

(2) Neuroblastoma: Neuroblastoma, which arises in specialized nervous tissue called the sympathetic ganglia, is the third most common solid cancer in children.

Incidence: Neuroblastoma accounts for 7-14% of all childhood malignancies. It is estimated to occur in 1 of 10,000-40,000 infants. The peak age incidence is 2 years and is rare in children over age 6 years. The tumor does have a higher occurrence rate in siblings and is associated with other hereditary disorders.

The most common sites of origin of Neuroblastoma are: the abdomen, mediastinum (see glossary), neck, pelvis and the eye.

Causes and Risk Factors: There are no known causes or risk factors for Neuroblastoma at the present time.

Signs and Symptoms: The most common clinical findings of Neuroblastoma are discovery of a mass in the abdomen or the neck by physical examination, or in the chest by x-ray examination. Pain produced by the mass is a very uncommon symptom which makes early detection difficult.

Other findings in Neuroblastoma are high blood pressure, which is otherwise unusual in infants and children. Some other nonspecific symptoms of Neuroblastoma may include fever, weakness, pale skin, weight loss, cough and shortness of breath.

Sadly, 55 -70% of cases of Neuroblastoma have already spread to distant sites by the time of the original discovery of the cancer, and these metastases manifest their own peculiar symptoms. Bulging of the eyes (exophthalmus) is the most frequent late symptom when the tumor arises in the eye.

Screening Tests: Screening blood tests or x-rays which are practical and cost effective for surveillance of large numbers of the childhood population are not yet available. However, the thorough history and physical examination, especially in newborn infants, is very useful and cost effective.

Diagnosis: A sample of tissue for pathological examination is required for the diagnosis of Neuroblastoma. When biopsy is technically feasible it should consist of excision of the entire cancerous mass at surgery. Occasionally, the diagnosis of Neuroblastoma can be established by biopsy of a metastatic deposit by a needle of such accessible sites as the bone marrow, a lymph node, and abdominal or chest mass.

Staging Systems and Tests: An anatomic staging system of Neuroblastoma is available and is based on; original cancer size, its extension to local structures and across the midline of the body, spread to local lymph nodes and remote organs such as bone, bone marrow, liver, soft tissue and to other distant lymph nodes.

Another important variable of Neuroblastoma, which can significantly alter the stage of disease, is whether or not the entire primary cancer mass can be removed surgically.

The categories of Neuroblastoma are designated as stages I, II, III and IV. A special category, designated as stage IV-S, indicates the same characteristics as stage I or II neuroblastoma plus distant spread limited to the liver, skin or to the bone marrow but not in the bone substance (cortex) itself.

Most of the accurate staging information needed for Neuroblastoma is obtained at surgery where the surgeon outlines and visualizes the degree of local extension of the tumor. Several other specific tests are required for staging prior to surgery. These include: the complete history and physical examination including blood pressure; complete blood count, blood chemistry profile and liver function tests; chest x-rays, bone scan and liver scan; computed tomography (CT) of abdomen and chest cavities; and a special urine test to detect the presence of a unique chemical produced by this tumor—it is called vanillylmandelic acid (VMA)—a derivative of epinephrine or adrenaline. This chemical is used in a serial manner to detect recurrences of neuroblastoma, or to identify unsuspected incomplete removal of the tumor at first surgery.

Prognosis: The outcome of therapy and survival in neuroblastoma are very much influenced by the stage of the cancer and the age of the child at time of diagnosis; and by the relatively high risk of mortality during or shortly after surgery.

Approximately 1/3 of all children can expect complete 'true cure' of neuroblastoma. Surgical or operative mortality is under 10%. About 2% of children under the age of two years experience regression of the tumor after treatment to a benign condition. Children over two years of age with Stage IV neuroblastoma will have an eventual fatal outcome. The following table gives prolonged survival rates according to anatomic stage of neuroblastoma:

Stage	**Survival Rates**
Stage I	86%
Stage II	70%
Stage III	44%
Stage IV	49%
Stage IV-S	about 100% (but 75-85% is more realistic).

The sites of spread of neuroblastoma has significant effect on survival rates. The presence of spread to the bone substance—but not to the bone marrow—has an especially poor prognosis.

Therapeutic Modalities: Surgery remains the mainstay of treatment of neuroblastomas with attempts at complete removal of the entire cancer mass considered the ideal procedure. If complete tumor removal is not technically possible then removal of as much tumor as possible (called debulking) is required. The other therapeutic modalities used for neuroblastoma after surgery are more effective when the maximum amount of tumor is removed (called debulking). However, some experts in the field have recently questioned this debulking concept.

Radiation therapy: Postsurgical radiation therapy is not given to all cases of neuroblastoma. The age of the patient and the amount of residual cancer remaining after surgery dictate whether this modality is used at all. Neuroblastoma is a relatively radiation sensitive cancer.

Chemotherapy drugs for neuroblastoma when studied in earlier years had little significant effect on survival rates in patients with distant spread but more contemporary agents are having a much greater impact. The chemotherapy agents are usually used in combination rather than singly and those combinations include: cyclophosphamide +DTIC+vincristine; cyclophosphamide+doxorubicin; or cis-platinum +VP-16 (etoposide).

Recommended therapeutic applications by stage of neuroblastoma follows:

Stage	**Treatment of Choice**
Stage I	Surgery alone
Stage II, under age 1 year	Surgery alone
Stage II, over age 1 year	Surgery+radiation
Stage III	Surgery if removable; Radiation+chemotherapy
Stage IV	Surgery if removable; Radiation+chemotherapy
Stage IV-S	Radiation+single agent chemotherapy

Management Team: The management team for neuroblastoma is similar in composition to the one recommended for RETINOBLASTOMA with the exception of the ophthalmologist.

Follow Up: Serial follow up examinations with special attention to urine tests for VMA and general physical examination are mandatory.

The majority of the more commonly encountered cancers in the United States and those with the highest fatality rates have been covered in the preceding sections of this book. However, some of the rarer types of cancer have not been touched upon, not because they are not important but because of the limitations of space and the magnitude of information their complete discussion would present. If the reader wants information about one of these rare forms of cancer, their physician, their local county or state medical societies, or the local American Cancer Society office can provide guidance to other sources of information.

Part Eight

Drug Therapy of Cancer

Introduction

Drug Therapy of Cancer

Strictly speaking, this section will deal with those chemical agents which are used to kill or damage the cancer cell. I emphasize this very important point to distinguish these agents from the many other ancillary medications used in cancer management but which do not attack the cell. These other ancillary medications are discussed in later pages.

These ancillary agents include those drugs used to treat the side effects of chemotherapy, the complications of the cancer and the general comfort measures for the patient. The agents referred to include: pain relievers, psycho-therapeutic drugs, sleep aids, sedatives, anti-vomiting aids, antibiotics, vitamins, hematinics (blood builders), and the like.

The anticancer agents discussed are divided into five main types: Cytotoxic agents, Hormonal Agents and Hormone antagonists, Immunotherapy agents, and Biological response modifiers. Some of the side effects are listed for each agent along with the symptoms produced by those side effects, and some of the cancers which are treated by each drug is given.

Some useful definitions are in order before beginning the discussion of the chemotherapy agents.

Chemotherapy Agents: A chemotherapy agent is any chemical, synthetic or natural, used to kill or eliminate cancer cells, impede their growth or stimulate their removal by the body. These drugs are also called anticancer, anti-tumor, anti-neoplastic agents and cytotoxic drugs.

Side Effect: A side effect is any unwanted and undesirable symptom or change which results from administering chemotherapy agents. Such side effects include: nausea, vomiting, diarrhea, bone marrow suppression, anemia, hair loss (alopecia), fatigue, decrease in appetite (anorexia), weakness, depression, suppressed immunity with increased infection risk, internal organ damage, etc.

Some clarification of the term side effects appears warranted here. When the side effects are listed for each agent they should be viewed as adverse reactions which *may* occur but do not necessarily have to occur. There is a common misconception that these side effects *must* occur in order for the chemotherapy to work against the cancer. This notion is incorrect. In fact, your physician should exert great effort to reduce or eliminate these side effects. They do not occur in all people nor do they occur with all agents. The likelihood of side effects is also unpredictable, except in a general, broad sense, and they can vary in their occurrence rate and severity.

Therapeutic/Toxic Ratio: The therapeutic/toxic ratio is that value or concept which your physician uses to weigh the risks of therapy against the hoped-for-benefit one is trying to achieve in treating your cancer. Your chemotherapist must carefully consider this ratio and thoroughly discuss it with the reader and your family before embarking on any treatment program which includes these powerful drugs. The ultimate decision, *to treat or not to treat* , and whether the benefits of therapy are worth the risks involved can only be made by you, the patient. The moral support of the family and the advice of the physician can help the patient make an informed, rational decision.

Chapter 45

The Chemotherapeutic Agents

The Cytotoxic agents: These compounds can be derived from natural products such as plants, minerals or bacteria, or they can be synthetically produced. In either case they all have in common the limiting property of damaging normal cells and tissues as well as cancer cells. By and large it is this property of the cytotoxic agents which accounts for most of the side effects they produce. In most cases these side effects are temporary, nonfatal and reversible. If they were irreversible the cytotoxic agent would be discarded as too highly toxic for clinical use in treating cancer.

The following is an alphabetical listing of those cytotoxic agents with some of their clinical characteristics.

ASPARAGINASE: Other names; Elspar®.

Uses: acute lymphoblastic leukemia in children.

Side effects: drowsiness, fever, skin rash, joint pain, itching, nausea and vomiting. Less common reactions are; difficulty in breathing, puffiness of the face, stomach pains. Minor side effects are headache, temporary loss of appetite (anorexia), sore throat, mouth sores, unusual thirst, frequent urination, leg pains.

Notify physician immediately if the following signs or symptoms occur: fever over 101 degrees, difficulty breathing, convulsive seizures, collapse or coma.

AZACYTIDINE: 5-azacytidine, 5 aza-C, ladakamycin.

Uses: acute non-lymphocytic leukemia.

Side Effects: suppressed blood counts-common and severe; nausea/vomiting-common; sore mouth/tongue-occasional; diarrhea-common; muscle pain/weakness/sleepiness/coma-uncommon; liver damage-rare; fever-occasional.

Symptoms due to side effects: fever/chills/infection; difficulty swallowing/eating/chewing; yellow jaundice.

BLEOMYCIN: Brand name Blenoxane®.

Uses: Cancers of: the testicles; head and neck; penis; cervix; vulva; anus; skin; lung. Hodgkin's Disease and non-Hodgkin's Lymphoma.

Side Effects: suppressed blood counts-uncommon; nausea/vomiting-occasional; hair loss/sore mouth and tongue/redness of skin/thickening of nails/darkening, scaling of skin-common; lung damage-dose related and rare; fever-common; sleepiness/headache/joint swelling-rare; pain at injection site-uncommon.

Symptoms: fever, chills, infection; difficulty in swallowing, eating, chewing; cough, shortness of breath.

BUSULFAN: Brand name Myleran®.

Uses: Chronic granulocytic leukemia.

Side Effects: suppressed blood counts-dose related; nausea/vomiting-rare; darkening of skin-occasional; lung damage-rare; adrenal gland damage-rare; gout-common; amenorrhea/irregular menstrual periods-common; second malignancies-very rare.

Symptoms: fever, chills, infection; cough, shortness of breath; muscle weakness, salt craving; sever joint pain.

CARBOPLATIN: Paraplatin®

Uses: Cancer of the ovary, lung, lymphomas, breast, bladder.

Side Effects: Nausea and vomiting; Bone marrow suppression; peripheral neuropathy (uncommon); hearing loss.

Symptoms: fever, chills, infection, bleeding; numbness and tingling hands and feet.

CARMUSTINE: other names: BCNU.

Uses: Cancer of lung, brain, colon, rectum, stomach; lymphomas, multiple myeloma, malignant melanoma.

Side Effects: Suppressed blood counts-common; nausea/vomiting-common; facial flushing, darkening of skin with direct contact by the drug-common; liver, lung, and kidney damage-uncommon.

Symptoms: fever, chills, infection; shortness of breath, cough, jaundice.

CHLORAMBUCIL: Brand name-Leukeran®.

Uses: Chronic lymphocytic leukemia; Lymphomas.

Side Effects: suppressed blood counts; nausea/vomiting-rare; liver damage-rare; second malignancy-rare; amenorrhea in females/male sterility-common; drug fever & rash-uncommon.

Symptoms: Fever, chills, bleeding.

CISPLATIN: Other names: Platinol®, DDP, CDDP, cisplatinum.

Uses: Cancers of the testicles, ovary, bladder, head/neck, lung, lymphomas, possibly breast and colon cancers.

Side Effects: Suppressed blood counts-common; nausea/vomiting-common; kidney damage-common but avoidable; high tone deafness-common but not incapacitating; acute allergic reactions-occasional; peripheral nerve damage-rare; gout-rare.

Symptoms: infection/bleeding; numbness of fingers and toes; acute joint pain.

CYCLOPHOSPHAMIDE: Cytoxan®, CTX.

Uses: Cancer of the breast, lung, ovary, testicle, bladder. Sarcomas of soft tissue and bone. Hodgkin's and non-Hodgkin's Lymphomas. Acute and chronic leukemias; and Wilm's Tumor of childhood. Multiple myeloma.

Side Effects: suppressed blood counts-very common; nausea/vomiting-very common; hair loss-common but reversible; darkening of skin and nails; sore mouth and tongue. Bloody urine-uncommon. Suppressed immunity, amenorrhea in women/sterility in men-common. Lung damage-rare.

CYTARABINE: Cytosine arabinoside, ara-C, Cytosar-U®.

Uses: Acute non-lymphocytic leukemia, lymphomas, primary and secondary brain tumors.

Side Effects: Suppressed blood counts; nausea/vomiting-common; sore mouth and tongue-occasional; flu-like symptoms and rash-occasional; liver damage-rare, mild and reversible.

Symptoms: infection/bleeding; fever, muscle aches and fatigue.

DACARBIZINE: DIC, DTIC, imidazole carboxamide.

Uses: Malignant melanoma, soft tissue sarcomas, lymphomas.

Side Effects: suppressed blood counts-common but mild; nausea/vomiting-common and severe; hair loss, redness of skin, hives and other rashes-uncommon; flu-like syndrome-common.

Symptoms: infection/bleeding; fever, muscle aches and fatigue.

DACTINOMYCIN: , act-D, Cosmegen®.

Uses: cancer of testicles, cancers. Wilm's Tumor, soft tissue sarcomas and Ewing's sarcoma of childhood.

Side Effects: suppressed blood counts-common and severe; nausea/vomiting-common; redness, darkening, scaling of the skin; sore mouth/tongue; hair loss-common; mental depression-rare.

Symptoms: Infection & bleeding. Difficulty swallowing/chewing.

DAUNORUBICIN: Daunomycin, rubidomycin, DNR, Cerubidine®.

Uses: Acute non-lymphocytic leukemia.

Side Effects: suppressed blood counts-common and severe; hair loss-common; sore mouth/tongue-rare; heart damage and heart failure-occasional but avoidable; urine discoloration-common; phlebitis in veins injected with drug-uncommon.

Symptoms: infection/bleeding; difficulty/pain swallowing and chewing; shortness of breath, swollen ankles.

DOXORUBICIN: ADR; Adriamycin®.

Uses: Cancer of the breast, bladder, esophagus, liver, lung, prostate, stomach, and thyroid . Sarcomas of bone and soft tissue. Hodgkin's and Non-Hodgkin's lymphoma. Acute lymphocytic and acute non-lymphocytic leukemias. Wilm's tumor, and rhabdomyosarcoma of children.

Side Effects: Suppression of blood counts-common; nausea/vomiting-common; sore mouth and tongue-common; hair loss-common but reversible; darkening of skin over veins used for injection-common.

Special Side Effects; Heart damage which is directly related to the total dose administered over a prolonged period of time. The total dose for adults should not exceed 500-850 mg. depending on the size of the individual. The damage can be irreversible if the total dose is not carefully monitored.

Red urine is common but not a sign of kidney or bladder damage.

Phlebitis of the veins used for injecting the drug is frequent. Fever and chills directly due to a reaction to drug is uncommon.

Symptoms: Infestation/bleeding. Difficulty swallowing and chewing, poor appetite. Shortness of breath, swollen ankles, cough. Swollen, red, painful veins.

ESTRAMUSTINE: Estracyt, Emcyt®.

Uses: Metastatic cancer of the prostate.

Side Effects: Suppression of blood counts-occasional; nausea/vomiting-common; skin rash and fever-rare; enlargement and tenderness of male breasts-occasional; heart failure-occasional.

Symptoms: Infection/bleeding; shortness of breath, cough, swollen ankles.

ETOPOSIDE: Epipodophyllotoxin, VP-16, VP-16-213, Vepesid®.

Uses: Small cell and Non-small cell cancers of the lung; acute non-lymphocytic leukemia, Hodgkin's and Non-Hodgkin's lymphomas.

Side Effects: Suppression of blood count-common; nausea/vomiting-uncommon; hair loss-common; sore mouth and tongue-rare; low blood pressure during injection-rare and preventable. Phlebitis of vein used for injection-rare.

Special: Severe drop in blood pressure if injected rapidly. Rare major allergic reactions with wheezing, shortness of breath and shock.

FLOXURIDINE: FUDR.

Uses: Cancer of the liver, both primary and metastatic. Can be given directly into an artery by infusion or it can be given systemically by intravenous injection.

Side Effects: Suppression of blood counts and nausea/vomiting-are both rare with infusion but can occur with intravenous infusion; sore mouth/tongue, inflammation of esophagus and colon-occasional; hair loss-uncommon; darkening of skin and nails are occasional; nerve injury-rare.

Symptoms: Infection/bleeding. Difficulty swallowing, chewing and diarrhea. Headache, visual disturbances, loss of balance and equilibrium.

FLUDARABINE: Fludara.

Uses: Chronic Lypmphatic Leukemia; Lymphoma.

Side Effects: see Cytarabine

FLUOROURACIL: 5-FU, Fluorouracil, Adrucil®, 5-fluorouracil.

Uses: Cancers of the breast, colon, rectum, stomach, pancreas, esophagus, liver, and gallbladder. Basal cell skin cancer—as an ointment.

Side Effects: suppressed blood counts-common; nausea/vomiting-common; sore mouth and tongue; partial hair loss-common; darkening of skin and veins; skin rash-uncommon; nerve injury-rare; excessive tearing of the eyes-rare.

Symptoms: Infection/bleeding; difficulty swallowing/chewing/loss of appetite/diarrhea; headache, vision disturbances, loss of balance and equilibrium.

GOSERELIN: Zoladex®

Uses: Prostate Cancer; Breast Cancer

Side Effects: Increase in bone pain; hot flashes; urinary obstruction in men with prostate cancer.

Symptoms: Inability to urinate.

HEXAMETHYLMELAMINE: HXM

Uses: Cancer of the ovary.

Side Effects: suppression of blood counts-uncommon; nausea/vomiting/diarrhea/abdominal cramps-occasional; hair loss, skin rash, itching-rare; nerve damage and brain damage-rare.

Symptoms: Infection/bleeding; difficulty swallowing/chewing; numbness of fingers/agitation; confusion/hallucinations/depression/tremors of fingers and hands.

HYDROXYUREA: Hydrea®.

Uses: Head and neck cancers; chronic granulocytic leukemia; acute lymphocytic and non-lymphocytic leukemias.

Side Effects: suppression of blood counts-common; nausea/vomiting-uncommon; soreness of mouth-rare; skin rash-uncommon; kidney damage-rare; brain damage-rare.

Symptoms: Infection/bleeding; difficulty urinating; headaches, visual disturbances and loss of equilibrium.

IFOSFAMIDE: Ifex®

Uses: Lymphomas, sarcomas, cancer of the ovary, breast, lung.

Side Effects: Nausea and vomiting; confusion; kidney damage; bone marrow suppression; bloody urine (cystitis); blurred vision.

Symptoms: fever, chills, infection, bleeding; confusion, hallucinations.

LOMUSTINE: CCNU, CeeNU®.

Uses: Lung and kidney cancer; Hodgkin's and non-Hodgkin's lymphomas; brain cancers, both primary and metastatic.

Side Effects: suppression of blood counts-very common; nausea/vomiting-very common; hair loss and sore mouth-rare; brain damage-rare; liver damage-rare; second malignancy-possible.

Symptoms: Infection/bleeding; confusion, lethargy and loss of equilibrium; yellow jaundice and tender liver.

MECHLORETHAMINE: Nitrogen mustard, HN2, Mustargen®.

Uses: Hodgkin's and non-Hodgkin's lymphomas; lung cancers; malignant fluids in lung space (pleura), abdomen (pertioneum), and around the heart (pericardium).

Side Effects: suppression of blood counts-universal; nausea/vomiting-common; sore mouth, and skin rash-rare; phlebitis of veins-common; amenorrhea and sterility in males-common; mild brain effects-uncommon; severe allergic reactions-rare; second malignancies-possible.

Symptoms: Infection/bleeding; difficulty chewing and swallowing; cessation of menstrual periods; weakness, sleepiness and headache; wheezing and shock.

MELPHALAN: Phenylalanine mustard, L-sarcolysin, L-PAM, Alkeran®.

Uses: Multiple myeloma, cancers of breast, ovary and testicle.

Side Effects: Suppression of blood counts-common; nausea/vomiting-rare; hair loss, skin rash and sore mouth-uncommon; lung damage-rare.

Symptoms: Infection/bleeding; shortness of breath, shortness of breath, cough.

METHOTREXATE: Amethopterin, MTX, Mexate®.

Uses: Cancers of the breast, head & neck, liver, colon, stomach, esophagus, lung, and cancers. Sarcomas of bone. Acute lymphocytic leukemia, leukemia involving the brain covering (meningeal).

Side Effects: Suppression of blood counts-universal; nausea/vomiting-occasional; soreness of mouth-common; red skin rash, hives, skin darkening-uncommon; hair loss-rare and mild; liver, kidney, and lung injury-uncommon.

Symptoms: Infection/bleeding; difficulty chewing/swallowing.

MITHRAMYCIN: Mithracin®; Plicamycin.

Uses: Cancer of the testicle; severely high blood calcium (Malignant Hypercalcemia).

Side Effects: Suppression of blood counts especially the platelets which aid the clotting of blood. Nausea/vomiting-common; blushing of face, darkening of skin, scaling of skin-occasional; soreness of mouth-common; hair loss-uncommon; colon irritation; brain injury; phlebitis-all uncommon; kidney injury-uncommon.

Symptoms: Infection/prolonged and severe bleeding. Diarrhea; headache, irritability, and lethargy.

MITOMYCIN: Mitomycin-C, Mutamycin®.

Uses: Cancer of the stomach, pancreas, esophagus.

Side Effects: Suppression of blood counts-common and can be severe; nausea/vomiting-common but mild; soreness of mouth and hair loss-common; kidney injury-uncommon; fever-common.

Symptoms: Infection/bleeding; difficulty chewing, swallowing; fever and chills.

MITOTANE: Lysodren®, o,p'-DDD,.

Uses: Cancer of the Adrenal glands.

Side Effects: Suppression of blood counts-never occurs. Nausea/vomiting-common; skin rash-occasional; brain injury-common but reversible; bloody urine, high blood pressure, black out spells, visual disturbances-are all uncommon.

Symptoms: Lethargy, sleepiness, dizziness/vertigo.

PENTOSTATIN: 2-Deoxycoformycin; Nipent.

Uses: Hairy Cell Leukemia; Non-Hodgkin's Lymphoma.

Side Effects: see under Cytarabine pg. 366.

PROCARBAZINE: Matulane®.

Uses: Cancers of the lung; Hodgkin's and non-Hodgkin's lymphomas, brain cancers.

Side Effects: Suppression of blood counts; nausea/vomiting-common; diarrhea-uncommon; soreness of mouth-uncommon; hair loss, itching and rash-uncommon; brain injury-occasional; visual disturbances, black out spells-rare.

Special: The use of alcohol, and certain medications and foods must be avoided when taking this chemotherapy agent.

Symptoms: Infection/bleeding; numbness of digits, headaches, dizziness, depression, anxiety, insomnia, nightmares, hallucinations, confusion, convulsions and coma.

SEMUSTINE: Methyl-CCNU.

Uses: Cancers of the rectum, colon and stomach. Brain tumors; Hodgkin's and non-Hodgkin's lymphomas; Malignant Melanoma.

Side Effects: Suppression of blood counts. Nausea/vomiting-common; kidney and liver injury-uncommon.

Symptoms: Infection/bleeding.

STREPTOZOTOCIN: Streptozotocin, Zanosar®.

Uses: Cancer of the pancreas.

Side Effects: Suppression of blood counts-uncommon and mild; nausea/vomiting-common and severe; kidney injury-common but mild and preventable; hypoglycemia (low blood sugar) occurs only with special kinds of pancreatic cancer; liver injury-uncommon.

Symptoms: Infection/bleeding; blood and protein in urine; weakness, tremor and coma reversible with food or sugar intake.

THIOGUANINE: 6-Thioguanine, 6-TG.

Uses: Acute non-lymphocytic leukemia; non-Hodgkin's Lymphoma in children.

Side Effects: Suppression of blood counts-common; nausea/vomiting-occasional; soreness of mouth and irritation of intestinal tract-uncommon; skin rash-rare; liver injury-rare.

Symptoms: Infection/bleeding; difficulty swallowing/diarrhea.

THIOTEPA: Triethylenethiophosphoramide.

Uses: Cancer of the urinary bladder; malignant effusions; cancers of breast and ovary.

Side Effects: Suppression of blood counts-universal; nausea/vomiting-uncommon; soreness of mouth-uncommon; brain injury-rare; fever-rare; amenorrhea and male sterility-common.

Symptoms: Infection/bleeding; dizziness/headache.

VINBLASTINE: VLB, Velban®.

Uses: Cancers of the testicle, kidney, breast; cancers; Hodgkin's and non-Hodgkin's Lymphomas.

Side Effects: Suppression of blood counts-uncommon and mild; nausea/vomiting-common but mild; hair loss-common but mild; soreness of mouth-common but rarely severe; nerve injury-common but mild and reversible; liver injury-uncommon; low blood pressure-rare.

Symptoms: Infections/bleeding; difficulty swallowing/loss of taste; numbness of digits/constipation/jaw pain; depression/headache/convulsions.

VINCRISTINE: VCR, Oncovin®

Uses: Cancers of the breast; Hodgkin's and non-Hodgkin's lymphomas; Acute lymphocytic leukemias; Wilm's Tumor, soft tissue sarcomas and Ewing's sarcoma of childhood; multiple myeloma.

Side Effects: Suppression of blood counts-rare and mild; nausea/vomiting-not seen; hair loss-common and severe; nerve injury-common and related to dose/reversible with reduction of dose.

Symptoms: Infections/bleeding; numbness of digits/constipation/abdominal pain.

VINDESINE: VDS.

Uses: Cancer of breast, lung, colon, rectum, esophagus; Hodgkin's and non-Hodgkin's Lymphomas; Acute lymphocytic and granulocytic leukemias; brain tumors (glioma); malignant melanoma.

Side Effects: Suppression of blood counts-common but mild; nausea/vomiting-occasional and mild; hair loss-common; nerve injury-common but dose related; chills and fever-occasional.

Symptoms: *Infections/bleeding; numbness of digits/muscle pains and weakness/ constipation; lethargy/confusion.

*Infection/bleeding-referred to above under symptoms of side effects indicates major infections such as; pneumonia, meningitis, blood stream infections (septicemia), abscesses of rectum, lung, abdomen, skin; kidney infections; tuberculosis, etc. It does not refer to mild infections such as the common cold or intestinal "flu." The bleeding referred to usually means major bleeding such as, uncontrolled massive nose bleeds, vomiting blood, massive bruises of skin, brain hemorrhage, rectal bleeding, gum bleeding, coughing blood, intra-abdominal bleeding, etc.

Chapter 46

Hormonal Agents and Hormone Antagonists

Hormonal agents and hormone antagonists are a group of diverse chemical agents—which were discovered either accidentally or logically—that are effective in treating a variety of different cancers. For example, it seemed logical to try to treat a cancer of a female organ—say, breast cancer—with a male hormone, such as testosterone. On the other hand there was no reason to expect that a pregnancy-type hormone—megesterol acetate—would be useful in treating cancer of the kidney, an incidental discovery.

The side effects of the hormone drugs are often exaggerations of otherwise normal effects which are magnified because the doses of the hormonal agent used are much greater than the amount of hormones naturally produced by the body.

AMINOGLUTETHIMIDE: Cytadren®, Elipten®. This agent's use in cancer resulted from its ability to destroy or ablate the human adrenal glands. For many years it had been observed that surgical removal of these glands produced temporary arrest of the growth of breast cancer.

Uses: Breast cancer and cancer of the adrenal glands.

Side Effects: Suppression of blood counts-rare; nausea/vomiting-uncommon; skin rashes-common but clears spontaneously in a short time; neurological side effects.

Symptoms: Lethargy, vertigo, loss of equilibrium, visual disturbances, facial flushing, swelling around the eyes.

ANDROGENIC HORMONES: Androgenic hormones are those which produce the natural effects of male physical appearance and masculinization. These agents include; Testosterone, Halotestin®, Testolactone, and Methyl-testosterone.

Uses: Breast cancer in women.

Side Effects: Blood counts-none; nausea/vomiting-rare and mild; acne-like skin rash; masculinization; liver injury-uncommon and reversible; fluid retention-common.

Symptoms: Masculinization, i.e., increase in facial, axillary and body hair, deepening of voice, acne, baldness. Liver injury-yellow jaundice, itching, nausea, loss of appetite. Fluid retention-swelling of ankles, high blood pressure, shortness of breath, and weight gain.

ESTROGENS: Estrogens are the naturally produced female hormones which produce feminine characteristics in females. Agents utilized include; Diethylstilbestrol, ethinyl estradiol, and other variants.

Uses: Cancer of prostate, cancer of the breast in women.

Side Effects: No effect on blood counts. Nausea/vomiting-common initially but stops spontaneously. Skin-darkening of breast nipples. Feminization in males. Menstrual irregularities in females. Fluid and salt retention, high blood pressure, phlebitis.

Symptoms: Fluid and salt retention leading to swollen ankles, high blood pressure, shortness of breath.

Feminization in men-loss of facial and body hair; enlargement of breasts; decreased sexual desires and performance; decrease in size of testicles.

HORMONAL ANTAGONISTS

ANTI-ESTROGENS: Tamoxifen - Nolvadex.®

Uses: Breast cancer, Ovarian cancers, Malignant Melanoma.

Side Effects: Hot flashes and other menopausal symptoms. Nausea/vomiting-rare. Skin rash and itching-rare. Menstrual irregularities; fluid retention; increased bone pain.

Symptoms: Hot flashes, emotional lability, vaginal bleeding. Lassitude, headache, leg cramps, and dizziness. Swollen ankles, shortness of breath, high blood pressure, weight gain. Increased bone pain when bone metastases are present but is a temporary problem.

LEUPROLIDE: Lupron®. This agent is active simply because of its central nervous system effects-uncommon; impotence and swollen tender breasts-uncommon; loss of appetite, constipation, nausea/vomiting-uncommon.

Symptoms: swelling of ankles/shortness of breath/high blood pressure; headache/dizziness/anxiety/lethargy/insomnia.

ANTI-ANDROGENS

FLUTAMIDE - see previous listing.

EMCYT- see previous listing.

PROGESTATIONAL AGENTS

PROGESTINS: Medroxyprogesterone, Provera®, Depo-Provera®, Hydroxyprogesterone, Delalutin®, Megestrol, Megace®.

Uses: Cancers of the breast, endometrium, kidney, and ovaries.

Side Effects: Blood count effects and nausea/vomiting-very rare. Hair loss and skin rash-rare. Fluid retention-occasional and mild; menstrual irregularities; liver injury-occasional and mild.

Symptoms: Swelling of ankles, slight weight gain, vaginal bleeding.

Chapter 47

Immunotherapeutic Agents

Simply defined, immunotherapy agents include those methods found to arouse or modify the bodies natural abilities to eliminate cancer cells through its very complex immune systems. It is worthy of mention that these same immune systems are useful in diagnosing, and treating cancers and, it is hoped, in the production of a preventative vaccine.

The agents discussed here are, in general, those which in a nonspecific and artificial way arouse the bodies immune mechanisms. The naturally occurring agents—the biological response modifiers—will be discussed in a separate section under that title.

Overall, however, the immunotherapeutic measures studied up to this time have had only a small impact on cancer therapy. However, its popular use in some foreign countries, and by unconventional cancer treatment 'peddlers' demands some discussion of the topic.

BCG VACCINE: Bacillus Calmette-Guerin Vaccine. This substance was originally developed as a vaccine against tuberculosis and is still used for this purpose in other parts of the world.

Uses: Malignant Melanoma, Superficial Bladder Cancers, Lung cancer.

BCG vaccine is used either by direct injection into visual skin cancers (melanoma); by escarification of the skin for systemic effect on disseminated cancers (metastatic malignant melanoma); injection into natural body cavities (the pleural space for lung cancer); or directly into the urinary bladder for control of superficial bladder cancers.

Side Effects: These are minimal with only an occasional case of fever and drug rash, and a rare case of disseminated tuberculosis.

Other Agents: DNCB, C. parvum and others have also been used to stimulate natural immunity in treating cancer but have had little utility.

A great deal of research remains to be done on these agents before generalized applications can be recommended.

LEVAMISOLE: Ergamisol®

This substance was originally used as an antihelmintic in domesticated animals; i.e., to kill parasitic worms. It is also believed that it stimulates the immune system.

Uses: Approved for adjuvant treatment of Duke's C colon cancer when used with 5-fluorouracil.

Side Effects: Gastrointestinal; nausea, vomiting, diarrhea, loss of appetite. Skin; rash, itching, hair loss (rare). Blood; anemia, infection, bleeding. Nervous System; insomnia, headache, fatigue, dizziness, blurred vision. Other; Flu-like symptoms, muscle aches, joint pain.

Chapter 48

Biological Response Modifiers

Biological response modifiers are a group of naturally produced substances which exert their anticancer effects by stimulating or modifying the bodies immune systems for removing cancer cells without necessarily producing direct cancer cell death. This definition serves to distinguish them from true chemotherapeutic, immunotherapeutic, and hormonal agents.

INTERLEUKIN-2 AND LYMPHOKINE-ACTIVATED KILLER CELLS: (IL-2 and LAK Cells). This complex method of immune manipulation is still considered investigational and not yet proven useful to the medical community at large. Although IL-2 alone has now been approved to treat malignant melanoma and kidney cancer.

Uses: The IL-2+LAK Cell method has had some minimal, preliminary effectiveness in cancers of the colon-rectum, malignant melanoma, kidney cell cancer, lung cancer, and the lymphomas.

Side Effects: Salt and water retention; low blood pressure-both are common but controllable. However, there is an occasional but real risk of fatal heart attack.

Symptoms: Swelling ankles, shortness of breath, high blood pressure; extremely low blood pressure and even shock and death.

OTHER INTERLEUKINS:Interleukin-3. Interleukin-6, etc.

INTERFERONS: The interferons, of which there are several types, are naturally occurring proteins isolated from human white blood cells which were initially studied for their antiviral effects. They were subsequently found to have anticancer properties. They are presently divided into three main groups: the alpha, beta and gamma interferons. The development of genetic engineering techniques have now made these agents more readily available in sufficient quantities to the medical community.

ALPHA-INTERFERON: Also known as IFN-2a, Roferon-A®, Intron-A® and others.

Uses: Hairy cell leukemia, chronic granulocytic leukemia, non-Hodgkin's Lymphomas, Cutaneous T-Cell lymphoma, Kaposi's Sarcoma (AIDS related), urinary bladder cancers (locally instilled into bladder).

Side Effects: "Flu" like symptoms-common but easily prevented; fatigue/loss of appetite-uncommon; suppression of white blood count-common; liver injury-uncommon; central nervous system injury-uncommon; nausea/vomiting/diarrhea-uncommon; heart injury-rare and reversible.

Symptoms: headache/fever/chills/muscle aches; infections; abnormal liver function blood tests; confusion/disorientation; abnormal heart rhythm/low blood pressure.

BETA-AND GAMMA-INTERFERONS: These two agents are among the newest of the interferons to be discovered and studied. Their precise utility and safety have yet to be clearly defined but they do hold some clinical promise. They are not yet generally available to the medical community.

MONOCLONAL ANTIBODIES: These agents are in essence antibodies which are produced against a single clone (ergo., monoclonal) of specific cancer cells or the protein products of those cells. Once the antibody is artificially produced in a laboratory animal it is harvested and purified. Then, the antibody is injected into the patient in an attempt to destroy those cancer cells. Although this system has shown some promise much research still needs to be done to determine its precise utility and safety.

OTHER AGENTS: There are many other agents of the Biological Response Modifier class which are still under research investigation. They are listed here for the sake of completeness. They include: Tumor necrosis factor (TNF); Transfer factor (TF); Macrophage Growth Factor (MGF); Colony Stimulating Factor (CSF; Transforming Growth Factor (TGF); and many other too numerous to mention here.

Acronyms Commonly Used To Indicate Combinations of Cancer Therapy Drugs

ABVD-adriamycin (doxorubicin) + bleomycin + vinblastine + dacarbizine

CHOP - cyclophosphamide+doxorubicin+vincristine+prednisone

CAF - cyclophosphamide + doxorubicin (Adriamycin®) + fluorouracil.

CMF - cyclophosphamide + methotrexate + fluorouracil.

CMF-T - same as CMF + tamoxifen

COPP - cyclophosphamide + vincristine + procarbazine + prednisone.

CVP - cyclophosphamide + vincristine + prednisone.

CY-VA-DIC -cyclophosphamide + vincristine + doxorubicin + dacarbizine.

FAC - fluorouracil + doxorubicin (Adriamycin®) + cyclophosphamide.

FAM - fluorouracil + doxorubicin + mitomycin.

MOPP - mechlorethamine + vincristine + procarbazine + prednisone.

MPL+PRED - melphalan + prednisone.

MTX+MP+CTX - methotrexate + mercaptopurine + cyclophosphamide.

VAC - vincristine + dactinomycin + cyclophosphamide.
VBP - vinblastine+bleomycin+cisplatin.

Part Nine

Questions to Ask Your Physician and Glossary of Terms

Questions

To Ask Your Physician and Glossary of Terms for Clear Communication

The following section will, it is hoped, help to guide the cancer patient and their family into the most practical, useful channels for discussion of their cancer and its management with their physicians. Of course, it is not always possible to anticipate the individual patient's questions since they are often based on their own concepts of cancer. Also, each patient has their own sets of values regarding the ideal goals to be accomplished with treatment. Points which are considered major factors to one person may be considered trivial to another. Nevertheless, your physician must never judge whether a question is trivial or significant to the reader since your values may not be the same as the care giver. If the patient feels the question is important enough to ask, your physician should consider it important enough to answer. Your physician may feel compelled to point out that the answer does not have a major impact on the treatment choice or the outcome but they should, nevertheless, answer the question.

Obviously, there are many questions which are applicable to some kinds of cancers and not to others. Other questions are based on the special needs of the individual as determined by their own set of circumstances and values be they personal, social, clinical, financial, psychological, medical, and so on. The following section will attempt to anticipate these questions and is based on the author's twenty years of experience in dealing with hundreds of cancer patients of all kinds. Therefore, some special areas maybe overlooked and for this the author apologizes. I hope your physician can help fill in the gaps for each of the readers.

At some point in the discussions with you and your family, however, your physician is obliged to interject the information which she knows is pertinent to your case even if the questions are not asked. It cannot be assumed since a specific, crucial point has not been raised that the individual reader does want to know those facts. The reader's lack of knowledge of the subject or the fear of hearing the answers often cause the individual to block out the obvious questions.

Questions to Ask: The following questions are designed to help the reader understand the significance of your cancer and how it may effect your future: (1) the diagnosis (and name of the cancer); (2) the stage of the cancer; (3) the treatments options available and the consequences of the treatment chosen; (4) and the prognosis of the cancer with and without the proposed treatment plan. These four points are all the reader needs to make a rational treatment choice although you may want more information. And, of course, the reader has the right to all the information they can comprehend. All of these points have been discussed in the preceding text but they will be summarized and clarified here.

Diagnosis:

The reader needs to know the name of their cancer even if the words themselves have very little meaning. The specific technical medical terms should be provided and then they should be translated into plain language without the use of technical jargon. For example, a diagnosis of "invasive carcinoma of the endometrium" conveys little or no information to the uninformed patient. However, when described as an aggressive, potentially fatal cancer of the inner lining of the uterus, the meaning is clearer to all. If it is not clear, more explanation is in order. If need be, the terms potentially fatal, aggressive, malignant, uterus, etc., should be explained and elaborated upon.

Questions Needing Answers

(1) **Diagnosis:** Is the diagnosis clearly established or only suspected?

• In other words, has a biopsy been obtained or some other form of tissue sample obtained to establish the diagnosis?

• If not, is a biopsy forthcoming? How is the biopsy to be obtained? What are the risks of obtaining the biopsy?

• Will the biopsy require major surgery, minor surgery, needle biopsy, etc.?

• Can the procedure used to obtain the diagnosis be fatal or cause spread of the disease?

• Is my general health good enough to withstand the biopsy?

• What are the alternative methods for obtaining the biopsy?

• What are the chances that the diagnosis is not cancer?

• What are the risks if I choose not to pursue the matter at all?

• Is there any danger in waiting for the disease to progress before taking action?

• What is the importance of early diagnosis and treatment?

• Will the procurement of the biopsy also be part of the treatment? If not, what treatment will be offered?

Most of these questions have been answered in prior portions of this book under the heading of the specific cancers or under the discussion of the 'biopsy' establishment of the diagnosis. However, all the questions cannot be answered in this work since special and unique factors may be involved in any individual case. If there are any doubts or unclear factors the reader must discuss them with their physician. Ask for clarification more than once if necessary to completely understand the meaning of the answers given. The readers have the right to know and to understand as much as is possible and practical regarding their cancer.

(2) **Staging:** The answers to questions regarding staging should not be given in vague, imprecise terms or with the use of jargon. They also should not be expressions of 'gut feelings,' they should be free of emotional melodrama, or reflect the physician's personal desires, unless designated as such. There are usually valid statistics available regarding survival rates, morbidity and mortality based on national or regional scientific study programs. But the patient should know that these statistics are influenced by clinical stage, age group, socioeco-

nomic factors, treatment methods, etc. This is not to say that the responses to the questions should be given by the physician in an aloof, unfeeling manner. The answers can be made precisely clear and still be given in a kind, considerate and compassionate way.

• What exactly is the stage of my cancer presented in accordance with the accepted standard systems of TMN, numerical, or others?

•What does the stage designation mean in terms of cancer size, location and distant organs involved?

• Does determining the stage of the cancer alter the choice of therapy, prognosis, morbidity, mortality, and so on.?

• What tests are done to determine the stage of the cancer? Are these tests relatively safe, low risk or high risk; and what is the chance of fatalities, morbidity?

• Is hospitalization usually necessary for testing or can staging be done as an outpatient? Does staging involve major surgery, minor surgery, needle biopsy, cytology? If necessary what is the usual length of the hospitalization, on the average?

• Do the testing procedures cause any pain? is it severe or mild?

Is my general health adequate to withstand the surgery or other means of staging?

• What are some of the possible complications and secondary effects of staging procedures?

• Why can't treatment be administered blindly without staging?

• Does the staging proceed in a logical, step wise manner or is it a general, blind group of tests which every patient receives?

• About how long will the total staging process last?

• Is there any danger in delaying treatment to complete staging process? What should I watch for to indicate progression of the disease during the staging process?

• What is the approximate cost of each test, total cost of entire process? Does my health insurance cover part or all of the staging procedures?

• Will staging have to be repeated after or during course of therapy?

Many, if not all, of these questions should have been answered in the preceding text of this book under the headings for each of the specific cancer types.

(3) **Treatment Options:** What is the primary form of treatment for the stage of the cancer in question? Will it be surgery, radiation therapy, chemotherapy or a combination of these?

• Are the treatments, if a combination, given in sequence, simultaneously or in a random, as needed, fashion?

• What is the therapeutic purpose of each treatment modality used? Is the goal total cure, prolongation of survival, or palliation of symptoms?

• Is the therapy modality part of the diagnosis, staging or other processes?

• What are the risks, side effects, dangers of the treatment plan adopted?

• Is there a chance of death, disfigurement, pain, morbidity, incapacitation due to the treatment plan? If so, how severe might it be? Are the complications treatable or reversible, temporary or permanent?

• What are the numerical (average) chances of each of these undesirable effects?

• What are the consequences if I choose no treatment at all or a modified form of treatment?

• What is the usually recommended treatment plan?

• Will there be a team of specialists involved in my care?

• Who will head the management team?

• What other specialists are involved?

• Are there any experts on the team in nursing, physical therapy, nutrition, psychology, social work, pastoral care, etc.

• If **surgery** is chosen as part of the treatment plan, exactly which organs or parts of organs will be removed?

• Can my cancer be completely removed or only partially excised? Why?

• Is this a major, high risk surgical procedure?

•Will the goal of the surgery be for treatment, diagnosis or staging purposes or all of these?

• What is the usual surgical mortality rate?

• Is my general health adequate to tolerate major surgery?

• Why is surgery chosen over other forms of therapy?

•What is your personal experience, as a physician, in this surgical procedure?

• Is it a commonly performed surgical procedure or an unusual surgery best performed by a surgical specialist in the field?

• Is it best performed at a major referral center?

• Does my community hospital have the staff, experience, support, equipment, etc. to obtain the best result?

• How do local results compare with national statistics?

• If radiation therapy is chosen as primary treatment form, why is it chosen?

• What are the risk and side effects of the radiation therapy plan?

• Are the side effects permanent, temporary, reversible, preventable, correctable, disfiguring? do the side effects alter the function of the organ treated?

• Will the radiation therapy be administered before, after or during surgery?

• Why is it given in that manner?

• What is the purpose of the radiation?

• Does the radiation therapy improve the 'true cure' rate, or remission rate?

• Is the radiation therapy given for palliation only?

• Is there any significant mortality associated with its administration? How are the results of the radiation therapy measured and monitored?

If **chemotherapy** is chosen as part of the treatment plan, why is it chosen?

• Will the chemotherapy be the primary therapy; secondary; combined with radiation, surgery or other therapies?

• Is it given before, after, or simultaneously with the other modalities? When does the chemotherapy begin?

• Who administers the chemotherapy? Will it be supervised by a chemotherapy specialist?

• Where are the chemotherapy treatments given? in or out of the hospital?

• How often will I receive the chemotherapy treatments?

•What chemotherapy drug or drugs will be given for my cancer? What are the common names of the drugs used?

• Why do you choose this one chemotherapy drug or this combination of drugs?

• What are the chemotherapy drugs suppose to accomplish?

• Do the chemotherapy drugs alter the cure rate, remission rate, control of disease, palliation, or spread of the cancer?

• What are the actual observed 'true cure' rates, remission rates? Are they partial or complete remissions?

• Will the therapy be given simply for palliation?

• Is the length of survival prolonged with therapy?

• What is the average duration of survival with and without chemotherapy?

• How are the chemotherapy drug(s) given; by injection, by mouth?

• Will I be able to work or remain active while taking chemotherapy?

• What tests are performed to monitor the side effects of therapy and/or the response of my cancer?

• What if I miss a dose or several doses of chemotherapy?

• What are the possible side effects of the chemotherapy?

• Is there any significant mortality from chemotherapy? what is the actual percentage rate of mortality?

• Are there any immediate effects or any long-term and late side effects?

• What should I do if I experience a side effect?

• Are there any special side effects I should report to my physicians; report then immediately or on my next office visit?

• Are there any medicines or remedies which can be used to avoid, modify, or counteract the side effects?

• Does the chemotherapy effect my ability to have children, my sexual performance, my sexual desires or my physical appearance?

• Does the therapy have any effect on my children born later after my chemotherapy is completed?

• Is my general health adequate to tolerate chemotherapy? Are my other medical problems capable of withstanding the chemotherapy and its side effects? How might the chemotherapy effect my other medical conditions (diabetes, high blood pressure, heart disease, etc.)?

• Can I continue to take my other medications during chemotherapy treatments?

• Are there any medicines which I should especially avoid? Are they proprietary or prescription drugs?

• Can I safely use alcoholic beverages during the period of my chemotherapy?

• If not, why not? What symptoms should I watch for?

•What happens if I forget and take some alcohol inadvertently? What should I do if this happens?

• Are there any special foods or diet to utilize or avoid during chemotherapy?

• Should I restrict or increase my fluid intake during chemotherapy? What kinds of fluids?

• Is there anything in the way of activities to avoid during chemotherapy?

• Is there another effective treatment available if the first treatment program fails? If there is, what does it accomplish? cure? remission? palliation?

• How much will the chemotherapy cost, generally speaking?

• How much of the cost is covered by the health insurance?

(4) **Prognosis:** The reader is advised to try to obtain as much information as possible regarding precise, statistical values for your type and stage of cancer. In most cases average cure rates, durations of survival, remission rates are available to your physician. Occasionally,

the information is not immediately at hand but it is obtainable. Your physician should be given a reasonable amount of time to look up the statistics for your particular cancer and the treatment plan you have jointly chosen. The other option is for your physician to consult a local or regional oncologist.

Unfortunately, valid statistics are not always available, anywhere in world, for certain rare or unusual cancers. This is especially true for the very rare types of cancer and for very new forms of therapy. If this is the case your physician should be willing to admit the fact and consult an expert.

The reader must not settle for vague, sentimental, platitudinous, ambiguous statements, such as; " I think you'll do all right"; "I think we can take care of it"; "You're a strong person I think you'll be okay"; "You've been a good person so I think you'll survive this"; or with a pat on the back and a, "Don't you worry about it. Leave it to me." Certainly, there are some readers who cannot face the true survival figures as they exist and they may prefer these vagaries. As I have stated elsewhere, this is the patient's choice. If that is the one they make. So be it.

Of course, the reader does not want just cold, dry figures thrown out at her as if from an unfeeling computer. However, a caring, compassionate physician needs no instruction on how to be considerate and reassuring without being callus or conveying false expectations. If your physician has not learned this technique by the time he begins treating people it is already too late for him.

To reemphasize the obvious, if there is any doubt about your physician's definition, or the reader's understanding of *true cure*, remission, duration of survival, quality of survival you must ask her for her working definition.

It is inappropriate to ask your physician, "How many months do I have to live?" or "How much time do I have, Doc?" or "What will the end be like?" or "Will I suffer at the end, will there be a great deal of pain?" However, your physician cannot possibly know the precise answers to these valid questions, nor can anyone else. If your physician gives the patient a chance of 'true cure' of, say, 65%, they cannot honestly tell you if you will be in the 65% who will be cured or in the 35% who will not be cured. This is just not possible by contemporary measures of prognosis. In addition, such precise predictions are not available at any medical center or any famous clinic or from any famous physician.

Questions regarding prognosis must include:

- What is the prognosis for my type and my stage of cancer if I choose not to have any treatment?
- How will the treatment change the prognosis for this type and stage of cancer?
- Is the prognosis significantly better or worse than when no treatment is given at all?
- If cure is not possible, is control (remission) possible?
- How long is the average duration of remission? What are the chances of complete versus partial remission?
- Is part of the therapy plan to alleviate distressing symptoms or just to make the cancer smaller in size?
- If cure or remission is not possible can relief be provide for pain or other symptoms (palliation) with chemotherapy or by other means?
- If cure or remission is not possible what is the average length of survival with and without treatment?
- If all available forms of treatment fail is there some 'experimental therapy' program which is available, or can my case be referred to a cancer center to receive the experimental therapy?

(5) **Follow Up Medical Examinations:** In this physician's and writer's viewpoint the reader should never be told, 'come back to see me only if you have any trouble,' Such a statement is true for all patients who have a chronic disease or a condition which has a significant likelihood of recurrence whether or not they are cancer patients. Much more definitive direction can and should be given by a careful, informed and caring physician. The reader should never settle for such vague advice. Not all cancer patients have to be monitored by the specialist who treated their cancer but they should be monitored by

some physician on a regular, periodic basis. The regular follow-up professional can be a family physician, general internist, pediatrician, general surgeon or whomever is available. But some physician must except the responsibility of follow up care and can assume that role.

Questions Regarding Follow Up:

• How are the side effects and results of the therapy program monitored and measured? What tests and x-rays are utilized?

• How often should these tests be performed?

• How much do these tests cost?

• Are they done in the hospital setting or as an outpatient?

• Are they different from the tests I originally received?

• Is a complete physical examination required periodically?

• Is it performed every year or more frequently? less frequently?

• What symptoms should the patient watch for to signal recurrence of disease or the side effects of treatment?

• Should patients examine themselves? How? How often? Should they call the physician immediately or as soon as practical?

• Are there any emergency signs to watch for?

• Are there any tests done to detect short-term/long-term ill effects of chemotherapy? Of Surgery? Of Radiation Therapy?

• What are those tests? How often are they performed? What do they cost? Will my health insurance carrier pay for them?

• Can I obtain a second opinion regarding all of the above decisions? Should my case be referred to a major cancer center or do the physicians on the team feel confident they can manage this kind of cancer?

• If the reader seeks another opinion is their physician willing to continue to manage my case when they return to this locality?

• Is there any value in the so called 'unconventional,' 'unofficial,' 'unapproved' treatment methods? Why not? Should I look into these? If not, why not?

Glossary of Useful Oncology & Medical Terms

Adrenal Glands - two small organs located just above the kidneys which are responsible for secreting normally occurring hormones.

Adrenalectomy - surgical removal or chemical ablation of the glands. Commonly used in treatment of breast cancer.

Adjuvant therapy - additional therapy, either chemotherapy or radiation therapy, given in concert with surgery and/or radiotherapy.

Alopecia - loss of hair from the body and/or scalp.

Androgen - a male hormone responsible for the physical characteristics of men. Commonly used to treat breast cancer.

Anemia - Low red blood cell count.

Anorexia - a term meaning general loss of appetite. Anorexia nervosa is only one type of this condition.

Antiemetic - drugs which control or prevent vomiting.

Antineoplastic Agent - a substance that kills or inhibits the growth of cancer cells. Syn: Anticancer agent.

Axillary Lymph Nodes - the lymph nodes found in the armpit.

Barium Enema - the introduction of a contrast substance—barium—into the large bowel (colon) to study the structure and detect disease in the large bowel. Syn: Lower G.I. Series, Colon X-ray.

Basal cell carcinoma - one type of skin cancer.

Benign - the opposite of malignant; used to describe a tumor that is not cancerous or does not have a tendency to spread.

Betatron - an instrument used to give radiation therapy to cancers located deep in the body.

Biological Response Modifier - a means of stimulating the body's natural defenses against cancer cells. Ex: Interferons, Interleukin-2.

Biopsy - the process by which a small piece of tissue is removed for diagnosis for microscopic examination by the pathologist.

Blood count - a laboratory test which actually counts the number of red blood cells, white blood cells, and platelets. Syn: CBC, Complete Blood Count.

Bone marrow - the major, central portion in bone that produces the red, white blood cells and the platelets.

Brachytherapy - radiation treatment whose source is applied to the surface of the body or a short distance from the body.

Bronchogenic Cancer - a type of lung cancer that arises in the lining of the bronchial tubes.

Cancer - a general, nonspecific term for a group of abnormally growing, potentially malignant cells.

Cancer in situ - a cancer that has not formed into a visible swelling or lump but is in a thin sheet on the surface of an organ. This type of cancer is often detected by the 'Pap smear,'

Carcinoma - a kind of cancer that arises from tissues of the skin or inner surface linings of organs.

Adenocarcinoma - cancer arising from the glandular cells.

Basal Cell Carcinoma - the commonest kind of skin cancer.

Cervical Carcinoma - cancer of the cervix (the neck) of the uterus.

Endometrial Carcinoma - cancer of the inner lining of the uterus.

Castration - surgical removal of the testicles in males and the ovaries in females.

Catheter - a tube placed into a vein—and other natural body canals or reservoirs—to withdraw fluids (blood, urine, etc.) and/or to inject medications.

Cell - the basic, microscopic unit of living tissues of all living things.

Cervical Lymph Nodes - the lymph nodes found in the neck.

Cervix - the anatomic designation for the neck of the uterus.

Chemotherapy - the treatment of disease with drugs or medicines, i.e.,

Cancer Chemotherapy - the use of drugs to treat cancer.

Combination Chemotherapy -the use of more than one drug simultaneously to treat cancer.

Cobalt 60 - a type of radiation therapy machine which contains a radioactive substance (Cobalt 60) which emits the radiation.

Colonoscopy - a procedure used to visually examine the colon through a flexible instrument called a colonoscope.

Colostomy - surgical procedure that allows the colon to open out through the anterior abdominal wall and empty its contents into a reservoir.

Complete Blood Count (CBC)-the measurement of all the blood cells.

Cryosurgery - a special technique in which cells and tissues are destroyed by exposure to extreme cold.

Cytology - the science of examining cells such as the cells obtained in a 'Pap smear,'

Cytotoxic Agents or Drugs - drugs that are capable of killing cells. A commonly used synonym for chemotherapy drugs.

Cyst - an accumulation of fluid or a gel-like substance within a sack. Cysts may be benign or malignant.

Diagnosis - the final microscopic description for identifying a medical disease or condition.

Dosimetrist - a non-physician specialist responsible for planning and calculating the radiation dose to be administered.

Dysphagia - difficult or painful swallowing.

Dyspnea - difficult or labored breathing, or shortness of breath.

Echocardiogram - a procedure which uses waves to produce a structural picture of the heart.

Edema -an abnormal collection of fluid in some part of the body, such as swelling (edema) of the ankles, hands or face.

Endoscopy - any procedure utilizing tubes to visually examine an internal part of the body.

EKG (ECG) - Electrocardiogram; a graphic tracing of the electrical activity of the heart.

Erythrocyte - the red blood cell, as defined below.

Estrogen - a hormone responsible for the female physical characteristics. Commonly used to treat prostate cancer.

Excision - the entire surgical removal or 'cutting out' of a part of the body.

External Radiation - the kind of radiation therapy which is given via a machine located outside the body.

Fistula - an abnormal channel or connection between two areas of the body.

Gamma Rays - the kind of radioactive rays given off by a chemical substance (i.e., Radium) instead of that produced by electronic devices (i.e.. x-rays).

Gastrointestinal (G.I.) - referring to the entire digestive tract which includes mouth, throat, swallowing tube (esophagus), stomach, small intestine, large intestine (colon), and anus.

Granulocyte - a type of white blood cell responsible for fighting infection.

Granulocytopenia - a decrease in the number of granulocytes in the circulating blood. It is commonly caused by chemotherapy.

Guaiac Test - a chemical test used to detect blood in the feces.

Hematology - the science of studying diseases of the blood and blood forming organs.

Hematologist - a physician that specializes in the study of Hematology.

Hodgkin's Disease (Lymphoma) - a kind of cancer of the lymph nodes which starts in the lymph nodes, liver or spleen.

Hormone - a naturally occurring chemical produced by the organs of the body which affect the growth and function of other distant organs and tissues.

Hysterectomy - Surgical removal of the uterus only. Often combined with removal of other female structures. See Oophorectomy and Salpingectomy.

Ileostomy - a surgically created opening from the small intestine (the ileum) and outside through the anterior abdominal wall.

Immunity - a complex part of the systems used by the body to resist diseases.

Immunotherapy - artificial means of stimulating the body's immune defenses in treating cancer. See: Biological Response Modifier.

Implant - a method of radiation therapy whereby a container of radioactive material is temporarily placed inside the body.

Infusion - a method of injecting drugs or fluids slowly into a vein by letting them drip at a fixed rate through a tube and needle.

Injection - any method using a needle and syringe to introduce drugs or fluids into the body; commonly known as 'a shot' or 'shots,'

Internal Radiation - a type of radiation therapy where the radiation source is implanted into the body (also called Intracavitary radiation).

Interstitial Radiation - a type of internal radiotherapy where a radioactive source is placed directly into the diseased tissue.

Intracavitary Radiation - a method of radiation therapy where the radiation source is placed inside a naturally existing body cavity; i.e., vagina, chest cavity, sinuses, etc.

Intramuscular (IM) - the injection of a drug into muscle tissue.

Intra-operative Radiation - a method of administering radiation directly to a cancer while the body is still open for surgery.

Intrathecal - injection of medications into a natural body cavity such as the spinal canal.

Intravenous (IV) - the injection of a drug into a vein.

Irradiation - the technique of using x-ray beams to treat disease. See: Radiation therapy.

Lesion - an abnormal change in a body tissue or organ indicating the presence of disease, injury or other malady.

Leukemia - a form of cancer of the blood or blood forming organs which results in production of abnormally appearing white blood cells (leukocytes) and, frequently, with in an increase in the number of the white blood cells in the circulation.

Leukocyte - a white blood cell.

Linear Accelerator - a machine which creates and delivers a certain kind of high-energy X-rays to treat cancer.

Lumbar Puncture (LP) -see spinal tap.

Lumpectomy - the surgical removal of a solitary cancerous growth without removal of the entire organ. See: Mastectomy.

Lymph Node or Gland - a normally invisible, small collection of cells (lymphocytes) that can become enlarged due to disease.

Lymphocyte - one of the white blood cells which helps to make up the lymph nodes as well as circulating in the blood to fight disease.

Lymphoma - a general term used to designate a cancer of the lymph system. Such as Hodgkin's Lymphoma (Disease) .

Magnetic Resonance Imaging (MRI) - a method of imaging and examining parts of the body without use of radiation but by measuring the different magnetic fields emitted by different organs and tissues.

Malignant - a term used to indicate the aggressive and potentially fatal properties of a growth or tumor.

Mammography and Mammogram - an x-ray examination of the breast for detecting small, early and non-feelable cancers.

Mastectomy - Surgical removal of the entire breast. Includes the following types:

Segmental Mastectomy or Lumpectomy-surgical removal of a cancerous tumor of the breast.

Radical Mastectomy-Surgical removal of the breast, lymph nodes and chest wall muscles under the breast.

Modified Radical Mastectomy-surgical removal of the breast and the lymph nodes only without the muscles.

Simple Mastectomy-surgical removal of the breast only.

Melanoma - a cancer of the pigment (melanin) forming cells of the body. Usually occurs in the eye or on the skin.

Metastasize - the process by which cancer cells break away from the original cancer and spread to other parts of the body via the blood stream or the lymphatic system.

Metastatic -the state of already spread cancer cells.

Metastasis -a single accumulation of metastatic cells.

Metastases -more than one accumulation of metastatic cells.

Mucositis - see Stomatitis.

Myelogram - an x-ray examination of the spinal canal performed by injection dye into the spinal canal.

Myeloma (Multiple Myeloma or Plasma Cell Myeloma) - a cancer of the protein forming cells (plasma cells) of the bone marrow.

Neoplasm - a new, abnormal growth of cells or tissue that is generally malignant. Syn: Tumor, Malignant Tumor, Cancer, A Malignancy.

Neuroblastoma - a malignant tumor of the nervous system. See text.

Neutrophils - another name for granulocytes (see above).

Neutropenia- a decrease in the number of neutrophils in the blood.

Non-Hodgkin's Lymphoma - an arbitrary means of distinguishing this cancer from Hodgkin's Disease. See text under Non-Hodgkin's Lymphoma.

Nuclear Medicine - a specialized method for imaging and examining parts of the body. Such as; Bone scans, CT scans or CAT scans, etc.

Oncologist - a physician who specializes in the management of cancer; i.e., medical oncologist, radiation oncologist, surgical oncologist, pediatric oncologist, gynecologic oncologist, etc.

Oncology - the science that studies the management of cancer.

Oophorectomy - surgical removal of the ovaries.

Osteoma - a benign tumor of bone.

Osteosarcoma - a malignant tumor of bone.

Palliative therapy - treatment administered to relieve pain and other distressing symptoms of disease without necessarily curing the disease.

Pathologist -a physician who specializes in examining cells and tissues (biopsy specimens) to determine if disease is present and what the type of disease is present.

Plasma cell - a cell of the bone marrow that produces proteins responsible for body immunity.

Platelet - a blood cell responsible in part for the clotting of blood.

Polyp - an excessive growth of tissue projecting into a body cavity or orifice. Polyps may be either benign or malignant.

Proctoscopy - a method of visually examining the lower bowel (colon) with the use of a rigid instrument (proctoscope or sigmoidoscope) and opposed to a flexible instrument (colonoscope).

Progesterone - one of the female hormones produced by the ovaries.

Prostate - a gland found at the base of the bladder in males.

Radiation Therapy - a treatment for cancer and other diseases which utilizes high energy x-ray beams (also known as radiotherapy, irradiation therapy, x-ray therapy [XRT], cobalt therapy, linear accelerator therapy).

Radiation Physicist - a person trained in calculating proper radiation doses.

Red Blood Cells - cells of the circulating blood which carry oxygen to the tissues; often referred to in the complete blood count as the 'red count,' 'hemoglobin,' or 'hematocrit,'

Remission - the elimination of the signs and symptoms of disease by therapy.

Partial Remission-elimination of at least 50% of measurable disease.

Complete Remission -elimination of all signs and symptoms of disease.

Salpingectomy - surgical removal of the fallopian tubes. Commonly removed during hysterectomy .

Sarcoma - a malignant tumor of bone, muscle, cartilage or other connective tissues.

Side Effects - an undesirable result of any treatment which is usually temporary and reversible.

Sigmoidoscopy - a method of visually examining a specific portion of the large bowel (the sigmoid colon) with the use of a rigid instrument. See also colonoscopy and proctoscopy.

Spinal Tap - a test performed by inserting a needle through the lower back into the spinal canal to remove fluid for analysis or to administer medication. Syn: Lumbar Puncture.

Sputum - mucinous substance produced in the act of coughing or clearing the throat.

Sputum Cytology - the examination of the sputum for cancer cells.

Stomatitis - inflammation of the membranes of the mouth by chemotherapy or radiation therapy which can cause sores or blisters in the mouth and difficulty in eating and swallowing. Also see Mucositis.

Teletherapy - the application of radiation therapy which is distant from the tissue being treated.

Tracheostomy - a surgically created opening between the windpipe (trachea) through neck to the outside air to make breathing easier.

Thrombocyte -a synonym for Platelet (see platelet above) .

Tumor - literally the term refers to any abnormal swelling or enlargement; i.e., an abscess, a mole, a lump, etc. Very frequently used interchangeably and synonymously with a cancerous growth. Commonly used as an evasive term in place of the word 'cancer' .

White Blood Cells - the cells of the circulating blood responsible for fighting infection. As part of the complete blood count often referred to as 'the white count,' 'the neutrophil count,' 'the granulocyte count,'

X-Ray - high energy particles and beams used to treat and diagnose disease.

Conclusion

Final Advice and Guidance

Before closing I have attempted to offer some advice and guidance to the reader in the utilization of this book. This advice does, of course, have to be adapted to each individual's needs. As has been the author's habit throughout this work, advice is offered on how not to use this book.

Firstly, this book is not a 'Bible' on the management of cancer. And, therefore, it contains no scriptures or gospel truths. Their is no such 'Cancer Bible' as their is no 'Cancer Jesus.' The practice of medicine, whether it is oncology or any other specialty field, is not a precise science. It is a much an art as a science. There are no persons, self-acclaimed or otherwise, who have the final word, or the only word on the management of any disease.

The art of medicine is an art of judgement. The physician is a highly trained professional who is called on regularly to make some judgement calls. It is much like being an official in any sports contest, except the stakes are much higher—in which there will be many judgement calls but without an instant replay system to review the calls in retrospect. There are certainly no gods or prophets in medical science who can, by divine revelation, state that their choice of treatment is the only choice or even the best choice. And my own judgements and statements are no different in this regard.

There are, of course, consensus opinions and general rules which are espoused by the general medical community. But most physicians honestly admit that there is, and must be, room for maneuvering and bending the guidelines to suit each individual case and its special needs. As such, it is not appropriate to quote from this work—chapter and verse—the opinions and generalizations written therein.

Equally inappropriate, is to present the writings of this book with open page to one's physician and demand or insist that the approaches recommended therein be adhered to assiduously. The information provided in this book is meant to function as a road map which contains several primary and alternate routes to a particular destination. And, as in any good road map, one often has to recognize and use these alternative paths and plan on contingency courses to follow when indicated. In this writer's humble judgement this philosophy should apply to all the words of advice espoused from any physician whether he is located at a world renowned institution of great medical acclaim or the author of widely recognized writings on cancer management. Only physicians who see themselves as an equal to the Messiah from Nazareth would consider themselves to be equally infallible, and are best avoided.

A wise physician recognizes these variations in the management of any given cancer case and points out to the reader what these alternate routes are and why they may apply to their case. The physician uses her knowledge and experience to formulate a plan of approach with built-in adjustments and must avoid being too rigid and dogmatic. Even the Holy Bible does not have any universal agreement on its translation and interpretation. The wealth of medical knowledge gathered over the centuries by humans and interpreted by humans can expect nothing better.

At best, what has preceded in this book would be most appropriately used to help supply the readers with the information and suggestions they need in order to ask applicable questions, to choose their physicians wisely, to obtain appropriate details which will help them to make intelligent, informed choices. It is my hope, also, that this book has pointed out the road hazards and sand traps which could lead desperate, vulnerable people to the 'lunatic fringes' of medicine containing its quacks, hucksters and profiteering mystics.

The second 'how-not-to' is not to use this work as if it were a cookbook containing 'precise recipes' designed to produce a promised result, every time, if the formula is followed to the letter. Just as there are national chili contests, apple pie contests and cake baking contests there are many and varied successful recipes in treating cancer. It is appreciated that the general public finds it hard to understand and accept that there is no so much magic formula or recipe. It has often been said, 'we can put a man on the moon but we can't cure cancer'. The fact is that it is technically easier to put a man on the moon because space science is a more precise than medical science. The situation is not the way the medical profession or medical researchers want it but that's just the way it is. And thousands of researchers and clinical scientists still devote their entire lives to changing the situation.

Some readers might think, there could not be any clearer end point to reach than to endeavor to avoid early death, and no clearer goal to achieve than prolongation of life and good health. Indeed, these are clear endpoints and goals. In the cooking contests the end result is judged on the taste of the finished product and, therefore, since tastes will vary the means of reaching the end result will vary. Therefore, in cancer management even though the end point is the same, to please the taster, the recipes and formulas are bound to vary. The variation in tastes will depend on one's definition of living, good health, mode of dying, and the prices one is willing to pay to achieve these goals. For these reasons the recipes to reach these goals will also differ.

Why then is there not one outstanding, universally accepted cancer authority for all of the medical profession to follow, some readers might ask? There are several reasons for this. The reasons fall into one of two major categories, i.e., the Scientific and the Subjective.

Scientific:

First and foremost is the concept of biological variability of normal human physiology and abnormal pathological physiology (disease). The biological variability concept emphasizes the idea that the same disease does not necessarily behave in the same way in each and every patient. By the same token, therefore, the response to treatment of the disease is not the same in all people. Throughout our years of medical education, specialty training and medical practice we physicians are constantly reminded to avoid two inflexible concepts: the concepts of always and never. Both of these concepts are fraught with many pitfalls and traps. These "always and never" concepts remind physicians that even if 99.99% of cases behave in a predictable manner one must constantly be on the alert and attentive to the remaining 00.01% which behave differently. These are the cases viewed too rigidly which burn our fingers and turn dreams into nightmares.

To make matters more difficult even so called normal physiology' is so extremely variable. Not every person suffering a gun shot wound to the brain dies of the wound, not every person has the same 'normal' body temperature—although they fall into an average a range—not everyone who free-falls from a height of 20,000 ft. without parachute dies on impacting the ground. History is replete with many examples of these deviations from the expected 'norm.' In other words, not all human beings are alike even if they are grouped together by similarity in age, sex, race, regional residence, nationality, ethnicity, dietary habits, life-styles, nutritional status, social status and all the other parameters medical science uses in an attempt to obtain a homogeneous group.

The second factor within the scientific realm falls under the broad heading of scientific and technical imperfections. Which is to say, in spite of our great technical sophistication there are no tests, x-rays, research systems, treatment modalities, statistical analysis systems which can boast pure, unfaltering perfection. In addition, there are no tests which are always abnormal or exclusively diagnostic for only one disease or medical disorder. At the same time, there isn't any one disease which always produces the same set of symptoms or signs. On the other hand, it cannot be stated that any disease never produces a particular sign or symptom. It is for these reasons that a physician's logic is given, predominantly, to lists of possibilities, likelihoods and statistical probabilities.

The same kind of variability is also the reason that technical medical language is so replete with vague qualifiers and modifiers such as; almost always, almost never, very rarely, frequently, not infrequently, occasionally, most likely and so on. These terms are not used in an attempt to be vague or evasive. They are used to avoid the universal taboos of never and always. The elimination of these imperfections of medical science and medical technology are what continuing medical research is all about. The same concepts are also what is embodied in the statement, "medicine is not a pure or and exact science."

Another fact which has become obvious to the public recently is the appearance or discovery of previously unknown, and completely new diseases. Such facts are obvious when the reader considers, for example, that diseases such as Legionnaire's Diseases and Acquired Immune Deficiency Syndrome (AIDS) did not exist prior to World War II. We in the United States have a tendency to believe that we can accomplish anything and everything with more money or more effort. Such a perception accounts for statements like, "we can land a man on the moon but we can't cure cancer."

Even, if and when, basic information such as the agent causing an illness is known it doesn't mean a cure is around the corner or in the very next test tube. When, for example, Poliomyelitis was the ravage of the developed countries of the world most major research centers were working on a cure or a vaccine for prevention of this terrible viral disease. In spite of the fact that the virus which causes Polio had been known, identified and characterized for decades a vaccine aluded the best scientific minds in the world for many years. In summary, there is now and continues to exist the realm of the unknown and, as history has demonstrated, when old diseases are conquered new ones, unfortunately, move in to fill the void.

It seems redundant to state that unexpected complications have an effect on statistical interpretations of research data since this also fits under 'the unknowns' mentioned above. However, it is an important point to elaborate upon and clarify. Although the complications of a treatment or test are known it does not mean they are always preventable or that they can be detected before they occur. Since all diseases begin at the cellular, or at the even lower molecular level, many of them can escape detection because of our still relatively crude techniques which are just beginning to probe to these molecular depths.

A wise man once observed that the human body is the most complex machine ever created. As a consequence, it is also the most difficult machine to decipher.

Subjective Variability:

Subjective variability refers to the concept of individual human fluctuation in its interpretation of biological data and its response to biological stimuli. Simply stated, it refers to the observation that all the people involved in medical care and medical research are fallible human beings. Not only are the care-providers and clinical performers included in the group but the subjects or patients add their own degree of inconstancy.

Even if one could exclude the scientific variables of the subjects of medical treatments and the research discussed above one still has to deal with differences in education, misinformation, religious beliefs, life styles, personality, character, individual choices, social preferences, fear of the unknown, ethnicity, inheritance and genetics, locality of residence, personal habits, nutritional habits, environment, and the ever nebulous but real factor called, 'the will to live.' The list is infinite and, most likely, there are many other factors which should be on the list which are still unknown.

The medical research minds which formulate and apply the medical principles are also fallible, changing, imperfect human beings. Most significantly, there is no one perfect "God" of medicine as there was in Greek and Roman mythology. There are many apostles and prophets, priests and priestesses and workers in the vineyard but there is no 'supreme being.' There is also no "Mecca" of cancer care but there are many excellent cancer centers scattered throughout the world.

Competent physicians formulate their treatment plans based on the current research reports and consensus recommendations from the cancer centers. They then combine these factors with their own professional training, knowledge and experience. They should maintain an open mind and be willing to accept new thoughts and changes in the grand plan. They must mold the individual plan to suit the particular circumstances, needs and desires of each patient but still maintain a degree of scientific consistency. When the patient has misconceptions and misinformation which can erroneously effect their choices the physician must gently and logically try to influence those decisions with reason and persuasion. They do not force their advice and recommendations on the patient or their family. And, while they are doing so, the physician must keep in mind the ultimate welfare of the patient and not their own ego or personal reputations. The satisfaction the physician derives from the practice of medicine must be predicated on their desire to provide the best treatment they believe will benefit the patient and not from a need to appear omniscience or to 'always be right.'

In conclusion, my advice is that the reader use this book as a source of reference on which to build a firm foundation for the understanding and insight needed to guide them in making informed, knowledgeable decisions and choices in regards to the prevention, early detection, diagnosis and treatment of cancer.

Index

A

B

D

E

Index

L

M

N

WANT TO KNOW MORE ABOUT AMERICA'S NUMBER TWO KILLER CANCER?

Here is a book that will tell you everything you want and need to know about the description and definition of cancer; all of its known causes, symptoms, means of prevention and early detection; and your options regarding its treatment and cure. This book has it all whether you are a cancer victim or just want to learn how to avoid becoming one.

ESPECIALLY FOR CANCER PATIENTS:

1. Information about which kind of doctor(s) or specialist(s) to consult.
2. The types of treatments available and their cure rates, remission rates, side effects and toxicities.
3. What tests should be done to evaluate your cancer status before, during and after treatment.
4. What questions to ask your doctors and what kinds of answers to expect and insist on.
5. How to obtain a second opinion, and about unconventional forms of treatment.
6. What your general rights are in making decisions in reference to your cancer's treatment.

Dr. R. Aigotti is the author of this book and is an expert in the diagnosis and treatment of cancer. He has practiced his art and science for over 30 years and has been a consultant to many other physicians in the Indiana-Michigan area.

Credit Card Orders see reverse side.

Belletrist Publishing Co., P. O. Box 11506. South Bend, In. 46634

ORDER FORM

Please send________ copies of **"THE PEOPLE'S CANCER GUIDE BOOK"** @ $29.95 per copy to:

NAME ____

STREET ADDRESS ______________________ APT.# ______________

CITY ____________________ STATE ________ ZIP ________________

Satisfaction Guaranteed or Your Money Back.

☐ CHECK ☐ MONEY ORDER

TOTAL for Books ________________

Please allow 4-6 weeks for delivery.
No CODs please.

INDIANA residents
Add $1.50 sales tax per copy ____________

SHIPPING& Handling
add $4.00 per copy ____________

Prices subject to change without notice.

TOTAL THIS ORDER ____________

[OVER PLEASE]

FOR CREDIT CARD ORDERS

VISA ☐ **MASTERCARD** ☐ **AMEX** ☐ **DISCOVER** ☐

Card No.____

Expiration Date - ___-___-___

Authorized Signature ______________________________

1. MAIL THIS FORM TO ADDRESS ON REVERSE SIDE,

2. or **CALL TOLL FREE** TO 1 - 800 - 477 - 7869,

3. or **FAX** TO 1 - 219 - 234 - 6860